# Anatomy and Physiology in a FLASH

## An Interactive, Flash-Card Approach

# Anatomy and Physiology in a FLASH!

## An Interactive, Flash-Card Approach

**Joy A. Hurst,** MATL, MFS, NCMA
*Former Professor*
Kaplan University
Frederick Campus

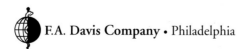
F.A. Davis Company • Philadelphia

F. A. Davis Company
1915 Arch Street
Philadelphia, PA 19103
www.fadavis.com

Copyright © 2011 by F. A. Davis Company

Printed in the United States of America

Last digit indicates print number: 10 9 8 7 6 5 4 3 2 1

*Acquisitions Editor:* Andy McPhee
*Manager of Content Development:* George W. Lang
*Developmental Editor:* Yvonne Gillam
*Art and Design Manager:* Carolyn O'Brien

As new scientific information becomes available through basic and clinical research, recommended treatments and drug therapies undergo changes. The author(s) and publisher have done everything possible to make this book accurate, up to date, and in accord with accepted standards at the time of publication. The author(s), editors, and publisher are not responsible for errors or omissions or for consequences from application of the book, and make no warranty, expressed or implied, in regard to the contents of the book. Any practice described in this book should be applied by the reader in accordance with professional standards of care used in regard to the unique circumstances that may apply in each situation. The reader is advised always to check product information (package inserts) for changes and new information regarding dose and contraindications before administering any drug. Caution is especially urged when using new or infrequently ordered drugs.

**Library of Congress Cataloging-in-Publication Data**

Hurst, Joy A.
  Anatomy and physiology in a flash : an interactive, flash-card approach / Joy A. Hurst.
     p. ; cm.
  Includes index.
  ISBN-13: 978-0-8036-2361-3
  ISBN-10: 0-8036-2361-5
  1. Human anatomy—Programmed instruction. 2. Human physiology—Programmed instruction. I. Title.
  [DNLM: 1. Anatomy, Regional—Problems and Exercises. 2. Physiological Phenomena—Problems and Exercises. QS 18.2]
  QM33.H87 2011
  612—dc22

                                    2010032344

# PREFACE

Human Anatomy and Physiology is often the most feared course among students. There are many reasons students dread the thought of an Anatomy and Physiology course being included in their program of study. Some students are intimidated by the considerable amount of material contained in the average anatomy and physiology text, others are anxious about their ability to understand the "foreign" words or memorize so many facts, while others are distressed by the hours of time needed to prepare and study for class. Another cause for alarm among students is that this course is often an introductory class in many programs. This fact may be as overwhelming for those students who are majoring in the sciences as it is for those students without science backgrounds.

As difficult and stressful as learning human anatomy and physiology may seem, it is not an impossible task. Study and preparation for this course does not need to be as time-consuming as one may think. Medical terminology seems like a foreign language to so many because in actuality it is a foreign language. Medical terms are derived from Latin and Greek words. In this text many of the more commonly used medical terms are translated into English to aid in understanding. This text provides flash cards so students do not have to find the time to make their own. Therefore, all study time can be focused on learning not on creating study materials. Memorization of key terms is always part of the learning the process for any course. This text has a variety of strategies that will make the task of learning and memorizing the structures and functions of the human body much easier.

## Textbook

This textbook has many features to support your learning:

- A **workbook format** assists your learning by allowing you to write directly in the book. The act of writing enhances learning by actively engaging your brain in a way that reading alone does not.
- **Chapter exercises** allow you to practice defining terms and labeling anatomical structures.
- **Full-color anatomical illustrations** of body systems are labeled with correct anatomical terms. At the end of each chapter there are exercises that allow you to label the anatomical illustrations. This will reinforce your learning of these body parts.
- **Key terms** are listed at the beginning of each chapter. These terms are bolded throughout the text and are found with the explanation of that term. An appendix of all key terms is included.

- **Color coding of important words.** You will notice that anatomical or physiological terms are coded blue and pathology terms are purple.
- **Pathological terms** are found throughout the text and an additional table is included in each chapter. These terms consist of common diseases and disorders of each body system. An appendix of all pathology terms is included.
- **Flashpoints** appear throughout each chapter to give additional facts about the information in the text.

## CD Exercises

The CD-ROM that accompanies this book contains activities and exercises that allow you to review anatomy and physiology in a variety of ways. You will have the opportunity to practice spelling key terms, complete knowledge building exercises, and label anatomical illustrations.

## Flash Cards

Flash cards that correspond to key terms in this textbook are available for your use. Most of these cards contain visual cues as well. By reviewing these cards often you will increase your ability to memorize the meanings of these terms.

# REVIEWERS

DEBORAH J. BEDFORD, CMA (AAMA)
*Instructor, Medical Assisting*
North Seattle Community College
Seattle, Washington

CAROLE BERUBE, MA, MSN, BS, RN
*Professor Emeritus, Nursing*
*Instructor, Health Sciences*
Bristol Community College
Fall River, Massachusetts

DANIEL S. BICKERTON, MS
*Instructor, Biology*
Ogeechee Technical College
Statesboro, Georgia

RACHEL BRADSHAW, CMA (AAMA)
*Clinical Instructor, Medical Assisting*
Western Piedmont Community College
Morganton, North Carolina

DEBRA BROWN, RN
*Practical Nursing Instructor*
East Central Technical College
Fitzgerald, Georgia

REBECCA BUELL, BS, LMT
*Instructor, Massage Therapy*
McIntosh College
Dover, New Hampshire

SONYA M. BURNS, CMA (AAMA), BBA
*Instructor, Medical Assisting*
Augusta Technical College
Waynesboro, Georgia

ANNE D. GAILEY, CMA (AAMA)
*Instructor, Medical Assisting*
Ogeechee Technical College
Statesboro, Georgia

TAMMY T. GANT, RHIT, CMA (AAMA),
 CAHI
*Program Director & Instructor, Medical*
 *Assisting*
Surry Community College
Dobson, North Carolina

KAREN JONES, BS, MS, EdD
*Department Head, Biosciences*
Wake Technical Community College
Raleigh, North Carolina

JACQUE KEENER, AAS, CMA (AAMA),
 PBT (ASCP)
*Adjunct, Regulatory Affairs*
St. Jude Children's Hospital
Southaven, Mississippi

DIANE M. KLIEGER, RN, MBA, CMA
 (AAMA)
*Program Director, Medical Assisting*
Pinellas Technical Education Center
St. Petersburg, Florida

PAT G. MOECK, PHD, MBA, BA, CMA
 (AAMA)
*Director, Medical Assisting*
El Centro College
Dallas, Texas

LISA NAGLE, CMA (AAMA), BS
*Program Director, Medical Assisting*
Augusta Technical College
Waynesboro, Georgia

LYNDA J. OVERKING, RN, BSN, MS
*Coordinator, Health Occupations*
Monongalia County Technical
 Education Center
Morgantown, West Virginia

ROGER SKUGRUD, MA
*Instructor, Science & General Education*
Minnesota State College—South East
 Technical
Winona, Minnesota

CATHY D. SOTO, PhD, MBA, BA, CMA
 (AAMA)
*Program Director, Medical Assisting*
Paso Community College
El Paso, Texas

ELIZABETH STINGO, BSN, RN
*Instructor, Nursing*
Fred Eberle School of Practical
    Nursing
Buckhannon, West Virginia

DEBORAH L. WHITE, CMA (AAMA),
    MS/HPE
*Program Coordinator, Medical Assisting*
Trident Technical College
Charleston, South Carolina

DIANNA ZOMETSKY, CMA (AAMA),
    CMM
*Instructor, Health Science*
Lorenzo Walker Institute of
    Technology
Naples, Florida

# ACKNOWLEDGMENTS

My special thanks and gratitude goes to Andy McPhee, Senior Acquisitions Editor, for giving me this opportunity and having the faith that I could do it even when I did not. I would like to give a huge thanks to Yvonne Gillam, Developmental Editor, for all her guidance and showing me how seemingly random written pages and doodles become a textbook. Many thanks go to Lisa Thompson, Production Editor, and Jodi Kohl, Project Manager, for their keen eyes and to George Lang for his advice and clarification of so many editorial facts. Thank you to Dartmouth Publishing, Inc. for the wonderful artwork. To the reviewers who took time from their busy schedules to read the manuscript and give positive feedback. It was much appreciated. And a final thank you to the editors, artists, and staff at F.A. Davis whose names I never knew but whose talents have contributed in some way to the creation of this textbook.

# CONTENTS IN BRIEF

# TABLE OF CONTENTS

# INTRODUCTION

## Learning Styles

Individuals learn information in different ways according to their unique abilities and traits. Therefore, although all humans are similar, the ways in which you perceive, understand, and remember information may be somewhat different from other people.

In truth, all people possess a combination of styles. You may be especially strong in one style and less so in the others. You may be strong in two or three areas or may be equally strong in all areas. No style is inherently good or bad. They simply indicate how you most effectively perceive and process new information. As you learn about the styles described in this chapter and come to identify your own, you will then be able to modify your study activities accordingly. This will aid you in making the very most of your valuable study time, will enhance your learning, and will support you in doing your very best in future classes.

### Visual Learners

Most people are strongly visual learners. To most accurately and quickly grasp new information, these people need to see it represented visually. The more complex the data, the more true this is. Visual learners especially like data that is colorful and visually striking.

If you are a visual learner, you may have already noticed that you are drawn to visual information. Unless you also are an auditory learner, you may have some difficulty remembering information that is shared only verbally. Consequently, you may ask others to repeat themselves, or better yet, to write it down. When looking through books, magazines, or instruction manuals, you are especially drawn to photos and any visual illustrations because they help you to more accurately "see" what is being discussed. Within the classroom, you may prefer instructors who use written outlines and lots of visual aids.

You generally have a good sense of direction, rarely get lost, and can easily interpret and use maps. Your office and home may be littered with lists and notes that you've written to organize yourself and to remember things. You love self-adhesive note pads. You find listening to a lecture without stimulating visuals to be boring and tedious. You need to take notes, draw, or doodle to keep from falling asleep. In fact, you may appear to other people as if you are distracted or daydreaming when doodling on paper. However, you know that it actually helps you listen better. Your work and hobbies include activities that make use of color, shapes, and design or visual art. Just a few examples include drawing, painting, quilting, photography, and scrap booking.

## Study Strategies for Visual Learners

If you are a visual learner, try using study or memory techniques that aid you in being able to visually see and recall information. You may find **mnemonics** (memory aids) especially helpful for remembering lists or sequenced pieces information. Generally speaking, the more creative, whimsical, funny, or absurd they are, the better you will remember them. There are many different types of mnemonics. Here are some examples:

- Children use the well-known alphabet song, a musical mnemonic, to learn their ABCs.
- Students in anatomy classes use one of several mnemonic variations to remember the 12 cranial nerves (olfactory, optic, oculomotor, trochlear, trigeminal, abducens, facial, acoustic, glossopharyngeal, vagus, spinal accessory, and hypoglossal). An example is: "On Old Olympus' Tower Tops, A Finn And German Viewed Some Hops." Note that the first letter of each word is the same as the first letter of each of the cranial nerves.
- Most people use this spelling mnemonic to remember where to place the i and e: "i before e, except after c."

Another form of commonly used mnemonics is the **acronym**. An acronym is an abbreviation created by using the first letters or word parts in names or phrases. Examples of acronyms include LASER (light amplification by stimulated emission of radiation), FAQ (frequently asked questions), and PIN (personal identification number). In addition, the seven warning signs of cancer can be explained in the acronym CAUTION (**C**hange in bowel or bladder habits, **A** sore throat that does not heal, **U**nusual bleeding or discharge, **T**hickening or a lump in the breast or other area, **I**ndigestion or difficulty swallowing, **O**bvious change in a mole or wart, and **N**agging cough or hoarseness).

### *Auditory Learners*

Many people are auditory (or aural) learners. To most accurately and quickly grasp new information, these people need to hear it spoken. The more complex the data, the more true that is. The most common example of auditory information sharing is during a classroom lecture. However, there are other ways to hear information. Examples include audiotapes, videotapes, computer tutorials (with audio content), and oral discussions.

If you are an auditory learner, you may have already noticed that you are drawn to information presented aloud. Unless you are also a visual learner, you may have some difficulty remembering written information without some verbal discussion or review. You may often ask others to elaborate on details orally or may ask them to repeat themselves so you can hear it again. When recalling events you can sometimes "hear" how someone else speaks. You notice subtle inflections that convey meaning.

## Study Strategies for Auditory Learners

If you are an auditory learner, try using study or memory techniques that allow you to hear information aloud whether it is the spoken word or data set to music or any other auditory format. Auditory learners also are usually verbal learners. If this is true for you, then you learn best when you have the chance for a verbal exchange. This allows you to speak to and listen to others. You find mnemonics helpful, especially if they include rhyming or are catchy and fun to *say out loud*. A common example is the following mnemonic used to help people remember the number of days in each month:

> *Thirty days hath September,*
> *April, June, and November;*
> *All the rest have thirty-one,*
> *Excepting February alone:*
> *Which has twenty-eight, that's fine,*
> *Till leap year gives it twenty-nine.*

### Verbal Learners

It is sometimes said that some people must think (first) in order to speak. For verbal learners, the reverse may be true. They feel compelled to speak in order to think. Speaking aloud helps them to process information and think things through. This is especially true when the information is complex or the situation feels stressful. These people often "talk to themselves." Such individuals may state that doing so helps to slow down their brain to help them focus and think more clearly.

If you are a verbal learner, you may seek out a trusted friend to act as a "sounding board." You do not expect this person to solve your problem. Rather you need him to listen as you "think aloud" and "bounce things" off of him. Most likely, you love to read and enjoy some type of writing. This could take a professional form such as becoming an author, writing poetry for your own enjoyment, or simply writing in a private journal. You enjoy learning new words and incorporating them into your vocabulary. You find rhymes and tongue twisters entertaining. You may enjoy reading poetry aloud because speaking it is more enjoyable that silently reading it.

### Study Strategies for Verbal Learners

If you are a verbal learner, try using study or memory techniques that allow you to recite data or explain concepts aloud. Like auditory learners, you find mnemonics helpful, especially if they are fun to say or include rhyming. You also may find writing to be very helpful. Writing important data such as outlines, summaries, or vocabulary helps you remember the content. You are very likely a social learner who benefits from studying with a partner or in a study group. This provides ample opportunity for discussion. You especially benefit from explaining challenging concepts or "teaching" your study partners about a given topic.

For example, the members of your study group may decide to teach one another about the four major joint types in the body: hinge, ball and socket, pivot, and gliding. Each person describes the appearance and function of their assigned joint and gives an example. One person may compare a hinge joint such as those found in the knee and elbow to a door hinge. As he does so, he describes how it moves back and forth like a door that swings open and shut. The next person may compare a pivot joint, such as the one in the neck, to a chair that turns back and forth in a 180-degree half circle. Other students go on to teach about their assigned joints and give examples. To maximize the value of this exercise for verbal learners, you can add a requirement that all members of the group must verbally repeat key information or phrases after the "teacher" states it.

## Kinesthetic Learners

Most people have some kinesthetic (tactile) aspects to their learning style even though it may not be their most dominant style. People who are strong kinesthetic learners need to use their bodies as they learn. They like to touch and manipulate objects. This is especially important when learning physical skills. When assembling things, they may forego reading the instructions and just assemble the product based on feel and instinct. They are usually successful. But if not, then they may check the instructions, which will now make much more sense to them after having become physically acquainted with the parts.

If you are a kinesthetic learner you may have already noticed that you are eager to get your hands on objects to do things yourself. When the information being learned is theoretical, you are still eager to move your body somehow, even if it is to draw a diagram or fidget in your chair. Sitting through lengthy lectures feels tedious and almost painful to you. You like to touch things, and very likely have hobbies that include manipulating objects or making things with your hands. You notice textures and like how they feel. Your most productive thinking time occurs when you are on the move in activities such as biking, hiking, walking, or even running on a treadmill. You get restless if you sit around too long and feel eager to "do" something. You are very physical when communicating and may use big hand and arm gestures. You may enjoy dancing, sports, and other physical activities.

### Study Strategies for Kinesthetic Learners

If you are a kinesthetic learner, try using study or memory techniques that allow you to move your body or touch objects. When learning skills or procedures, your best strategy is to actually get your hands on the needed supplies and practice the procedure. For example, consider again the study group in which you and your friends are each describing major body joints. In addition to verbally describing the joints and giving examples, add a requirement that each person must somehow act out or physically mimic the joint movement; something like a charades game with talking allowed. The person describing the hinge joint now must physically get up and find a door to open and shut while he describes its function. Better yet, he might play the part of the door himself and move his body back and forth in an open doorway. The next person compares a pivot joint, such as the one in his neck, to a chair that turns back and forth in a 180-degree half circle. As he describes this, he literally turns his head back and forth and then turns the chair back and forth in a 180-degree circle. After each person performs his physical demonstration, other members of the group must perform the same physical movement. This gives everyone full kinesthetic value from the activity.

When actual physical practice of a skill is not possible, visualization is a great alternative. Play learning games, use flash cards, complete activities included in your textbook, use the student activity disc that accompanies many textbooks (including this one), and interact with a study partner or group.

## Social Learners

Many people are social learners. They learn most effectively when they are able to interact with other people. They enjoy the group **synergy** (enhanced action of two or more agents working together cooperatively) and are able to think things through with the verbal exchange that occurs during a lively discussion.

If you are a social learner, you may have already noticed that you are drawn to social situations and don't like to study alone. You communicate and interact well with others. You enjoy listening to and helping others. You may also be a verbal-auditory learner and may enjoy discussions and "bouncing ideas" off other people. You are drawn to social situations and may stay after class to talk with others. If you are athletic, you may prefer group sports to solo activities. You also enjoy social activities such as dancing and board games. You like working through problems with a partner or a group. Work activities may include teaching, coaching, or working in a people-oriented setting such as a restaurant or retail store.

### Study Strategies for Social Learners

If you are a social learner, you may find that you feel restless and have difficulty staying focused when you try to study alone. You need to seek out opportunities to study with one or more additional people. If there isn't a study group available, consider starting one. Group activities can include discussion, learning games, role playing, and creating mnemonics together.

### *Solitary Learners*

Many people are solitary learners. They learn most effectively when they are able to study alone without distraction from others. They are often somewhat private and enjoy time alone where they can ponder and reflect. They are strongly independent and know what works for them. Trying to conform to the group can be a source of frustration.

If you are a solitary learner you may feel frustrated trying to study with a partner or a group. You may feel like they are wasting your time and believe you would do better by yourself. You focus and concentrate best when alone. You are somewhat analytical and goal-oriented. You are also a self-starter and don't need anyone else to prompt you or to provide structure. You have learned to enjoy your own company, and enjoy solitude. Many people, especially your social friends, may find this difficult to understand because they may not like being alone. You may be known to travel alone, dine out alone, and go to movies or concerts alone. You don't feel that you are missing out when you do this. In fact, you may prefer it because you don't have to negotiate with anyone else about what to do or where to go.

### Study Strategies for Solitary learners

There are many ways that solitary learners study. The important thing is that they do it alone. They may read, review notes, and listen to taped lectures (if they are also auditory), or incorporate other strategies noted in this chapter, but alone.

### *Global Learners*

Global learners, sometimes called holistic learners, generally see the big picture first and later pay more attention to details. For example, when studying the human body, global learners first sees it as a whole, complete organism. With that picture in mind they are then able to begin studying the parts. This is true even when studying individual body systems, such as the cardiovascular system. Global learners first grasp the big picture of the entire system as it circulates blood throughout the body. With further study and thought, they appreciate how the system delivers oxygen and nutrients and eliminates wastes through a complex network of vessels including veins, arteries, and capillaries.

If you are a global learner, you may often respond based on intuition or emotion and are able to grasp symbolism. You may be able to accept rules, such as a math equation, without necessarily understanding how the steps work. You are probably good at recognizing relationships and "reading between the lines." You are flexible and do well with multitasking. When studying new concepts, you usually compare them with concepts you already understand. For example, when first learning about the lymphatic system, you may think, "This is very similar to what I know about the vascular system. They both have a complex network of vessels that convey fluid through the body." As you study the lymphatic system in detail, you then begin to distinguish the important differences.

## Study Strategies for Global Learners

If you are a global learner, you are probably also a visual/auditory learner, so try the study and memory techniques previously described. If you find studying details to be tedious and boring, try to find other, more creative and fun ways to learn the same material. For example, you may prefer drawing your own colorful diagrams or may enjoy using audio/visual tutorials or other activities that are often on the student disks that accompany textbooks or are available online.

Use your strengths. You are flexible. You are a multitasker. Don't be afraid to mix it up a bit to make your study efforts more lively and enjoyable. You are good at seeing the big picture and recognizing relationships. Therefore, begin each study session by identifying the relationship between what you are currently studying and your future career ambitions.

While reading, make note of terms, concepts, or sections that you skipped over or did not understand. You can do this by highlighting these areas in a specific color or by writing notes in the margins. After you've completed the initial read-through, force yourself to return to each of these areas and investigate them further.

### Analytical Learners

Analytical learners, sometimes called logical, linear, sequential, or mathematical learners, generally need to see the parts before fully comprehending the whole. For example, when studying the human body, analytical learners prefer to study in a methodical fashion beginning with the smallest parts and working up to the whole. Such people will prefer to take classes such as chemistry and cellular biology before taking classes like anatomy and physiology. As they continue learning about each of the body systems, they begin to appreciate how each relates to the other and comprises the whole organism.

Analytical learners readily identify patterns and like to group data into categories for further study. They love to create and follow agendas, make lists with items ranked by priority, and approach problem solving in a logical, methodical manner. They like to create and follow procedures and may grow impatient with others who do not. Analytical learners are often linear and orderly in their thinking and seek to quantify things whenever possible. They often pursue careers in accounting, sciences, computer technology, engineering, law enforcement, and mathematics.

## Study Strategies for Analytical Learners

Put your organizational talent to work to make your study efforts productive. Make an agenda or create a list of topics to be studied. Prioritize topics to ensure that you address the most important things first. This is your Must Know list. Set and follow time limits but don't overanalyze your plan. It is most important to get busy studying. Rather than getting sidetracked with interesting but low-priority items, make another list of topics as you go along, titled, It Would Be Nice to Know. Come back to this list later if, and only if, time permits.

Use your gift for identifying patterns by noting patterns within the material you are studying. This can be useful when you prepare for examinations because test questions often focus on features that are similar and those that are different. For example, a myocardial infarction (MI, also known as a heart attack) and angina both cause chest pain. In both cases, the pain is caused by inadequate blood supply to the heart. These are two important and similar features when comparing these disorders (chest pain and lack of oxygen). On the other hand, an MI causes actual death of heart muscle tissue but angina does not. This is an important difference.

To make the most of some study strategies, give yourself permission to be illogical or even silly. If a technically "inaccurate" mnemonic or silly song will help you remember something, then why not use it? Your global-learner classmates can help you with this if you will let them.

As you continue through this book you will find study tips included in every chapter. These tips suggest study techniques for all learning styles. Keep an open mind as you move forward and be willing to try any that you believe may be helpful. Make notes as you do so about what did and did not work well and anything you might do differently next time.

## Resources

Please visit http://davisplus.fadavis.com and search for keyword "Joy Hurst" for pertinent websites to aid in your studies.

# ANATOMICAL ORGANIZATION AND DIRECTION

1

Study of the human body allows us to understand how the body reacts to different stimuli and gives us a basis to understand disease processes. Anatomy and physiology are like two sides of the same coin: You need both to gain an understanding of the human body and how it operates.

*Anatomy* is the study of the structure of the body and how the structures relate to one another; included are features such as composition, size, and shape of the body. *Physiology* is the study of how the body functions; this includes how different structures of the body work, why they work, and how they relate to other bodily functions.

Anatomy and physiology are studied together because the structure of a body part often determines its function and how it relates to other body parts. For example, capillaries are needed for gas exchange throughout the body. These structures are only one cell thick. The thinness of the capillary allows an easy exchange of oxygen and carbon dioxide. A thicker blood vessel such as a vein cannot let gases flow in and out.

This chapter describes structural organization, the body systems, functions of living things, homeostasis, and directional terms.

## Structural Organization

The body is studied at six different structural levels: chemical, cellular, tissue, organ, system, and organism (see Fig. 1–1). Each level becomes more complex as it incorporates the structures and functions of the level before it.

First is the *chemical level.* This level describes how atoms become molecules. Atoms are the building blocks of matter, which is anything that has weight and takes up space. When similar atoms combine, they create an element. Hydrogen and oxygen are examples of common elements. When different elements combine, they form molecules. If the elements hydrogen and oxygen combine, they create the molecule called water. Molecules can combine to make even more complex forms such as cells. Everything has a chemical level because all things, including you and this textbook, are made of atoms.

The second structural level is the *cellular level.* Even though *cells* are formed from molecules, for the purposes of anatomy and physiology they are considered to be the first functional level for living things. The human body contains billions of cells that are responsible for various tasks that keep the body alive.

At the third structural level, similar cells work together to perform a common function and create structures called *tissues.* There are four basic body tissues types: epithelial, connective, muscle, and nerve.

## Key Terms

abdominal cavity

abdominopelvic cavity

anatomical position

anatomy

cell

cellular level

chemical level

cranial cavity

*Continued*

*Flashpoint*

There are several branches of the study of anatomy. Comparative anatomy is concerned with the structural similarities and differences between plants and animals. Histology studies only the tissues of living things. Embryology is concerned with the developmental aspects of plants and animals.

*Flashpoint*

The human body is composed of 63% hydrogen atoms, 25.5% oxygen atoms, 9.5% carbon atoms, and 2% nitrogen atoms.

*Flashpoint*

The largest cell in the human body is the female ovum or egg. The smallest is the male sperm cell.

## Key Terms—cont'd

dorsal cavity

epigastric region

frontal plane

homeostasis

hypochondriac region

hypogastric region

iliac region

lumbar region

median plane

organism

organ

pelvic cavity

physiology

plane

quadrant

region

sagittal plane

spinal cavity

system

thoracic cavity

tissue

transverse plane

umbilical region

ventral cavity

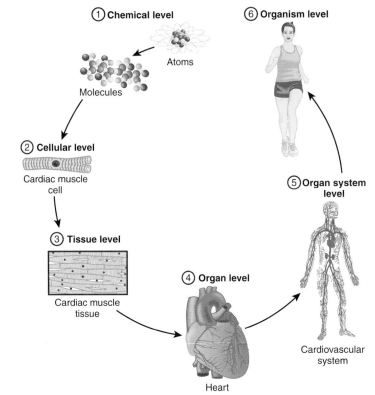

FIGURE 1-1  **Structural levels.**

Two or more different tissues that perform the same function create the fourth structural level, called an ***organ.*** An organ can perform complex functions that are essential to life. For example, the heart is the pump that keeps blood moving throughout the body to provide oxygen and other nutrients to the cells.

When several organs perform a common function, they create a structural level called a ***system.*** Each organ has its own task, but is dependent on the other organs in the system to complete a process. For example, the organs of the urinary system include the kidneys and urinary bladder. The task of the kidneys is to produce urine, and the urinary bladder stores the urine before it is released from the body. The kidney and bladder have different functions, but they work together to remove fluid waste from the body.

All organ systems working together form the highest, or sixth, structural level, which is the whole ***organism.*** The human organism comprises 11 systems that interact to create and maintain the functions that keep us alive. These systems are integumentary, muscular, skeletal, lymphatic, cardiovascular, respiratory, digestive, nervous, urinary, endocrine, and reproductive (see Fig. 1–2).

*Flashpoint*

Gross anatomy is the term used to describe the study of the organs and organ systems of organisms.

## Overview of Body Systems

- The integumentary system is the external covering of the body and comprises skin, hair, glands, and nerve receptors. The skin protects and cushions the body and regulates body temperature.
- The muscular system is responsible for body movement. The muscles are the main structures of this system, which also includes the tendons, which connect the muscles to bone.

*(text continues on page 6)*

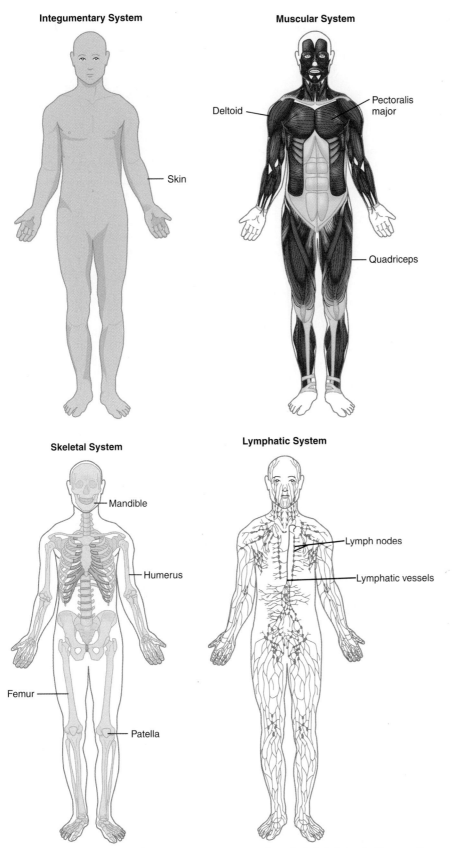

**Integumentary System**

Skin

**Muscular System**

Deltoid

Pectoralis major

Quadriceps

**Skeletal System**

Mandible

Humerus

Femur

Patella

**Lymphatic System**

Lymph nodes

Lymphatic vessels

FIGURE 1–2  The body systems: integumentary, muscular, skeletal, lymphatic, cardiovascular, respiratory, digestive, nervous, urinary, endocrine, and male and female reproductive.

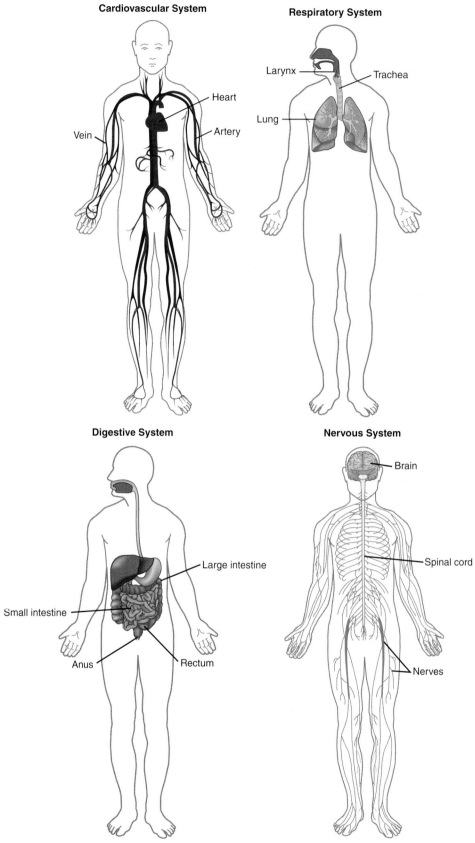

FIGURE 1-2  cont'd

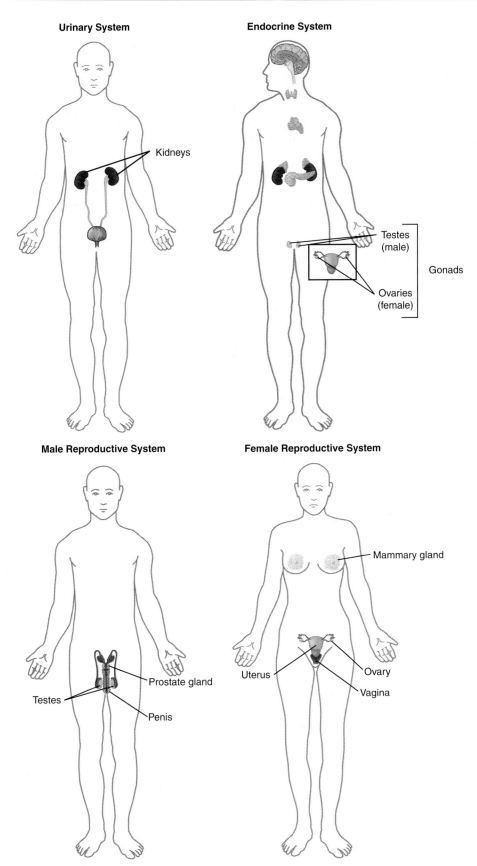

**FIGURE 1-2  cont'd**

- The skeletal system comprises bones, cartilage, ligaments, and joints. Bones support the body and hold it upright. This system also stores minerals and is responsible for the creation of blood cells.
- The lymphatic system cleanses the blood and aids in protection from foreign substances. This system includes the lymph nodes, thymus, spleen, tonsils, and other related tissues.
- The cardiovascular system is responsible for pumping blood throughout the body. The heart is the organ that along with the blood vessels brings oxygen and nutrients to the cells.
- The respiratory system provides gas exchange for the body. It constantly supplies oxygen to the cells and removes the waste product carbon dioxide. This system includes the nasal and oral passages, the larynx, trachea, bronchi, and lungs.
- The digestive system breaks down food into its basic forms called nutrients that can be absorbed and used by the body. The esophagus, stomach, small intestine, and large intestine are the organs of this system.
- The nervous system conducts and interprets sensory information from inside and outside the body, which then responds as needed. The organs of this system are the brain, spinal cord, and connecting nerves.
- The urinary system removes liquid wastes from the blood and regulates blood pressure. This system includes the kidneys and bladder.
- The endocrine system uses hormones to control the functions of the body systems. It includes the pituitary gland, thyroid gland, ovaries, and testes.
- The reproductive system produces cells that carry the genetic material for the purpose of creating a new organism. This system includes the ovaries and uterus in the female and the testes and penis in the male.

## Functions of Living Things

*Flashpoint*

A population is a group of the same living organisms, and a habitat is the place in which they live.

Organisms, or living things, no matter how different, all share common life functions. One trait of all organisms is that they have and maintain boundaries that separate them from the environment. They have a shape or form that distinguishes them from others. In humans, this boundary is created by the skin. Organisms can also increase in size or grow. Another trait all living things share is the ability to reproduce to create new organisms like themselves. All organisms engage in some type of movement and respond to internal and external stimuli. Organisms also have some means to ingest and break food down into nutrients. They use the nutrients to produce energy. Living things also can excrete waste material.

### Homeostasis

Another common trait of living things is that they attempt to maintain a stable or balanced state called **homeostasis.** This is the organism's response to constant changes in the internal and external environment. When the body is in homeostasis, it is considered to be healthy, and when the body is not in homeostasis, the result is illness or disease.

The body's response to a change in the internal environment occurs after eating and digesting a meal. After food has been broken down or digested in the stomach, the nutrients from that food are absorbed by the small intestine. The nutrients then enter the bloodstream. One of these nutrients is a sugar called glucose, which is used by the cells to make energy. In response to the presence of glucose in the blood, an organ called the pancreas releases a substance called insulin. Insulin carries glucose to the cells. The level of insulin produced by the pancreas depends on the level of glucose in the bloodstream; when the glucose level is high, more insulin is produced, and when the glucose level is low, less insulin is produced. The reaction of the pancreas to the presence of glucose is a healthy routine response.

An unstable or unhealthy state changes the ability of the body to maintain homeostasis. For example, if the pancreas is unable to produce insulin, the glucose in the bloodstream has no way to get to the cells, so the glucose levels continue to increase in the blood. Too much glucose in the blood is **hyperglycemia.** When hyperglycemia occurs, not only are the cells deprived of the nutrient they need to make energy for the body, but it also causes other symptoms, such as dehydration, fatigue, and nausea. Long-term effects of hyperglycemia are blindness, kidney failure, mental confusion, and coma. Each of these results changes the functions of several systems, placing the body out of homeostasis.

## Directional Terms

Directional terms show the relationship of body parts to each other (see Table 1–1). These terms are always used to refer to anatomical position. The body when standing erect with the face front and arms at the side with palms facing forward is said to be in **anatomical position** (see Fig. 1–3). Directional terms are always used to refer to anatomical position regardless of the actual position of the body. This is helpful to remember because the body cannot remain in anatomical position. For example, when the body is relaxed, the hand turns over, and the thumb points inward. Also, when a person is reclining, all body parts are on the same level, so there is no "up" or "down."

Table 1–2 presents the common positions that the body can be placed in for medical examinations and procedures. If a patient is moved into a position for an examination, such as sitting upright or lying face down, the directional terms remain the same regardless of the position of the patient. Proximal means the end closest to where the body part joins or attaches to another body part. For example, the proximal end of the arm is where it attaches to the shoulder. Even if you were standing on your head, the proximal end of the arm would remain the same because it would still be closest to its point of attachment.

Each directional term has a term with an opposite meaning. Superior means above or toward the head, and inferior means below or away from the head. Because of anatomical position, each term can refer to any body part. For example, the head is superior to the neck, and the knee is superior to the foot. Another way of thinking is that the neck is inferior to the head, and the foot is inferior to the knee.

**TABLE 1–1**

**DIRECTIONAL TERMS**

| Term | Definition | Example |
| --- | --- | --- |
| Inferior | Away from the head or toward the lower part of a structure | The intestines are inferior to the lungs |
| Superior | Toward the head or upper part of a structure | The heart is superior to the stomach |
| Anterior (Ventral) | Toward the front of the body | The eyes are located on the anterior skull |
| Posterior (Dorsal) | Toward the back of the body | The spine is posterior to the umbilicus |
| Distal | Farther from the attachment of a body part | The fingers are distal to the wrists |
| Proximal | Close to the attachment of a body part | The thigh bone is proximal to the hip |
| Medial | Toward the midline of the body | The umbilicus is found at the medial abdomen |
| Lateral | Away from the midline, on the outer side | The ribs are lateral to the sternum |
| Superficial | Toward or at the body surface | A paper cut is a superficial wound |
| Deep | Away from the body surface | A stab wound is a deep wound |

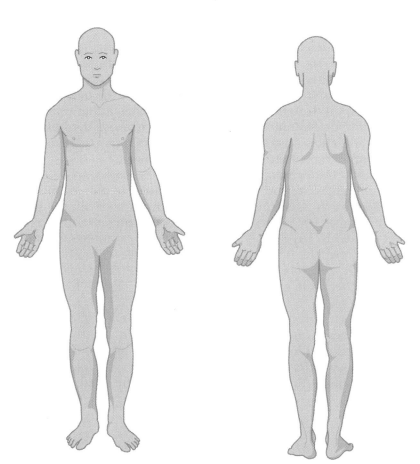

FIGURE 1–3  Anatomical position.

## TABLE 1–2
### PATIENT EXAMINATION POSITIONS

| Term | Definition | Common Use |
|---|---|---|
| Dorsal recumbent | Patient's legs are bent at the knees and feet are resting on the table | Gynecological examinations |
| Fowler's | Patient is in the sitting position | Examinations of head, neck, and chest |
| Lithotomy | Patient's feet are placed in stirrups | Gynecological examinations and PAP smears |
| Prone | Patient is lying face downward | General examinations of the dorsal body |
| Sims' | Patient lies on the left side with the left arm behind the body, and the right arm and right leg are sharply flexed on the table | Colonoscopy or rectal examinations |
| Supine | Patient is lying face upward | General examinations of the ventral body |

*Continued*

**TABLE 1–2**

**PATIENT EXAMINATION POSITIONS—cont'd**

| Term | Definition | Common Use |
|---|---|---|
| Trendelenburg | Patient's legs are raised above the head | Patients in shock |

## Planes of the Body

**Planes** are imaginary flat surfaces that pass through an object. For the purpose of anatomy, the body has three planes (see Fig. 1–4). These planes separate the body into sections. (1) The **sagittal plane** runs vertically through the body. The **median plane,** or mid-sagittal plane, is a sagittal plane that divides the body into equal right and left halves. (2) The **transverse plane,** or horizontal plane, separates the body into superior and inferior sections. (3) The **frontal plane,** or coronal plane, divides the body into anterior and posterior sections.

## Body Cavities

*Flashpoint*

When using diagnostic imaging, such as computed tomography (CT) scan, magnetic resonance imaging (MRI), or positron emission tomography (PET) scan, the planes of the body are referred to using X-Y-Z coordinates. The sagittal plane is the X-Z plane, the transverse plane is the X-Y plane, and the frontal plane is the Y-Z plane.

The human body contains many cavities, or hollow spaces. The ones that contain the internal organs are the dorsal cavity and ventral cavity (see Fig. 1–5).

The **dorsal cavity** actually contains two cavities: cranial and spinal. The **cranial cavity** is within the skull and contains the brain. The **spinal cavity** is within the spinal column and contains the spinal cord.

The **ventral cavity** is divided into three cavities. The **thoracic cavity** (chest) is located under the rib cage and above the diaphragm. The **abdominal cavity** is below the diaphragm and under the abdominal muscles. The **pelvic cavity** is the space within the pelvis. Because the abdominal and pelvic cavities are not physically separated, they are sometimes referred to as the **abdominopelvic cavity**.

## Divisions of the Abdominopelvic Cavity

Because the abdomen and pelvis contain most of the internal organs, a way to narrow down the location of a pain, injury, or trauma is by dividing the abdomen. The abdominal cavity can be separated into four sections or nine sections depending on how specific the location needs to be. Different organs or parts of organs are found in each section.

### Quadrants

The abdominal cavity can be divided into four sections called **quadrants**. These quadrants are formed by a transverse plane and a sagittal plane crossing at the

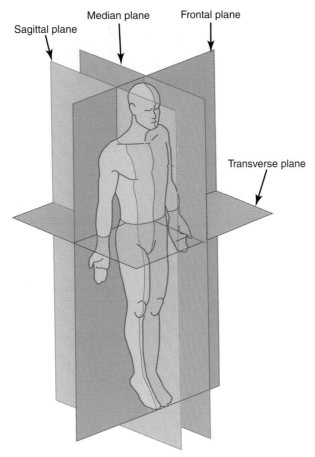

Sagittal plane     Median plane     Frontal plane

Transverse plane

**FIGURE 1–4  The body planes.**

umbilicus or navel. These quadrants give a general location of the internal organs and are referred to as upper right, lower right, upper left, and lower left. The upper right quadrant contains the liver and part of the small intestine and large intestine. The upper left quadrant contains the stomach, spleen, and portions of the intestines. The right lower quadrant contains the small and large intestines and the appendix. The lower left quadrant contains a portion of the small intestine and the colon.

## Regions

To give a more specific location of organs, the abdomen can be divided further into nine sections called *regions*. The regions are formed by the crossing of two transverse planes and two sagittal planes so that the sections resemble a "tic-tac-toe" grid. The center section covers the umbilicus and is the *umbilical region*. Directly above is the *epigastric region* (on the stomach), and directly below is the *hypogastric region* (below the stomach). Lateral to the umbilicus are the right and left *lumbar regions*. Above these regions are the right and left *hypochondriac regions* (below the ribs), and below the lumbar regions are the right and left *iliac regions*. Figure 1–6 shows the quadrants and regions of the body.

Flashpoint
The integumentary system is the only body system not located in a body cavity.

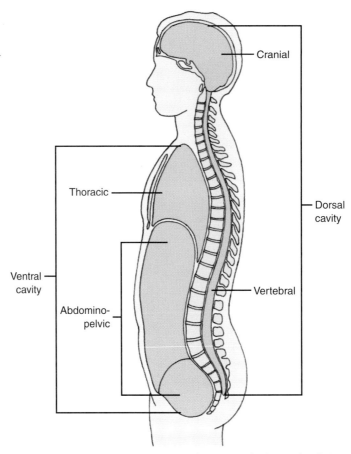

**FIGURE 1-5  The dorsal and ventral cavities.** (From Eagle S. *Medical Terminology in a Flash!* Philadelphia, PA: FA Davis; 2006:13.)

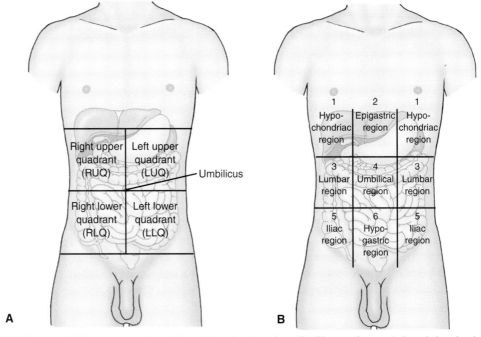

**FIGURE 1-6** *(A)* **The quadrants of the abdominal cavity.** *(B)* **The regions of the abdominal cavity.** (From Eagle S. *Medical Terminology in a Flash!* Philadelphia, PA: FA Davis; 2006:13.)

# Practice Exercises

## Multiple Choice

1. The position used when a patient is in shock is the _____.
   a. dorsal recumbent
   b. ventral recumbent
   c. Trendelenburg
   d. lithotomy

2. Similar cells working together form a(n) _____.
   a. tissue
   b. organ
   c. system
   d. membrane

3. The term dorsal means _____.
   a. front
   b. side
   c. above
   d. back

4. An organ of the integumentary system is the _____.
   a. heart
   b. kidney
   c. skin
   d. lung

5. The opposite meaning of the term distal is _____.
   a. proximity
   b. proximal
   c. superior
   d. supra

## True or False

1. True   False     Anterior and ventral both refer to the front of the body.

2. True   False     Dorsal and medial have opposite meanings.

3. True   False     The lithotomy position can be used for childbirth.

4. True   False     The abdomen is divided into six regions.

5. True   False     The left lower quadrant contains the heart.

6. True   False     Anatomical position describes the body when reclining.

7. True   False     Tissues are the basic functional level of living things.

8. True   False     Homeostasis is the stability of the body in response to change.

9. True   False     The chemical level describes how atoms combine to make molecules.

10. True   False    The ventral cavity contains the cranial and spinal cavities.

## Fill in the Blank

1. The _____ plane separates the body into equal right and left halves.

2. A patient lying face down is in the _____ position.

3. A wound near the skin surface can be described as _____.

4. A position above another is called _____.

5. An example of a _____ wound is a puncture.

6. _____ is the study of how the body works.

7. Two or more organs working together form a _____ level.

8. A _____ plane divides the body into superior and inferior sections.

9. The center region of the abdomen is the _____ region.

10. _____ is the study of the structure of the body.

## Short Answer

1. **Name the two positions that can be used for gynecological examinations.**

2. **Name the body cavities.**

3. **Define an organism.**

4. **Define a plane.**

5. **Define anatomical position.**

## Labeling

*Fill in the blanks with the appropriate anatomical terms.*

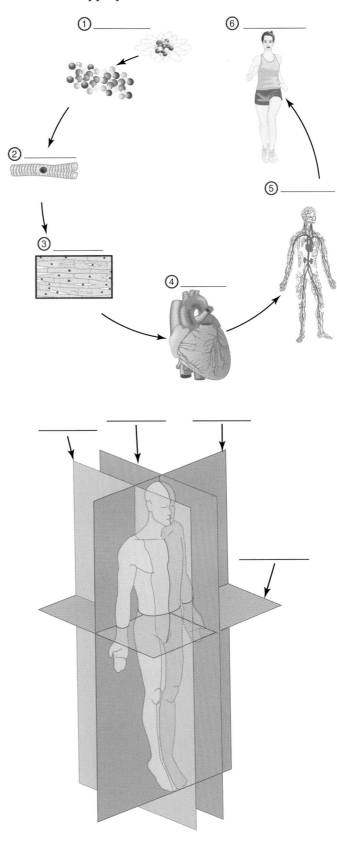

① _____

② _____

③ _____

④ _____

⑤ _____

⑥ _____

_____     _____     _____

_____

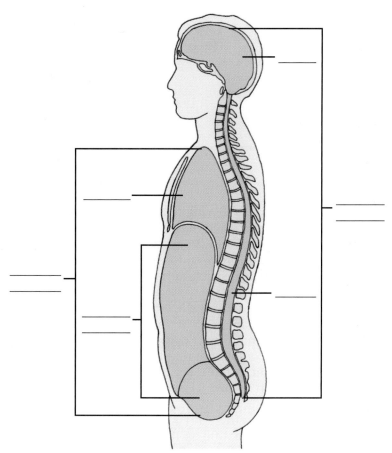

(From Eagle S. *Medical Terminology in a Flash!* Philadelphia, PA: FA Davis; 2006:20.)

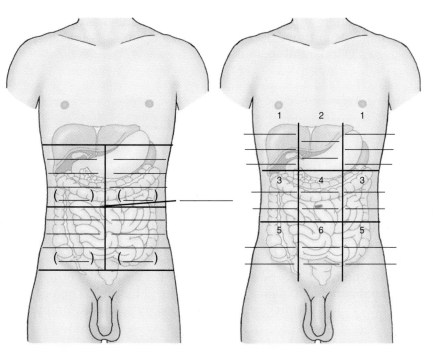

(From Eagle S. *Medical Terminology in a Flash!* Philadelphia, PA: FA Davis; 2006:21.)

# CELLS AND TISSUES

## Key Terms

active transport

ATP

bulk transport

cell membrane

cellular transport

chromosome

cilia

codon

concentration gradient

cytoplasm

cytosol

diffusion

DNA

endoplasmic reticulum

equilibrium

*Continued*

The **cell** is the basic structure of all living things. In the human body, cells are too numerous to count, but it is estimated that there are approximately 100 trillion cells in each one of us. These cells vary in size, shape, and function. Most cells are so small that a microscope is needed to view them. Cells can be round, rectangular, or irregular, and some cells can even change shape as they move. Cells have the ability to function alone or to work in groups. Each individual cell can alter its functions to meet the needs of the group.

A group of similar cells working together forms a **tissue**. Four different types of tissue are found in the human body: epithelial, connective, muscle, and nervous. These tissues are the component of all organs and their surrounding structures. Because of the variation in organ function, tissues also vary in their function, appearance, and structure. Tissues are responsible for different tasks such as protection, movement, secretion, absorption, conduction of electrical current, and transportation of other substances. In appearance and structure, tissues can be just as varied, existing as thin sheets, fine weblike strands, or dense ropelike bands. Tissues can be solid, semisolid, or fluid.

This chapter discusses cells and tissues. The cell section gives an overview of the general characteristics of a cell and special cell structures. It also describes the different types of cellular transport and the processes of DNA replication, protein manufacture, and cellular division.

The tissue section of the chapter outlines the four different tissue types, describes the cells of those tissues, and gives examples of each. This chapter also discusses glands and membranes of the body.

## Cells

Individual cells have many features that are similar to the features of an organism. Many organisms, such as bacteria and amebae, are only one cell. Because cells vary in function, size, and shape, there is no one cell type that is representative of them all, but all cells share some common features. All cells have a covering or membrane, house organelles, transport substances, contain genetic material, make protein, and divide to create new cells.

Because a cell is a living thing, it maintains a boundary to separate itself from the environment. The boundary of a cell is a skinlike outer covering called the **cell membrane**, or plasma membrane (see Fig. 2–1). The cell membrane is two layers thick and is made of phospholipids, cholesterol, and protein.

### Flashpoint

Cells can be classified as prokaryotic, which are simple cells that do not have a nucleus, but only a region where genetic material is located, and eukaryotic, which are cells that do contain a nucleus. Bacteria are an example of prokaryotic cells. Animal and plant cells are eukaryotic.

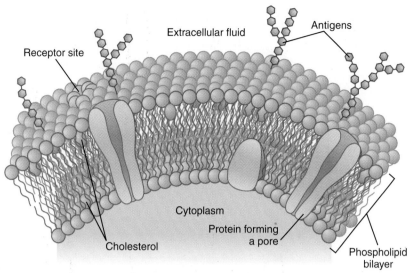

Receptor site · Extracellular fluid · Antigens · Cholesterol · Cytoplasm · Protein forming a pore · Phospholipid bilayer

FIGURE 2–1  **The cell membrane.**

Key Terms—cont'd

facilitated diffusion

filtration

flagellum

gene

gland

Golgi body

lysosomes

matrix

meiosis

membrane

microvilli

mitochondria

mitosis

nucleus

organelle

osmosis

peroxisomes

protein synthesis

ribosomes

RNA

selectively permeable

transcription

translation

Phospholipids are the main component of the cell membrane. The individual phospholipids create a barrier, but it is not solid, so it allows some substances to pass through, while keeping other substances out. Phospholipids are similar in appearance to a lollipop. The round heads prefer to be in a fluid environment, and the tails prefer a dryer environment. To create a perfect environment for both sides, the tails of the two layers join to form the dry inner membrane, and the heads are in the outer membrane, which is exposed to fluid. The head of one side of the membrane lines the inner cell, and the head of the other side of the membrane touches the external environment. Cholesterol lines the underside of the phospholipid barrier and acts as support for the membrane.

Scattered throughout the membrane are large proteins that aid in transport and act as receptors. These proteins are embedded in the membrane. Some form pores, which allow substances that are too large to pass through the membrane to enter. The other proteins are specialized and are called receptors. These receptors have several different functions. They can be places for enzymes to pass through the membrane or sites for hormones to bind. Receptors can also be antigens, which act as surface markers. A surface marker is a unique shape that acts as identification for that the cell.

When the cell membrane allows some substances to pass through while keeping other substances out, it is being **selectively permeable** or semipermeable. This ability of the cell membrane provides protection for the cell. It also provides a means of allowing only the substances the cell organelles would use inside, while excess materials are kept outside.

Solid and fluid structures are found within the cell membrane (see Fig. 2–2). Collectively, everything inside the cell membrane is the **cytoplasm** (cell material). The solid structures are **organelles** (little organs) that resemble our organs. Each organelle has a specific function and works with the other organelles to perform activities that keep the cell alive. An average cell has the following organelles: a nucleus, mitochondria, ribosomes, endoplasmic reticulum, Golgi bodies, lysosomes, and peroxisomes.

All organelles are suspended in the clear gel-like fluid of the cytoplasm called **cytosol**. The main component of cytosol is water, but it also contains enzymes, salts, and proteins. Not only does the cytosol hold up the organelles, but also its proteins control many activities of the organelles.

*Flashpoint*

Plant cells have an extra covering surrounding the cell membrane called the cell wall. This is a rigid membrane that protects the cell and aids in life functions.

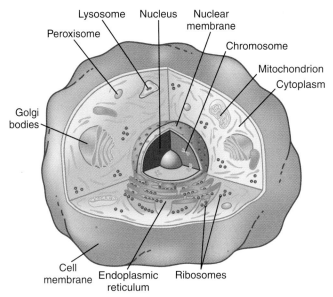

FIGURE 2-2  Generalized cell showing the organelles.

The largest cell organelle is the **nucleus**. This organelle contains chromosomes, which are the genetic material of the cell. This genetic material is deoxyribonucleic acid, or **DNA**. Similar to the cell itself, the nucleus is surrounded by a double-layered membrane called the nuclear membrane. This membrane separates the chromosomes from the other organelles.

**Mitochondria** are sausage-shaped organelles that are called the "power-house" of the cell. Mitochondria take oxygen and glucose and turn them into an energy source called adenosine triphosphate, or **ATP**. This energy source is used to power the cell itself and the whole organism. Mitochondria are plentiful in cells that need extra energy. For example, muscle cells need a constant supply of ATP to be able to shorten or contract to produce movement. Muscle cells need more ATP than other cells even when at rest because the muscles always maintain a slight contraction or tone to keep the body upright.

Proteins are needed by the individual cell and the whole organism. Each cell contains organelles that act like tiny protein factories called **ribosomes**. Some ribosomes, which resemble grains of sand, float within the cell, whereas others are scattered along another organelle called the endoplasmic reticulum. The more ribosomes a cell contains, the more protein it makes. Cells that produce proteins for delivery to other cells have a higher number of ribosomes than the average cell. For example, the pancreas needs to transport digestive enzymes to the stomach. Many ribosomes are needed by the pancreas to package and send those enzymes when they are needed. Cells in the spleen would have fewer ribosomes because they do not transport materials to other cells.

The **endoplasmic reticulum**, or ER, is a series of canals that weave around the cell. These canals are a transportation system or roadway. This organelle moves proteins produced by the ribosomes and other substances the cell may need to other places within the cell. The sections of the ER covered with ribosomes are referred to as rough ER, and the sections without ribosomes are referred to as smooth ER. Rough ER transports the proteins made by the ribosomes attached to it. Smooth ER is responsible for not only transportation, but also the breakdown of cholesterol and fat.

Flashpoint

The DNA in mitochondria is maternally inherited, meaning it is passed on by the mother with no mixture with the DNA of the father.

The processing of proteins, carbohydrates, and other substances the cell may need to secrete is done by the **Golgi bodies**, or Golgi apparatus. This organelle has the appearance of several flattened bags stacked together and acts as the "Fed Ex" of the cell. Golgi bodies package proteins in membrane and send them to wherever they are needed either inside or outside the cell. These proteins are needed to repair and maintain the cell membrane and are used by organs such as the pancreas, which needs protein to transport digestive enzymes to the stomach.

Other organelles called **lysosomes** move freely inside the cell. They are round baglike membranes that can vary in size. Lysosomes act like trash collectors and ingest debris. Cell debris can be substances such as dead or worn cell parts or bacteria. These organelles contain enzymes that digest or break down the debris. Leukocytes or white blood cells contain numerous lysosomes because the job of a leukocyte is to clear the body of bacteria and other harmful microorganisms.

**Peroxisomes** are another freely moving organelle. Similar to lysosomes, they are membranous bags containing enzymes. These enzymes cleanse the cell by breaking down fatty acids and detoxifying alcohol. In addition, they break down free radicals, which are molecules that are a normal by-product of cell metabolism. These by-products are capable of damaging proteins, which leads to the breakdown of the cell or tissue. Free radicals contribute to the changes that occur in our skin and organs as we age. The enzymes in the peroxisomes convert these free radicals to hydrogen peroxide, which is converted to water. These organelles are numerous in liver cells because they assist the organ with detoxification of the body.

## Special Cell Structures

Some cells have additional needs and specialized structures such as cilia, flagella, or microvilli to aid them (see Fig. 2–3). **Cilia** are long hairlike projections on the surface of some cells that move substances across the outside of the cell. The fallopian tubes are lined with cilia that help an egg cell move down the tube to the uterus. A **flagellum** is a single projection that moves a cell, such as sperm, by propelling it forward. **Microvilli** are also found on the surface of cells, but in contrast to cilia they are thicker and fingerlike in appearance. Microvilli increase the surface area of a cell and aid in absorption of substances. The cells that line the small intestine contain microvilli to absorb the nutrients from digested food.

## Cellular Transport

Certain substances need to pass through the cell membrane to supply the cell with materials it needs to survive. Also, many cells make substances that the body needs to live. Because the cell membrane is selectively permeable, some substances can flow in and out of the cell without any effort. Other substances are too large to pass through and need the cell to change to accommodate them.

Moving substances back and forth between the cell and the environment is known as **cellular transport**. There are several ways that a cell can transport substances into and out of the cell membrane. These types of transport are diffusion, osmosis, facilitated diffusion, filtration, and active transport (see Fig. 2-4). Some of these means of transport use no energy, but some require energy expenditure by the cell to transport materials in and out.

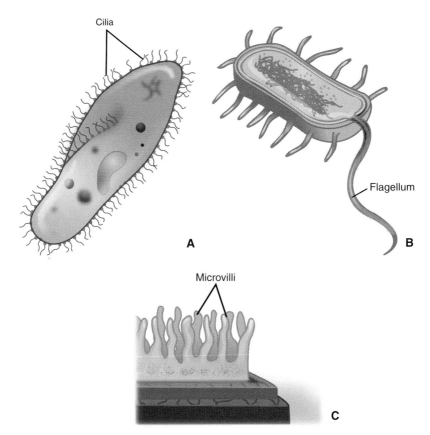

FIGURE 2–3  Specialized cell structures. *(A)* Cilia. *(B)* Flagella. *(C)* Microvilli.

The simplest form of cellular transport is **diffusion** (see Fig. 2–4A). Diffusion occurs when molecules move from an area of greater concentration to an area of lesser concentration. This range of concentrations is referred to as a **concentration gradient**. The molecules move along the gradient until an equal amount is dispersed throughout the area and there is no longer a higher concentration of one substance or another. When this state is reached, it is called **equilibrium**.

Diffusion occurs whenever you drop a sugar cube into a glass of tea. The concentrated sugar cube is in an environment without sugar. To change, the cube breaks down and releases the sugar particles into the solution. The molecules continue to disperse until an equal amount of sugar is found throughout the solution.

An example of diffusion in the body occurs in the capillaries. Blood returning from the lungs is high in oxygen and low in carbon dioxide. Blood leaving the cells has a higher carbon dioxide level, but low oxygen concentration. Oxygen and carbon dioxide are gases. When these gases meet at the capillaries, oxygen diffuses into the cell where there is a lesser concentration of oxygen, and carbon dioxide diffuses out also to a place of lesser concentration. This process is gas exchange, and it enables cells to receive the oxygen they need to live and provides a means of expelling the waste product carbon dioxide from the body.

**Osmosis** is similar to diffusion, but it involves the flow of water from a place of more water to a place of less water (see Fig. 2–4B). Similar to diffusion, the water moves only until a balance is achieved between both places. This type of transport is used by the kidneys to prevent dehydration in the body. The kidneys have the ability to reabsorb water from the body to offset the amount lost during urination.

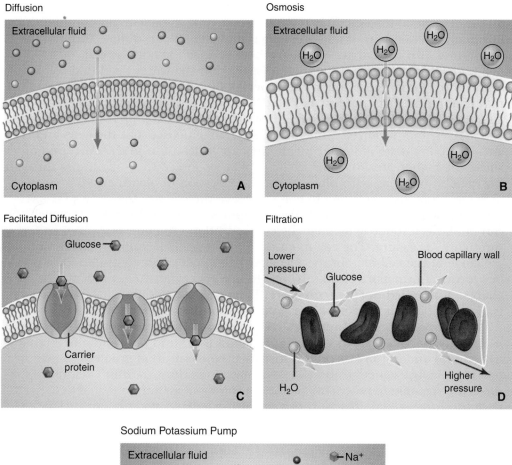

Diffusion

Extracellular fluid

Cytoplasm          A

Osmosis

Extracellular fluid

Cytoplasm          B

Facilitated Diffusion

Glucose

Carrier
protein          C

Filtration

Lower
pressure          Glucose          Blood capillary wall

$H_2O$          Higher
pressure          D

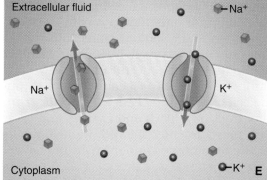

Sodium Potassium Pump

Extracellular fluid          Na$^+$

Na$^+$          K$^+$

Cytoplasm          K$^+$     E

FIGURE 2–4  Transport mechanisms. *(A)* Diffusion. *(B)* Osmosis. *(C)* Facilitated diffusion.
*(D)* Filtration. *(E)* Sodium-potassium pump.

The amount of water reabsorbed depends on the amount lost so that homeostasis
is maintained.

Some other substances need to move from a place of higher concentration to a
place of lower concentration, but cannot flow through a membrane. To bring
these substances in and out of the cell, they need to be assisted. This type of
transport is ***facilitated diffusion*** (see Fig. 2–4C). Facilitated refers to something
that is aided.

Glucose is a sugar needed for cells to create energy, but glucose molecules
cannot cross the cell membrane. To enter the cell, glucose must use facilitated

diffusion. Glucose molecules bind to enzymes, called carrier enzymes, located on the surface of the cell. These enzymes are able to pass freely through the membrane. When bound to the enzyme, the glucose can diffuse through the membrane with the carrier enzyme and be released inside the cell.

If both water and the substances dissolved in the water need to cross a membrane, force is needed to push the water along with the substances through that membrane. This process is ***filtration***, and it uses pressure to create movement (see Fig. 2–4D). In the body, filtration creates blood pressure. Capillaries carry gases and dissolved substances, such as glucose, that the cells and tissues need. Pressure is higher inside the capillaries than in the surrounding tissues. The higher pressure inside the capillaries forces the substances through the membrane along with plasma, the fluid portion of blood, into the tissues.

Some substances needing to enter or leave the cell are too large to pass through the membrane, do not have receptors on the cell surface to which they can bind, need to move against the concentration gradient, or cannot be forced through by pressure. The cell must accommodate these substances by creating a change in the cell membrane. Because this process, in contrast to the previous forms of transport, needs the cell to use energy, or ATP, to create the change, it is called **active transport**. There are two different means of active transport: the sodium-potassium pump and bulk transport.

The first type of active transport, the ***sodium-potassium pump*** (see Fig. 2–4E), is an active process because the ions sodium ($Na^+$) and potassium ($K^+$) must be moved into and out of the cell against their concentration gradient. A cell needs to have a higher concentration of potassium ions than sodium ions inside for the cell to be able to rest. This results in more potassium ions inside the cell than there are outside the cell. The cell also has fewer sodium ions on the inside of the cell than exist outside the cell. These two ions diffuse freely through the cell membrane so that the potassium wants to flow out and the sodium wants to flow in to reach equilibrium. Because the cell needs the potassium concentration to be higher than the sodium, it must find a way to work against the natural diffusion process. The solution is the sodium-potassium pump, which continuously pumps excess sodium outside to its higher concentration and pumps potassium back into the cell also to its higher concentration.

If a substance wanting to enter the cell cannot enter through any other transportation method, the cell can use a process called **bulk transport** (see Fig. 2–5). There are two types of bulk transport: endocytosis and exocytosis.

If a large substance needs to enter the cell, it positions itself against the cell membrane. Because the membrane cannot break to allow entry, the membrane wraps itself around the substance in a process called ***endocytosis*** (into the cell). By forming a mouthlike cavity, the two sides of the membrane envelop the substance until the sides meet (see Fig. 2–5A). When the membrane meets, it seals itself creating a vesicle or sac with the substance trapped inside. When the vesicle is sealed, the substance is fully inside the cell. The vesicle detaches from the membrane and floats freely in the cytoplasm. A lysosome finds it and attaches itself to the vesicle and uses its enzymes to digest the contents of the vesicle.

If a package for export is too large to leave the cell, the opposite of endocytosis occurs. The membrane-wrapped substance, usually mucus, hormones, or cellular waste, attaches to the cell wall. It pushes against the wall until it pushes past the wall and forms a budlike projection (see Fig. 2–5B). This process is called ***exocytosis*** (outside the cell). The bud breaks and releases the substance into the body. The membrane packaging is left behind to act like a plug, and it fuses to the wall so that the cell membrane is maintained.

Endocytosis can also be specialized in some cells. If a cell performs endocytosis to rid the body of bacteria and dead cells, it is called ***phagocytosis*** (cell eating)

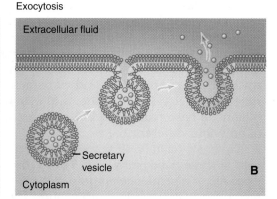

Endocytosis

Exocytosis

Phagocytosis

Pinocytosis

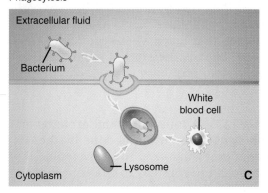

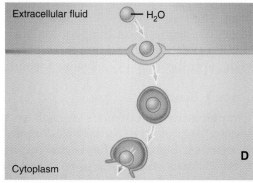

FIGURE 2–5 **Bulk transport.** *(A)* Endocytosis. *(B)* Exocytosis. *(C)* Phagocytosis. *(D)* Pinocytosis.

(see Fig. 2–5C). There are several different phagocytes in the body. One is a white blood cell that patrols the body searching for and engulfing bacteria and other microorganisms that may be harmful to the body.

If a cell is responsible for taking in fluid, the process is called ***pinocytosis*** (cell drinking). Just as a cell surrounds a bacterium, it surrounds and engulfs a fluid droplet (see Fig. 2–5D). Cells that are needed for absorption, such as the cells in the small intestine, perform pinocytosis routinely.

## Protein

The DNA of each chromosome inside the nucleus of a cell is a blueprint with instructions to make every protein within that cell. Proteins have many functions in the cell and in the body. They are needed to build and maintain structures and to control many activities inside and outside of the cell. Regardless of the function of the protein, all proteins are made by a combination of 20 different amino acids. The process of making a protein begins with the replication, or copying, of the DNA sequence. After a copy of the protein sequence is made, it is transcribed and then translated in a manufacturing process called protein synthesis.

### DNA Replication

A human cell contains 46 chromosomes; each carries a specific code created by the sequence of the DNA. Within this DNA sequence are genes. A ***gene*** is a specific section of the code that is responsible for the creation of a protein.

*Flashpoint*

Human beings are 99.9% genetically identical.

**Chromosomes** are the carriers of the sequence that makes all the proteins that form every cell, tissue, organ, and system in the human body.

DNA resembles a spiral ladder called a double helix. The rungs of the double helix are made of nucleotides or nitrogenous bases. Each rung is a pair of complementary bases that are formed by the following nucleotides: adenine (A), thymine (T), guanine (G), and cytosine (C). When these nucleotides bind, adenine always joins to thymine, and cytosine always binds to guanine. All the billions of base pairs found in our chromosomes are created by the arrangement of only four different bases.

The basic form of all proteins is an amino acid. The genetic code for an amino acid is three base pairs long. These three base pairs are called a **codon**. For example, if a sequence contained AAA, it would be the codon for the amino acid lysine, and GCA would be the codon for the amino acid alanine. Each protein is formed by a sequence of codons or amino acids. Different proteins vary in the number of amino acids and the number of codons they contain. If a protein contains 100 amino acids, it contains a sequence of 300 base pairs. Also found along the sequence of the gene code are codons that mark where each individual protein code starts and stops. The codon AUG signals the start of a new protein code, and the codon UGA shows where the protein sequence ends.

## Protein Synthesis

Changing the genetic code in each sequence of DNA into individual proteins is known as protein manufacture, or **protein synthesis**, and it is done by the ribosomes. Before synthesis can occur, some problems need to be overcome. First, proteins cannot be made until the code is interpreted, so ribosomes need a way to decode the sequence. Second, the DNA is located in the nucleus and does not leave. The ribosomes are located in the cytoplasm or on the endoplasmic reticulum, and they cannot move to the nucleus. So not only do the ribosomes need a decoder, but they also need a means of getting the code from the nucleus to the ribosomes.

To solve these problems, another nucleic acid called ribonucleic acid, or **RNA**, assists the DNA (see Fig. 2–6). RNA is similar in structure to DNA, but it is only single-stranded. Because it is a nucleic acid, it is also made from nucleotides. Similar to DNA, it uses the individual bases adenine, cytosine, and guanine, but instead of thymine it uses uracil. RNA is found outside the nucleus and comes in three forms: messenger RNA, which carries the blueprint for DNA from the nucleus to the ribosomes; ribosomal RNA, which helps to build proteins; and transfer RNA, which brings amino acids to the ribosomes.

Protein synthesis involves two processes: transcription and translation. Transcription refers to changing information from one form to another. An example of transcription is when a long form document is written from notes taken by shorthand. In protein synthesis, **transcription** is the process of changing the sequence of DNA into information that RNA can deliver to the ribosomes. For transcription to occur, each DNA strand unwinds one section at a time. As it unwinds, the base pairs separate, and the strands pull apart so that the DNA resembles an open zipper. Messenger RNA (mRNA) goes to the open strand and creates a complementary sequence or a negative of that sequence. A DNA sequence of AAA-GCA-TCC would have a complementary mRNA of UUU-CGU-AGG. When all the bases are copied, mRNA leaves the nucleus and carries the negative to the ribosomes.

The second process of protein synthesis begins when mRNA attaches to a ribosome. The next process is translation, which means to take one language and change it to another. In the case of DNA, **translation** of a gene sequence is

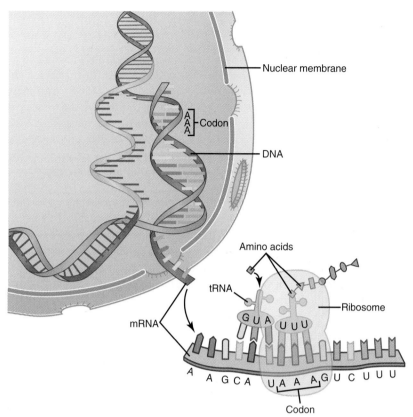

FIGURE 2–6  Protein synthesis.

changing it from nucleic acid bases into amino acids. When the mRNA attaches to the ribosome, transfer RNA (tRNA) brings amino acids from the cytoplasm and matches them to the corresponding codon similar to matching puzzle pieces. After the amino acid is bound to the strand, tRNA is released, and it returns for another amino acid. Each piece of the strand is translated until tRNA recognizes a stop codon. When one is encountered, tRNA stops delivery of the amino acids. The newly made protein is released from the ribosome, and the next is translated (see Box 2–1).

## Cellular Division

All cells reproduce to create new cells using a process known as cell division. Within the body, two different types of reproduction exist. One is mitosis, or asexual reproduction, and the other is meiosis, or sexual reproduction.

### Mitosis

Most cells replicate or copy themselves by **mitosis**, or asexual reproduction. The purpose of these phases is to divide the cell and make two new identical cells. Division by mitosis increases cell numbers for growth or repair of a cell and replaces cells that have died. Mitosis has the following different phases: interphase, prophase, metaphase, anaphase, and telophase (see Fig. 2–7). Cells replicate themselves only for a limited number of times, although the number is different for different cells. At this point, the cell becomes specialized, so it does not need to divide further, such as a nerve cell, or it dies.

## Box 2–1 Mutations

Sometimes when typing the wrong key is pushed and a word is misspelled, or a stitch is dropped when knitting, or a color in a sequence of beads is skipped. We call these errors mistakes, but when a mistake is made during protein synthesis, it is called a mutation.

DNA is the template for all the proteins in the body. During translation, the transfer RNA brings nucleic acids to the copy of a gene to create the protein that gene represents. Sometimes the wrong nucleic acid is placed in the sequence, or more than one nucleic acid can be brought to the same place. The nucleic acid itself could be damaged or even skipped.

If only one mistake is made in a sequence, it is called a point mutation, but often several bases are rearranged, skipped, or damaged. Mutations can also be caused by ultraviolet radiation, exposure to chemicals, or some viruses that can cause a change in the gene structure.

Mutations can cause severe effects, some mutations are beneficial, and some mutations have no effect at all on the organism. Some mutations can be passed on to offspring, and these are called inherited traits. An example of an inherited trait that has a detrimental effect is a disease called sickle cell anemia. If a child inherits a mutated gene from both the mother and the father, the child has a disease of the red blood cells. This disease causes the red blood cells to be shaped like the letter "C" (see figure), and they are unable to transport oxygen correctly. A gene can also be passed on that has no effect on the health of the individual. An example of this type of mutation is red hair. To have red hair, the person has to inherit the mutated gene from both the mother and the father.

Some inherited mutations can be advantageous or helpful to the individuals who have them. Having a mutation that causes someone not to be susceptible to a virus is an advantage. It ensures that the offspring with the mutant gene would be more likely to survive than the offspring without it. Advantageous mutations help species to evolve by making them stronger or fit to survive in their environment.

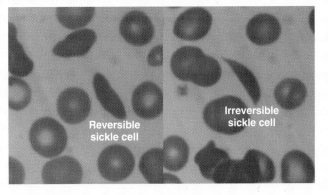

Reversible sickle cell

Irreversible sickle cell

### Phases of Mitosis

The first phase of mitosis is *interphase*. This is the time that the cell is preparing itself for division. Because the cell divides itself in two, there needs to be two sets of organelles present within the cell before it replicates. During interphase, all organelles including DNA in the nucleus are duplicated.

The chromosomes in the nucleus are usually in a shapeless form. To replicate, they need to reform. During interphase, the chromosomes take shape and become visible in the nucleus. The chromosomes are two strands of DNA that have temporarily joined in the center at a place called the *centromere*. This form resembles the letter "X." The cell is now in the second stage called *prophase*. At this time, microtubules called *spindle fibers* appear at either

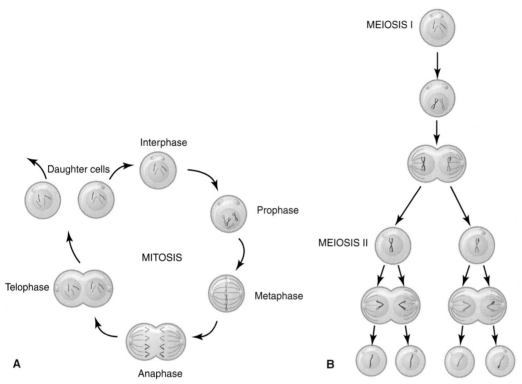

MEIOSIS I

MEIOSIS II

Interphase

Daughter cells

MITOSIS

Prophase

Metaphase

Telophase

Anaphase

**A**

**B**

FIGURE 2–7  *(A)* **Phases of mitosis.** *(B)* **Meiosis.**

side of the cell and attach themselves to the chromosomes. The spindle fibers look like ropes, and they begin to pull the chromosomes to the center of the cell.

*Metaphase* is the third or middle phase of mitosis. At this time, the chromosomes have lined up in the middle of the cell. There is a spindle fiber attached to both strands of the chromosome, one on each side.

To make two new cells, the chromosomes must separate. The spindle fibers attached to the centromeres shorten. As they shorten, they begin to tear the centromeres apart. When full separation occurs, the cell is now in the fourth stage, called *anaphase*. The individual chromosome strands continue to be pulled in opposite directions as the spindle fibers retract.

When the chromosome strands have reached the opposite sides of the cell, the cell is now in *telophase*, the fifth and final stage of mitosis. At this time, a nuclear membrane reforms around the chromosomes. The two copies of the organelles arrange themselves so that one copy of each is on either side of the cell. When the organelles are arranged, the center of the cell contracts, and the cytosol pulls to either side, taking one copy of the organelles with it. The cell membrane pushes inward until two cells are created, and the membrane continues to push inward until the cells fully separate. The result is two cells called daughter cells that are identical to the original. When these cells need to replicate, mitosis occurs again.

### Meiosis

*Meiosis* is sexual reproduction, and it is how sex cells, or gametes, are created. Gametes carry the genetic material of the organism. In the human body, male gametes are called sperm, and female gametes are called ova or eggs. Through the process of meiosis, the gametes that are produced carry half the number of the original chromosomes. A gamete merges with the gamete of the opposite gender, and the chromosomes of both combine to create another organism.

*Flashpoint*

Heredity is the act of passing genes from parents to offspring.

# Body Tissues

Groups of cells with a similar structure and function form tissues. The tissues of the human body perform many diverse functions, such as protection, support, transportation, movement, and conduction of electrical impulses. The four basic body tissues are epithelial, connective, muscle, and nerve.

## Epithelial Tissue

*Epithelial tissue* acts as a covering or a lining. It surrounds the external body and the internal organs. It is also found lining the insides of organs and the body cavities. Epithelial tissue always has one free surface. The other side is called the basement membrane and connects the epithelium to the tissue beneath it. No blood vessels are found in epithelial tissue. This is why a superficial wound such as a paper cut does not bleed. Oxygen and nutrients are received from the connective tissues beneath the epithelium.

The cells of epithelial tissues multiply rapidly and grow tightly packed together. This fast reproduction ensures that epithelial tissue is continuously replaced. The tightness of the cells of the skin and mucous membranes creates a protective barrier. In addition to protection, epithelial cells can perform other functions, such as secretion, absorption, excretion, and sensory reception. In the body, the mucous membranes secrete a substance called mucus. Absorption of nutrients is done by the epithelial cells of the small intestine. The tissues of the kidneys excrete fluid waste. Sensory receptors are found in the skin and detect environmental stimuli.

### Classification of Epithelial Tissue

Epithelial tissues (see Fig. 2–8) are classified by shape and number of cell layers. Thin, flattened epithelial cells are called *squamous*. Cells that are thicker and cube-shaped are called *cuboidal*. Cells that are longer and more rectangular are called *columnar*.

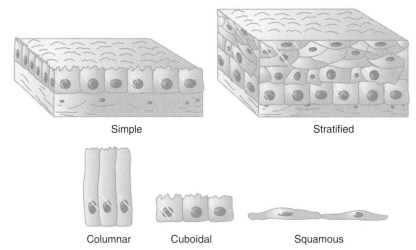

Simple            Stratified

Columnar      Cuboidal            Squamous

FIGURE 2–8 **Types of epithelial tissue: squamous, cuboidal, columnar, simple, stratified.**

A single layer of epithelial tissue is described as *simple*, and two or more layers are *stratified*. Simple epithelial tissues are most often found in organs that need to secrete or absorb substances, such as the lining of the small intestine. Stratified epithelial tissues, being thicker, act as protection for the organs in which they are found. Figure 2–8 shows examples of these cell shapes and layers.

These shapes and layers combine to form different types of epithelial tissue: simple squamous, stratified squamous, simple cuboidal, simple columnar, transitional, and ciliated (see Table 2–1).

*Simple squamous epithelial* tissue is one layer of flattened squamous cells. This tissue is very thin and smooth. It is found where gas exchange needs to occur, such as in the alveoli of the lungs and the capillaries of the body.

*Stratified squamous epithelial* tissue is many layers of flattened cells on the surface and more rounded squamous cells in the lower layers. This type of tissue is found in the epidermis of the skin. The lowermost layer produces new cells, which get pushed toward the outer surface. The cells flatten and harden, or keratinize, as they surface. Other locations for stratified squamous epithelium are the oral cavity and esophagus. These are mucous membranes, so the outer layer of cells is not keratinized. The tightly packed cells of this tissue act as a barrier to microorganisms.

*Simple cuboidal epithelium* is one layer of cube-shaped cells. This tissue is found in structures called glands. These cells arrange themselves in a circular pattern and secrete substances into the cavity they form. An example of a gland is the sudoriferous gland, which secretes perspiration.

*Simple columnar epithelium* tissue is a single row of columnar cells. These elongated cells are responsible for secretion and absorption. These cells are found lining the stomach and small intestine. In the small intestine, the columnar cells are called microvilli and are responsible for the absorption of nutrients broken down by the secretion of digestive enzymes by the columnar cells of the stomach.

*Transitional epithelium* is a multilayered tissue. This tissue is specialized to change shape so it can stretch and retract. It is found in the urinary bladder

**TABLE 2–1**

**TYPES OF EPITHELIAL TISSUES**

| Epithelial Tissue | Function | Location in the Body |
|---|---|---|
| Simple squamous | Filtration and diffusion | Wall of capillaries, air sacs of the lungs |
| Simple cuboidal | Secretion and absorption | Surface of the ovaries, lining of the ducts of some glands |
| Simple columnar | Absorption, secretion, protection | Lining of gastrointestinal tract |
| Stratified squamous | Protection | Outer layer of the skin, lining of mucous membranes |
| Stratified cuboidal | Protection | Lining of sweat glands and salivary glands |
| Stratified columnar | Protection and secretion | Male urethra and vas deferens |
| Transitional | Protection and flexibility | Inner lining of urinary bladder and uterus |

and the ureters. When the bladder is empty, the cells of the membrane appear stratified, and the superficial cells have a rounded appearance. As the bladder fills and stretches, the cells slide against one another causing them to become thinner and more squamous in appearance.

*Ciliated epithelium* describes columnar cells with cilia on the free surface. The cilia sweep materials across the surface of the cells. This tissue is found in the respiratory tract, where it lines the surface of the nasal cavity, larynx, trachea, and bronchial tubes. It is responsible for sweeping mucus filled with trapped particles, dust, and microorganisms toward the pharynx so that it can enter the stomach and be destroyed by the digestive juices.

### Glands

Glands are cells or organs that secrete a substance that has some effect on another cell or organ. These substances can work at the site of secretion or at a distant location. Glands can be either unicellular or multicellular.

Unicellular glands are only one cell thick. These cells are called *goblet cells* and are columnar cells that line the digestive and respiratory tracts. They secrete mucus. The secretion is *mucus*, whereas when referring to a membrane, it is *mucous*.

Multicellular glands comprise many similar cells working together. These glands can be either exocrine or endocrine glands. *Exocrine glands* have ducts or tubes that take the secretions away from the gland to be used at another location. The sudoriferous glands or sweat glands within the skin are exocrine glands that use ducts to carry sweat to the skin surface. *Endocrine glands* are ductless glands. These glands secrete chemicals called hormones directly into the bloodstream. The thyroid gland located in the throat secretes hormones into the blood supply that control metabolism and calcium absorption in the body.

## Connective Tissue

*Connective tissue* is the most common tissue in the body and performs various functions. Primarily as the name implies, it supports and adheres other tissues together. Connective tissues can also aid in protection, act as a framework for other structures, fill hollow spaces, store fat, produce blood cells, repair tissue damage, and fight infection. Because connective tissue is found throughout the body, the appearance of connective tissue and the cells within it varies depending on the function of the tissue (see Table 2–2). This tissue can also be found in various forms from fluid to semisolid to solid.

### Types of Connective Tissue

Connective tissues differ in appearance and function, but all connective tissues share one common trait; the cells of the tissue live in a *matrix*. A matrix is a substance made of nonliving materials in which the cells are suspended. The components of a matrix are mainly water, fibers, and proteins that bind the cells to the fibers. Three different types of fibers can be found in a matrix: collagen, elastic, and reticular. *Collagen* fibers are strong yet flexible. *Elastic* fibers have the ability to be stretched and return to their original state. *Reticular* fibers are a variation of collagen and are very thin fibers that form a weblike mesh to support other tissues. Each type of connective tissue has its own matrix. The types of connective tissue in the body are cartilage, dense connective, areolar, adipose, bone, blood, and reticular.

## TABLE 2–2

## TYPES OF CONNECTIVE TISSUE

| Connective Tissue | Description |
| --- | --- |
| Adipose | Also called fat, found below the skin and in spaces between muscles; cushions and protects organs and tissues |
| Areolar | Soft weblike fibers that hold organs in position and underlie the mucous membranes; responsible for tissue edema |
| Blood | Fluid that transports materials throughout the body |
| Bone | Rigid tissue that stores minerals such as calcium and phosphorus and supports the body |
| Cartilage | Attaches bones to bones and muscle to bone, protects tissues, and provides structure for bone development |
| Dense connective | Tightly packed elastic fibers that form tendons and ligaments |
| Reticular | Mesh of fibers found only in the lymphoid tissue to support lymphocytes |

*Cartilage* is a type of connective tissue that provides protection and support to other tissues. This tissue has a firm yet flexible protein matrix made of collagen fibers and is formed from chondrocytes (cartilage cells). Cartilage is found on the surfaces of bones that form joints to prevent friction. It is also found between the bones of the spine to prevent shock and in the trachea to keep the airway open. Our ears and the tips of our noses are also formed from cartilage. A fetal skeleton begins as cartilage, but it is replaced by bone as the fetus ages.

There is no blood supply to cartilage, so to receive nutrients it uses diffusion from the surrounding tissues to obtain nourishment. Because this process is slow, the healing of damaged cartilage takes a long time, much longer than that of a bone.

The three types of cartilage are hyaline, fibrocartilage, and elastic. Hyaline cartilage is the most abundant type of cartilage in the body. It supports the larynx, attaches the ribs to the sternum, and covers the ends of bones that create joints. Fibrocartilage forms the intervertebral disk of the spinal column. Elastic cartilage is pliable and forms the outside of the ear.

*Areolar* (open space) or loose connective tissue is distributed throughout the body; it holds organs in place, and lies beneath the mucous membranes. The cells of this tissue are fibroblasts, which are fixed or nonmoving cells that secrete proteins to create a matrix of collagen, elastic, and reticular fibers. These fibers form a soft, pliable, cobweb-like tissue with many areas of open space. Within the open space is fluid composed of water and salts. The wastes of cells and tissues are released into the fluid and then transferred to the blood. This tissue is also responsible for edema or tissue swelling because it soaks up the excess tissue fluid produced by inflammation.

*Adipose* is a connective tissue that stores fat. The cells of this tissue are called adipocytes (fat cells). These cells compose the bulk of the tissue, so the matrix consists of only a few collagen fibers and tissue fluid. Adipose tissue connects the dermis of the skin to the muscles beneath. It can also be found surrounding the internal organs. This fat layer acts as protection and a cushion to prevent shock. Adipose tissue also acts as insulation and keeps the body at an even temperature.

*Flashpoint*

Adipose tissue is a source of adult stem cells that have the potential to form into a limited number of other cells.

The amount of fat tissue in the body varies. Fat stores exist to provide energy if glucose is unavailable. If an individual takes in more nutrients than are used, the body converts these nutrients to fat and adds it to the adipose layer.

*Bone* is a hard connective tissue, often referred to as osseous tissue, which supports and protects the body. It also provides a storage area for calcium and phosphorus and a place for blood cell production. The cells found within bone are called osteocytes (bone cells), and they reside in a matrix of calcium salts and collagen.

*Blood* or vascular tissue is a fluid connective tissue that provides a means of transportation for nutrients and wastes. Three different cells are found in blood: erythrocytes, which carry oxygen; leukocytes, which fight infection; and thrombocytes, which cause blood to clot. The fluid matrix is called plasma.

*Dense connective* or fibrous tissue is formed from fibroblasts, and the matrix in which they reside is collagen. This tissue is similar to cartilage, but the fibers form tough yet flexible ropelike structures called tendons and ligaments. Tendons join muscle to bone, and ligaments join bone to bone. Similar to cartilage, this tissue has a poor blood supply and lacks nutrients, so the healing of a damaged tendon or ligament is a slow process.

*Reticular connective* tissue is a mesh of reticular fibers created by cells called reticulocytes. This tissue is found only in the lymphoid tissues, such as the spleen, lymph nodes, and bone marrow. Reticular tissue forms a bedding to support lymphocytes within the lymphoid tissues.

## Muscle Tissue

Muscle tissues are able to contract or shorten to create movement. The type of movement depends on the muscle tissue and its location in the body. There are three types of muscle tissue in the body: skeletal, smooth, and cardiac (see Fig. 2–9), and each has its own function.

*Skeletal muscle* is also called voluntary muscle. It is attached to bones and is consciously controlled. These muscles cause body movements by pulling on the sites where the muscles attach to the bones as they contract. Skeletal muscle has several nuclei in each cell and markings called striations (stripes). The striations give muscle cells the appearance and texture of an elastic band. These cells have the ability to contract and release quickly.

*Smooth muscle*, or visceral muscle, is also called involuntary muscle. It is found in the organs of the body and is not consciously controlled. These muscle cells have a single nucleus and are pointed at the ends. Smooth muscle is found

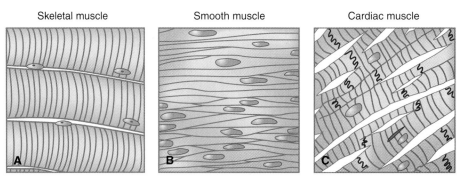

FIGURE 2–9  **Types of muscle tissue.** *(A)* **Skeletal.** *(B)* **Smooth.** *(C)* **Cardiac.**

in the walls of hollow organs, and contracts and releases to create movements that push substances along a path. An example is the wavelike movement of the esophagus that propels food to the stomach. Smooth muscle contracts more slowly than the other types of muscle.

*Cardiac muscle* is found only in the heart. Its appearance is a mixture of skeletal and smooth muscle. It has striations similar to skeletal muscle, but has one nucleus and is more pointed at the ends similar to smooth muscle. Cardiac muscle is involuntary, but needs to be able to contract rapidly similar to skeletal muscle.

## Nervous Tissue

*Nervous tissue* is composed of cells called neurons and is found in the brain, spinal cord, and peripheral nerves (see Fig. 2–10). This tissue responds to changes or stimuli in the internal and external environment. It responds to stimuli by conducting or transmitting electrical impulses from one neuron to another. This communication process coordinates and regulates many body functions, such as heart rate, blood pressure, and breathing.

Flashpoint
The human body has about 45 miles of nerves.

## Membranes

*Membranes* are thin layers of tissues that cover structures and line cavities. They consist of epithelial and connective tissues. The two types of membranes are mucous and serous.

*Mucous membranes* line body cavities that open to the outside environment, such as the nasal cavity and the digestive tract. They secrete a substance called mucus that keeps the tissue moist and acts as a barrier to trap foreign particles.

*Serous membranes* line cavities and cover organs with no opening to the outside. They secrete serous fluid that acts as a lubricant to prevent abrasion when organs rub together. Serous fluid is named for its location. Serous fluid found in the pleural cavity is called pleural fluid, and serous fluid surrounding the heart is called pericardial fluid.

For information about diseases and disorders of the cells and tissues, see Table 2–3.

Flashpoint
Spinnbarkeit is a medical term used to describe the thick, stretchy quality of mucus and saliva.

Nerve cell

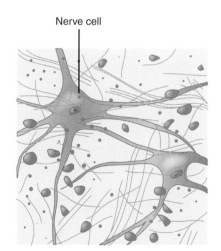

FIGURE 2-10  **Nervous tissue.**

## TABLE 2–3
## PATHOLOGY TERMS

| | |
|---|---|
| Ascites | Accumulation of serous fluid in the peritoneal cavity; most often caused by liver disease or trauma |
| Contracture | Decrease in mobility of connective tissue because of fibrosis or thickening of the tissue |
| Hemothorax | Collection of blood in the pleural cavity that prevents the lungs from expanding during inhalation; most often caused by trauma |
| Ischemia | Loss of blood supply to a localized area of tissue; associated with coronary artery disease |
| Pleural effusion | Collection of fluid in the pleural cavity that prevents the lungs from expanding during inhalation; most often caused by heart failure or kidney failure |
| Pneumothorax | Collection of air in the pleural cavity that prevents the lungs from expanding during inhalation; most often caused by smoking, lung disease, or trauma; also called a collapsed lung |

# Practice Exercises

## Multiple Choice

1. _____ brings amino acids to the ribosome for protein manufacture.

   a. mRNA

   b. tRNA

   c. rRNA

   d. dRNA

2. Membranes that line body cavities that open to the outside are _____.

   a. serous

   b. synovial

   c. mucous

   d. pleural

3. Connective tissue found in lymphoid organs is called _____.

   a. alveolar

   b. fibrous

   c. cartilage

   d. reticular

4. The middle phase of mitosis is _____.

   a. telophase

   b. anaphase

   c. metaphase

   d. prophase

5. Connective tissue cells are suspended in a nonliving _____.

   a. matrix

   b. membrane

   c. tissue

   d. fluid

6. The manufacture of protein is called _____.

   a. synovial

   b. transverse

   c. synthesis

   d. transport

7. Visceral muscle is also known as _____ or involuntary.

   a. striated

   b. skeletal

   c. smooth

   d. serous

8. The fluid portion of cytoplasm is called _____.

   a. cortisol

   b. cortisone

   c. cortical

   d. cytosol

9. A _____ secretes substances that affect other cells or organs.

   a. muscle

   b. neuron

   c. membrane

   d. gland

10. Sexual reproduction is known as _____.

   a. meiosis

   b. ketosis

   c. mitosis

   d. myosis

## Fill in the Blank

1. The organelle that produces energy is the _____.

2. Ribosomes are responsible for production of _____.

3. _____ are organelles that package protein.

4. Skeletal muscle is also called _____ muscle.

5. _____ tissue acts as a covering or lining.

6. _____ fibers are flexible and found in ligaments and tendons.

7. Thin flattened epithelial cells are called _____.

8. The process of changing nucleic acids to amino acids is _____.

9. Several layers of epithelial tissues are called _____.

10. The largest cell organelle is the _____.

## Matching

1. _____ The basic cell of nervous tissue

2. _____ Specialized cell structure that increases surface area

3. _____ Another name for loose connective tissue

4. _____ Organelle that produces energy

5. _____ The process of substances moving through a cell membrane

6. _____ Cells that find and clear debris

a. endoplasmic reticulum

b. lysosomes

c. osmosis

d. neuron

e. diffusion

f. peroxisomes

g. flagellum

h. endocytosis

i. microvilli

j. active transport

k. macrophage

7. _____ Hairlike structures on the surface of some cells

8. _____ Transport that cells use to envelop substances outside the cell

9. _____ Organelle that contains enzymes that digest cell debris

10. _____ Organelle that acts as a transportation system

11. _____ When particles move from a higher concentration to a lower concentration

12. _____ Specialized cell structure that aids in movement

13. _____ Transport that uses energy

14. _____ Organelle that detoxifies alcohol

15. _____ Transport that uses pressure to create movement

l. cilia

m. areolar

n. mitochondria

o. filtration

## Short Answer

1. **List the different types of tissue and give an example of each.**

2. **What is the difference between a mucous and a serous membrane?**

3. **Discuss the different types of bulk transport**

## Labeling

*Fill in the blanks with the appropriate anatomical terms.*

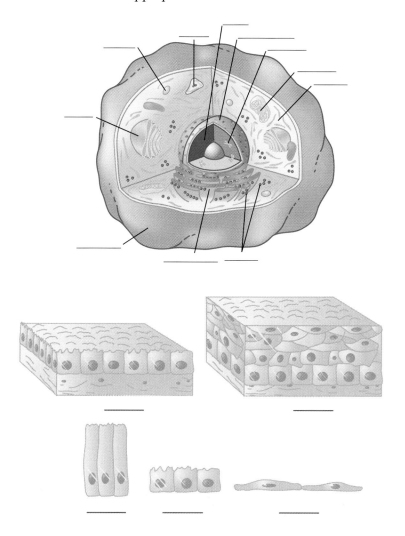

# THE INTEGUMENTARY SYSTEM

# 3

## Key Terms

adipose

basal cell carcinoma

dermis

epidermis

full-thickness burn

keratinize

malignant melanoma

melanin

melanocyte

partial-thickness burn

rule of nines

sebaceous gland

sebum

squamous cell carcinoma

stratum basale

stratum corneum

subcutaneous

sudoriferous gland

superficial-thickness burn

The largest organ of the body is the one you look at every day. The skin is the covering of our bodies, and it is the organ that, along with its accessory structures such as sweat glands and hairs, makes up the integumentary system. This covering has many functions, including protection from microorganisms and trauma, prevention of dehydration, regulation of body temperature, insulation, vitamin production, and sensory reception.

The skin aids in prevention of infections by forming a protective seal that keeps out harmful microorganisms. This protective covering also prevents damage to the body by trauma, ultraviolet (UV) radiation from sunlight, harsh chemicals, and extremes in heat and cold. Because this seal is waterproof, it keeps the body hydrated by preventing water loss. Skin aids in regulation of body temperature by producing sweat to cool the skin. It acts as insulation that cushions the internal organs. Cholesterol in the skin is converted by sunlight to vitamin D, which is needed for calcium absorption in the bones. Sensory receptors for pain, touch, cold, heat, and pressure are located in the outer layer of skin. These receptors transmit information about the external environment to the nervous system.

This chapter describes the layers of the skin and their structure and function. It also discusses the structure of hair and nails, describes the types and extent of burns, and explains the identification of skin cancers.

## Layers of the Skin

The skin comprises three layers: the epidermis, the dermis, and the subcutaneous. Each layer is composed of a different type of tissue, and each layer performs different functions (see Fig. 3–1). Skin thickness and depth are similar for all humans differing only slightly between ethnic groups and gender. Even though the skin is what we see every day, and what we most often use to identity and recognize ourselves and others, it is actually the underlying structures that give us our individual appearance.

### Epidermis

The outermost layer of the skin is the **epidermis**, and it is made of stratified squamous epithelial tissue. The cells of this tissue can harden, or **keratinize**, making this layer tough but flexible so that it is able to stretch and retain its shape. There are no blood vessels or glands in the epidermis. This is why a

*Flashpoint*

The integumentary system maintains homeostasis by regulating body temperature, preventing dehydration, and protecting the body against infection from microorganisms.

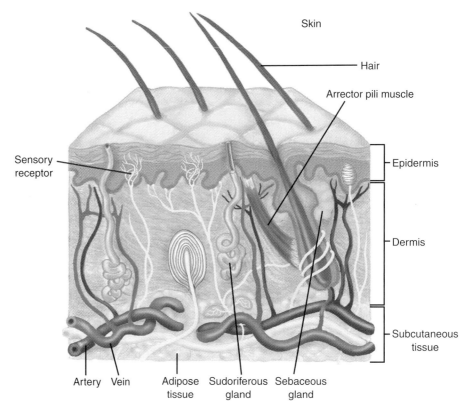

**FIGURE 3-1 Cross section of the layers of the skin.** (Adapted from Eagle S. *Medical Terminology in a Flash!* Philadelphia, PA: FA Davis; 2006:25.)

superficial wound such as a paper cut does not bleed. The epidermis is composed of five individual layers. Each layer is referred to as a stratum. From the innermost layer to the outermost layer they are the basale, spinosum, granulosum, lucidum, and corneum.

The **stratum basale**, also known as the germinativum or basal layer, is closest to the dermis and receives nutrients from the blood vessels in the dermis. The stratum basale is the source of epithelial cells. Millions of new cells are made by this layer every day. As new cells are created, the older ones get pushed upward away from the nutrient source. The epithelial cells are pushed through the middle layers of the epidermis first through the **stratum spinosum** and then through the **stratum granulosum**. As the cells move through these layers, they flatten, thicken, and harden as they fill with the protein called keratin.

The extra-thick and hairless skin found in certain places, such as the palms of the hands and soles of the feet, contains an extra epidermal layer called the **stratum lucidum**. The cells of this layer are flat and keratinized, or full of keratin. At this layer, the epithelial cells are dead and appear clear. This extra layer adds strength to the epidermis where more friction occurs.

The outermost layer of the epidermis is the **stratum corneum**. The corneum comprises about 20 to 30 cell layers, and it accounts for about three-quarters of the thickness of the skin. Cells of this layer are configured like roof shingles with one cell slightly overlapping another. All of these cells are dead and completely keratinized. Another term for keratinized is cornified, which is the how the stratum corneum got its name. These dead cells constantly fall off and get replaced by the cells beneath as the basale layer creates new ones.

Flashpoint
The skin sheds about 50,000 epithelial cells a minute.

The protein keratin gives skin its protective properties. Keratin is waterproof and forms the seal that prevents evaporation of water from our bodies and keeps outside water from entering. Keratin also helps protects the body by forming a barrier to keep out microorganisms, chemicals, and other substances. Unless the skin is broken, most bacteria and harmful microorganisms cannot penetrate the surface of the skin.

Another type of cell found in the lower epidermal layers is the **melanocyte** (black cell). These cells produce a pigment called **melanin**, which can appear black, brown, yellow, or any variation of these colors. This pigment gives color to the skin, hair, and iris of the eyes. The more melanin produced by the melanocytes, the darker the color of the skin, hair, and eyes. Very light-skinned and light-haired people produce melanin, but in smaller amounts. People with blue eyes do not produce any melanin in the iris, however. Blue eyes are a mutation, and blue is the natural color of the empty iris, not of a pigment.

Melanin production can be artificially increased. UV rays found in sunlight are damaging to the stratum basale. These rays can cause damage or mutations to the epithelial cells. In response to sun exposure, melanocytes produce more melanin to protect the skin from the UV rays. Darker skin has some natural protection against UV light, but can darken further with prolonged exposure to the sun. Tan skin is often equated with health. Actually, tan skin is skin that has been forced to protect itself from harmful light. Melanin is only a weak protection, and long-term exposure to UV light can result in permanent damage to the skin.

## Dermis

The second layer of skin is the **dermis**. It is composed of fibrous connective tissue containing collagen and elastic fibers. This layer gives skin its strength and elasticity, or the ability to stretch and return to its original shape. As we age, collagen and elastic fibers break down, and skin loses its elasticity and becomes loose and fragile (see Box 3–1).

All the accessory structures of the integumentary system are found in the dermis of the skin. It consists of blood vessels, nerves, hair follicles, and glands. The area of the dermis just below the epidermis is called the **papillary** layer. This layer is rich in capillaries to nourish the dermis and the stratum basale of the epidermis. The papillary layer also forms ridges that appear as various swirls and loops on the fingertips and toes. These patterns are formed during fetal development and act as friction pads to aid with picking up smooth objects such as paper and to prevent slipping when walking barefoot on smooth surfaces. Papillary ridges are individual to each person; not even identical twins have the same pattern. The patterns on the fingertips are commonly called fingerprints.

### Glands

Glands are made of epithelial tissue that has the ability to excrete substances. There are two types of glands in the body: endocrine and exocrine. **Endocrine** (secretions within) glands secrete substances directly into the bloodstream, and **exocrine** (secretions without) glands produce secretions that reach the skin surface via ducts. Where the ducts open into the external environment they form openings called pores. The two exocrine glands found in skin are the sebaceous and sudoriferous glands.

## Box 3-1 Skin Disorders

The skin is our largest organ and the one most visible to others. There are many common skin disorders that are not part of a disease process, but cause much distress to individuals affected by them.

Stretch marks form when the elastic fibers of the skin are stretched too far resulting in reddish scars that eventually fade to white. They are caused by rapid weight gain or loss and pregnancy. There is no true cure for stretch marks, although laser treatments and skin removal are effective.

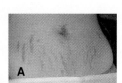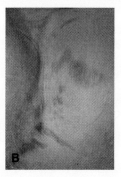

Stretch marks. (From Barankin B, Freiman A. *Derm Notes: Clinical Dermatology Pocket Guide*. Philadelphia, PA: FA Davis; 2006:155.)

Wrinkles are the creases or lines in the skin found most commonly on the face, neck, and hands, and are due to aging of the skin. Premature wrinkling comes from sun exposure and smoking. Treatment for wrinkles can range from use of moisturizers to injections of filler into the wrinkles or injections of muscle-paralyzing agents to smooth the skin. The most aggressive treatment is a facelift, or cutting into and pulling the skin to remove excess tissue.

Cellulite is dimpling of skin caused by the distribution of fat and connective tissue under the skin. It is more common in women and is most often found on the thighs, buttocks, and hips. At this time, the only true cure for cellulite is liposuction, or the surgical removal of the fat, although several lotions can cause a temporary smoothing of the area.

Dandruff or seborrhea is a form of dermatitis that commonly appears as thick scales on the scalp that flake off. There is no known cause for dandruff. Treatment includes products that reduce the inflammation.

Warts are a noncancerous growth caused by human papillomavirus, which causes an increase in cell production on the skin surface resulting in a grainy flesh-colored bump. There are many types of warts. More common warts appear most often on the fingers and hands. They often heal on their own, although treatment may be needed to stop them from spreading.

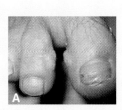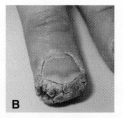

Warts. (From Barankin B, Freiman A. *Derm Notes: Clinical Dermatology Pocket Guide*. Philadelphia, PA: FA Davis; 2006:171.)

## Sebaceous Glands

**Sebaceous glands** produce oil and are found all over the skin except for the lips, palms of the hand, and soles of the feet. This is why the skin on these areas tends to be dry and can even crack. The oil produced by these glands is called **sebum** and is taken from the glands by ducts to the surface of the skin. The sebum keeps the skin and hair moist to prevent drying and aids in preventing bacteria from invading the body through cracks in the skin. During adolescence, sebaceous glands increase the output of sebum causing acne by blocking bacteria in the pores and hair follicles. Sebum production decreases with age, causing the skin to become dryer and more fragile.

## Sudoriferous Glands

**Sudoriferous glands** are sweat glands. The body contains 2 to 4 million sweat glands. There are two types of sweat glands: eccrine and apocrine. The **eccrine** glands aid in heat regulation by cooling the body. They produce sweat, which is mostly water, some salts, and metabolic wastes, that is secreted onto the skin surface and cools the body by evaporation.

The **apocrine** glands are found in the axillae and genital areas. These glands produce a secretion that is similar to sweat, but also contains fatty acids and protein. When these secretions are broken down by the bacteria that live naturally on the skin, a distinctive odor is produced. These glands begin to function at puberty. Other animals use scent to identify one another and to identify those who are different. Humans no longer use scent as identification, although we can tell the difference between the individual scents of people, such as the scent of a particular child on clothing.

The secretions of the apocrine glands are theorized to contain pheromones, which are chemicals that cause a behavioral response to attract the opposite sex. This theory has not been proved conclusively, but many studies have shown that we tend to prefer the scent of our partners to that of others (see Box 3–2).

*Flashpoint*
The organisms that live in and on the body are called normal or natural flora.

## Subcutaneous Layer

The innermost layer of the skin is the **subcutaneous** layer, also called the subdermis or hypodermis. This layer is made of **adipose**, which is a type of connective tissue containing adipocytes and collagen and elastic fibers. This tissue anchors the skin to the muscle beneath.

Adipose tissue stores fat, which can be a potential source of energy should the body be without glucose. It cushions bones, especially those that push against surfaces, such as the pelvis when sitting and the bottoms of the feet when standing or walking. Adipose also provides a limited insulation from cold.

## Structure of Hair

Hair is found all over the body except the lips, palms of the hands, soles of the feet, and inner labia of the female genitalia. The millions of hairs on the human body have little function now, but at one time they acted as insulation and protection against the cold. Hairs such as eyelashes and nose hairs still have a limited protective function by keeping particles out of the eyes and respiratory tract.

## Box 3-2 Pheromones

Pheromones are chemicals secreted by many different species that trigger a physiological or behavioral response in another member of the same species. Pheromones have been found in insects, plants, and mammals.

Insects use pheromones for many purposes. They use them to attract a mate, to signal readiness to mate, for marking territory, to sound an alarm in response to the presence of a predator, and to mark trails. Ants in particular use trail pheromones to mark the way back to the nest when gathering food. If you have ever seen ants traveling in a single line, they are using pheromones to guide each other.

Plants use scent as protection from insects and other predators that may eat or damage them. Plants also use scent to attract insects, especially bees, so that the insects can take pollen to another plant for pollination or fertilization.

Mammals also use pheromones to mark territory, to alert a male that the female is fertile, and as identification. Dogs and cats use the pheromones in urine to mark territory. If you have ever noticed a dog urinating in several places as he walks through the yard he is creating a boundary showing his territory to other dogs.

Humans are difficult when it comes to determining if pheromones change behavior. The sense of smell in humans is not as strong as that of insects and other mammals, so it is more difficult to test the effects of odors on human subjects. Research has shown, but not proven, that pheromones have an effect on the menstrual cycle, in identification, and on sexual attraction.

Studies have shown that menstruating women who share living space have menstrual cycles that occur at the same time. These studies have found that women who did not previously live together but are now doing so, such as in a dormitory room, eventually have their differing cycles become more synchronized. For identification, it has been shown that humans can differentiate people by scent and can recognize the smells of their children and their spouse. This ability is not strong in everyone, and humans are unlikely to recognize someone who is not always in close contact by scent. If humans use pheromones to create sexual attraction, it has not been proved, but studies do show that people do prefer the scent of their partner to that of others. They also describe people with scents they prefer as more attractive. Pheromones are also believed to be responsible for sexual chemistry that is felt strongly between some people and not at all with others.

Hairs are produced in structures called *hair follicles*. The rounded bottom section of the follicle is the *hair bulb*. The part of the hair inside the hair bulb where hair cells grow is called the root. This root anchors the hair in place. Hair that grows freely from the root is called the *shaft*. Figure 3-2 shows the structure of hair.

Similar to skin cells, hair cells are epithelial cells composed of a basale layer at the root. As the cells are produced, they are pushed upward, and as the cells get farther from the growth region, they thicken and keratinize. The hair shaft is made of dead epithelial cells and protein.

All hair shafts have a core called a medulla. The medulla contains melanin. As with skin, the combination of this pigment gives hair its color. As we age, the melanocytes in the medulla stop producing melanin, and the hair appears gray or white. The age of hair whitening is individual. Most people start to gray in their 30s, although some can start as teens or not until their 50s. An individual can be born with gray hair if the melanin in the medulla was never produced.

Around the medulla is a thick layer called the *cortex*, which gives hair its bulk or thickness. Surrounding the cortex is a single layer of overlapping cells

*Flashpoint*
Red hair is the result of a mutation that causes the production of a pigment called pheomelanin instead of melanin. People with this mutation also have a higher sensitivity to pain.

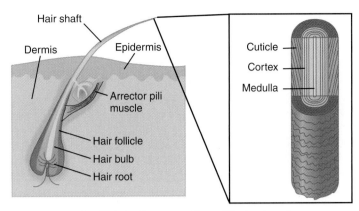

**FIGURE 3–2  Cross section of hair strand.**

called the *cuticle*. The cuticle is fully keratinized and provides strength to the hair shaft.

Hair comes in many shapes and sizes. Different body areas grow hairs of differing lengths and thicknesses. The shape of a hair is determined by the shape of its hair shaft. Hair with an oval-shaped shaft is smooth and wavy. When the shaft is round, the hair is straight and coarse. A flat shaft results in curly hair.

Each hair follicle has a tiny muscle called an *arrector pili* muscle attached to it. These muscles contract in response to cold or fright causing the hair to be pulled upright and the skin to dimple. Commonly we call these dimples "goose bumps." For humans, this action has lost its purpose, but in animals it helps to insulate the body and make an animal appear larger to frighten another animal.

## Structure of the Nail

Nails are a modification of the epidermis (see Fig. 3–3). Growth of each nail occurs in the basale layer, which lies beneath the *nail body*. The *nail matrix* is the portion of the basale where cell growth occurs. Similar to skin and hair, as nail cells leave the matrix, they keratinize and push forward forming the body of the nail. The *free edge* of the nail is the portion of the nail growing past the fingertip. The nail is attached to the finger laterally by skin folds and proximally by the *cuticle*, and it is anchored to the dermis beneath. Nutrients for the nail are received from blood vessels in the dermis. Nerves are also found beneath the nail, which why it is so painful to pull the nail away from the skin.

Nails are transparent, but appear pink because of the blood supply under the basale layer. The area of the nail that covers the nail matrix appears white and is called the *lunula* (crescent). Nails that appear blue are a sign of *cyanosis*. This is an indication of a lack of oxygen in the blood.

Flashpoint

If a fingernail is lost, it takes about 150 days to grow a new one.

## Classification of Burns

A burn is tissue damage caused by UV radiation, intense heat, chemicals, steam, or electricity. When a burn occurs, the body becomes dehydrated and loses electrolytes. When this occurs, the kidneys may cease making urine to

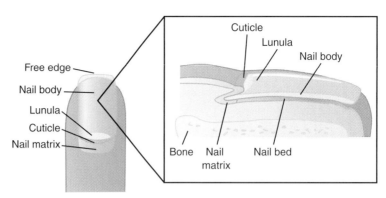

FIGURE 3-3   Cross section of nail structure.

prevent further dehydration. The heart may be unable to provide a sufficient blood supply because of reduction in blood volume. Electrolyte changes can also impair the ability of the heart to conduct properly, resulting in heart failure. In addition, changes may occur in the rate of metabolism, the response of the immune system, and the ability of the cardiovascular system to deliver adequate oxygen to the tissues.

Burns are classified into three different types based on severity (see Fig. 3–4). The least severe is the first-degree burn, also called a ***superficial-thickness burn***. It is red, sore, and hot. Only the epidermis is damaged. A sunburn or steam burn is the most common type of superficial-thickness burn.

A moderate burn is a second-degree burn, or ***partial-thickness burn***. The epidermis and dermis are damaged. This type is red and painful, and fluid-filled blisters form on the surface of the skin.

The most severe burn is a third-degree burn, or ***full-thickness burn***. The skin appears blackened and charred, and damage can go to the muscle and bone. Because the protective layer of skin is gone, the body is now open to invasion from microorganisms, and infection is common. Individuals with third-degree burns also have dehydration because the seal is gone, and fluids seeps from the wound. Both of these conditions are life-threatening.

Tissue regeneration with a full-thickness burn is impossible because the stratum basale is gone, so skin grafts must be done to cover the exposed tissues. These burns are not painful because the sensory receptors in the dermis are also destroyed. If the nerves are able to regenerate, pain occurs as the skin heals.

Some burns are considered critical, and medical attention is needed immediately. Second-degree burns that cover more than 25% of the body and third-degree burns that cover more than 10% of the body are critical burns. Any second-degree or third-degree burn to the face is critical because the respiratory system may be damaged, preventing breathing and causing possible suffocation. Also, any second-degree or third-degree burn to the genitals, hands, feet, or joints is considered critical. Any burn covering more than 10% of the body in a child is critical. Because of small body mass, children do not regulate their body temperature as well adults, and dehydration and fluid loss occur quickly. A child can easily go into shock and die from a burn. Elderly people are similar to children when determining a critical burn. Any burn except a minor burn can affect temperature regulation and cause dehydration and infection in an elderly person.

*Flashpoint*

Do not use butter, margarine, or lard to treat a burn. Cooking oils retain or increase the heat in the burn.

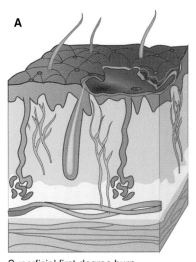

Superficial first-degree burn
• Involves top layer of epidermis only

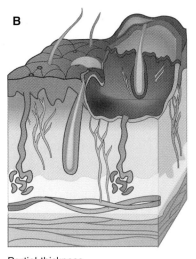

Partial-thickness
Second-degree burn
• Skin blister
• Involves all of epidermis and
  into the dermis

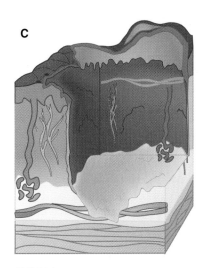

Full-thickness
Third-degree burn
• May extend to the bone

FIGURE 3–4  **Classification of burns.** *(A)* **Superficial-thickness.** *(B)* **Partial-thickness.**
*(C)* **Full-thickness.**

## Rule of Nines

The determination of how much of the body surface is burned is made using the
***rule of nines***. This method for determining the extent of burns divides the body
into 11 areas. Each area accounts for 9% of the total body surface. Because the
arm is about half the size of a leg, it accounts for 4.5%, as does the face. The
genitals represent 1% (see Fig. 3–5). For example, if the front of the arm was
burned, it would be 4.5% of the body; if the body was burned on the ventral and
the dorsal sides from the waist down, it would be 37% of the body.

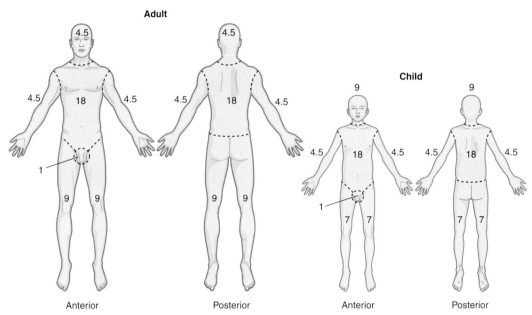

FIGURE 3–5 **Rule of nines for an adult and a child.**

# Skin Cancer

The skin may have many variations or lesions. These lesions may be as simple as a freckle or a scratch or more serious such as a tumor (see Fig. 3–6). **Neoplasms** (new growths) or tumors may form anywhere on the skin (see Table 3–1). Most are benign and do not spread to other areas of the body. Other neoplasms become malignant and invade other areas. These malignant neoplasms on the skin's surface are called **skin cancer**. Skin cancer is most commonly due to overexposure to UV radiation found in sunlight and tanning beds.

There are three types of skin cancer: basal cell carcinoma, squamous cell carcinoma, and malignant melanoma (see Fig. 3–7). The location, treatment, and survival rate depend on the type (see Table 3–2).

**Basal cell carcinoma** is the most common type of skin cancer, accounting for 80% of all cases worldwide. This cancer is a result of basale cells that cannot keratinize and push to the surface forming a shiny nodule. Because the face is more often exposed to sunlight, this type is of cancer is commonly found on the face or ears. This tumor is slow growing and rarely spreads to another site. Treatment includes removal of the nodule, and survival rate is 99%.

**Squamous cell carcinoma** is the second most common form of skin cancer in the United States; about 250,000 new cases occur each year. This cancer affects the middle layers of the epidermis. The result is scaly patches that ulcerate and scab over. They appear most often on the face, lips, and ears. This tumor grows quickly and spreads to other areas of the body. If caught early, survival rate is about 95%.

**Malignant melanoma** is the third most common skin cancer; about 160,000 new cases occur each year worldwide. This cancer is a result of damage to the melanocytes. It appears as a rapidly spreading black or brown splotch. The damaged cells often spread to the lymph glands or blood vessels. It is a rare

**PRIMARY LESIONS**

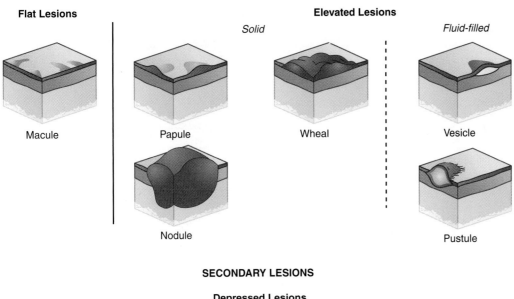

**Flat Lesions**

Macule

**Elevated Lesions**

*Solid*

Papule

Nodule

Wheal

*Fluid-filled*

Vesicle

Pustule

**SECONDARY LESIONS**

**Depressed Lesions**

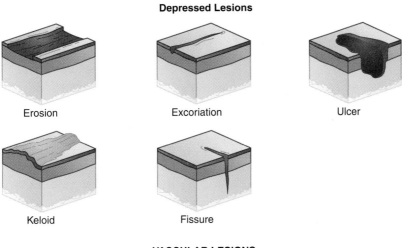

Erosion

Excoriation

Ulcer

Keloid

Fissure

**VASCULAR LESIONS**

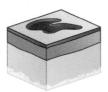

Ecchymosis

FIGURE 3-6 **Common lesions of the skin.**

tumor, but the most deadly, accounting for 75% of skin cancer deaths. Even with treatment, the survival rate is only 50%.

The American Cancer Society recommends all moles and spots be checked periodically. They have developed the ABCDE rule for detecting malignant neoplasms and recommend any changes be examined by a medical professional.

## TABLE 3–1
## COMMON LESIONS OF THE SKIN

| Lesion | Characterizations |
|---|---|
| Comedo | Discoloration created by sebum plugging an excretory skin duct; blackhead |
| Erosion | Loss of or wearing away of the epidermis |
| Excoriation | Scratch or abrasion |
| Fissure | Crack in the surface of the skin that extends into the dermis; hands and feet are the most common places of occurrence because of dry skin |
| Keloid | Overgrowth of scar tissue; occurs more commonly in darker complexions |
| Macule | Flat, pigmented patch of skin <1 cm in diameter; freckle |
| Nevus | Pigmented skin blemish; birthmark or mole |
| Nodule | Raised, solid mass >1 cm in diameter; can occur in any skin layer |
| Papule | Raised, solid mass <1 cm in diameter |
| Pustule | Small collection of pus usually <1 cm occurring frequently in the sweat glands or hair follicles |
| Ulcer | Crater-like wound that extends to the dermis |
| Vesicle | Small fluid-filled blister <0.5 cm in diameter |
| Wheal | Firm, elevated, often red and itchy swelling on the skin that usually lasts 24–48 hr; hives |

- *A* is for *Asymmetry*. Benign neoplasms are the same on both sides. An asymmetrical mole or spot is one that is not the same on both sides.
- *B* is for *Border irregularity*. The edges of the spot or mole are not smooth or even.
- *C* is for *Color*. Normal moles or spots are black, brown, or red. A spot with more than one color is abnormal.
- *D* is for *Diameter*. A spot is larger than 6 mm in diameter (size of a pencil eraser).
- *E* is for *Evolving* or *extending*. The mole or spot has changed or grown quickly.

For more information about diseases of the integumentary system, see Table 3–3.

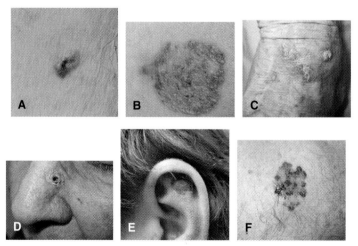

FIGURE 3–7 *(A, B)* **Basal cell carcinoma.** *(C, D)* **Squamous cell carcinoma.** *(E, F)* **Melanoma.** (From Barankin B, Freiman A. *Derm Notes: Clinical Dermatology*)

## TABLE 3–2
### TYPES OF SKIN CANCER

| | |
|---|---|
| Basal cell carcinoma | Most common; affects the stratum basale so cells cannot keratinize; the cells then spread into the dermis; appear as shiny dome-shaped nodules most commonly on face; slow growing and seldom spread; cure rate is 99% after removal |
| Squamous cell carcinoma | Affects middle strata of epidermis; appear as scaly, red bumps that form an ulcer on scalp, ears, and lip; grows and spreads rapidly; if detected early and removed, survival is good |
| Malignant melanoma | Rare cancer of the melanocytes; appears as a spreading brown or black splotch; spreads rapidly to lymph nodes and blood vessels; survival rate is 50% |

## TABLE 3–3
### PATHOLOGY TERMS FOR INTEGUMENTARY SYSTEM

| | |
|---|---|
| Abscess | Localized collection of pus; occurs when bacteria have entered skin through a wound and cause infection |
| Acne | Inflammation of the skin resulting in pustular eruptions; caused by overproduction of sebaceous glands in skin; more common in adolescents |
| Alopecia | Partial or complete absence of hair; baldness; can be hereditary, due to a skin condition, or a side effect of a drug |
| Cyanosis | Blueness of the skin usually caused by lack of oxygen |
| Dermatitis | General term for inflammation of the skin because of an irritant, such as soap, perfume, fabric, detergent, sunlight, or medications |
| Ecchymosis | Black-and-blue mark on the skin caused by blood vessel injury; also called a bruise |
| Erythema | Redness of the skin usually because of injury or inflammation |
| Impetigo | Inflammatory skin disease that results in pustules that crust over and rupture; highly contagious and occurs most often in children |

Impetigo. (From Barankin B, Freiman A. *Derm Notes: Clinical Dermatology Pocket Guide.* Philadelphia, PA: FA Davis; 2006:104.)

| | |
|---|---|
| Jaundice | Yellowness of the skin usually a result of liver malfunction |
| Leukotrichia | Loss of pigmentation to the hair; whitening of the hair; most often due to age |
| Pallor | Paleness of the skin |
| Pediculosis | Lice infestation |
| Pruritus | Itching |
| Tinea pedis | Fungal infection of the feet; athlete's foot |

*Continued*

### TABLE 3–3
### PATHOLOGY TERMS FOR INTEGUMENTARY SYSTEM—cont'd

| | |
|---|---|
| Urticaria | Allergic skin reaction that causes itchy, red, elevated patches; also called hives. |

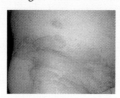

Urticaria. (From Barankin B, Freiman A. *Derm Notes: Clinical Dermatology Pocket Guide*. Philadelphia, PA: FA Davis; 2006:166.)

| | |
|---|---|
| Vitiligo | Localized loss of skin pigmentation resulting in white patches |

## Practice Exercises

### Multiple Choice

1. A cancer that occurs because epithelial cells cannot keratinize is called _____.

   a. squamous cell carcinoma

   b. basal cell carcinoma

   c. malignant melanoma

   d. malignant carcinoma

2. A full-thickness burn is also called a _____ burn.

   a. first-degree

   b. second-degree

   c. third-degree

   d. fourth-degree

3. The glands found in the skin are _____ glands.

   a. endocrine

   b. exocrine

   c. epithelial

   d. epimysium

4. The _____ is the outer layer of the hair.

   a. medulla

   b. shaft

   c. cortex

   d. root

5. The skin can use sunlight to make vitamin _____.

    a.   C

    b.   D

    c.   E

    d.   A

## True or False

1.  True   False      Melanin is the pigment that gives hair and skin its color.

2.  True   False      Sebaceous glands produce sweat.

3.  True   False      A first-degree burn is the most severe burn.

4.  True   False      In the rule of nines, the genitals equal 5% of the body.

5.  True   False      The epidermis contains blood vessels and glands.

6.  True   False      Fingerprints are formed during fetal development.

7.  True   False      The subcutaneous layer of the skin is made of adipose.

8.  True   False      The hair bulb holds the hair root.

9.  True   False      Malignant melanoma has the highest survival rate.

10.  True   False      Only a third-degree burn on a child is considered critical.

## Fill in the Blank

1. Hardened cells of the epidermis are said to be _____.

2. The _____ describes the extent of burns.

3. The core of the hair is called the _____.

4. _____ muscles cause goose bumps.

5. Nails grow from the part of the basale called the _____.

6. A(n) _____ spot is not the same on both sides.

7. The sebaceous glands produce _____.

8. The white crescent shape on the nail bed is the _____.

9. The _____ and _____ glands are sudoriferous glands.

10. A first-degree burn is also called a _____ -thickness burn.

## Short Answer

1. **Describe the layers of the skin.**

2. **Define the rule of nines.**

3. **Define the ABCDE rule.**

## Labeling

*Fill in the blanks with the appropriate anatomical terms.*

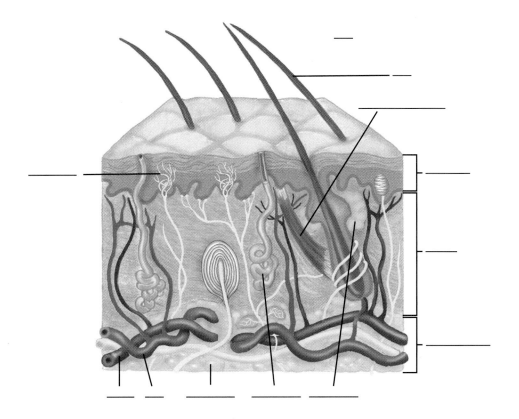

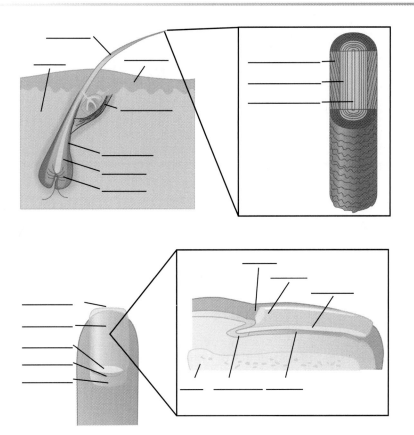

# 4

# THE MUSCULAR SYSTEM

## Key Terms

action potential

aerobic respiration

anaerobic respiration

antagonist

cardiac muscle

cellular respiration

contract

depolarization

fixator

insertion

isometric contraction

isotonic contraction

ligament

muscle fiber

muscle tone

origin

polarization

prime mover          *Continued*

There are approximately 650 muscles in the human body. Muscles create movement of the body, hold the body upright to maintain posture, produce heat, and regulate overall body temperature.

Some muscles attach to bones, and by pulling on these bones movement is achieved. Each muscle has the ability to **contract**, or create tension by shortening. The contraction creates the pull on the muscles that causes body movement. When referring to contraction of a muscle, it does not mean only to shorten but also to lengthen or stay the same. A slight contraction is always maintained, and this tension holds the body upright. The energy used to create tension also generates the heat needed to regulate body temperature. If the body becomes cold, the muscles shake or shiver to create more heat and warm the body.

This chapter discusses the different types of muscles, their structure, and their location in the body. How muscle movement occurs and the energy source for this movement are also described. In addition, the different types of exercise and their benefits to the body are discussed. Finally, an overview of the names and location of the larger muscles is provided.

## Types of Muscle

Within the human body, there are three different types of muscle: skeletal, smooth, and cardiac (see Fig. 4–1). These muscles differ in structure, function, and location.

### Skeletal Muscle

**Skeletal muscle** is also called voluntary muscle. This type is called skeletal muscle because it is attached to bone, and it is called voluntary because it is consciously controlled. Skeletal muscle is responsible for all body movement. The cells of skeletal muscle are elongated and cylindrical, and they have markings called striations that resemble elastic cord. The striations allow the muscle to stretch and spring back. Skeletal muscle cells are also multinucleate, meaning they have more than one nucleus in each muscle cell.

Muscle cells are also called muscle fibers. There are two different types of skeletal muscle fibers in the body: slow twitch and fast twitch. Slow twitch fibers have more mitochondria than fast twitch fibers and use oxygen to create

*Flashpoint*

The muscular system maintains homeostasis by maintaining body temperature. When the body is cold, the muscles spasm creating heat to cause an increase in temperature.

Skeletal                    Smooth                     Cardiac

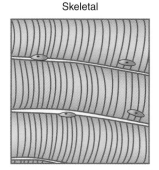 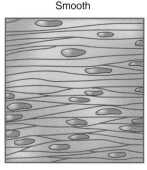 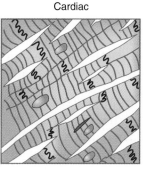

FIGURE 4–1  **Types of muscle: skeletal muscle, smooth muscle, cardiac muscle.**

energy. These fibers are called slow twitch because they produce enough energy to maintain contraction for a long time. Slow twitch fibers are associated with endurance.

Fast twitch fibers produce quick bursts of energy because they create energy without oxygen and so they have less energy available. Because of the shorter energy supply, they contract faster than slow twitch fibers. Fast twitch fibers are associated with strength.

The ratio of slow twitch to fast twitch fibers differs among muscles and among individuals. People who run long distances easily may have more slow twitch fibers, and people who find weight lifting easier may have more fast twitch muscles. Training for any activity can allow a person having a lesser amount of either type of fibers to be competitive with persons who have more.

Skeletal muscles have four functions:

- *Contractility*—the ability to shorten
- *Excitability*—the ability of muscle to respond to stimuli
- *Extensibility*—the ability to stretch and lengthen
- *Elasticity*—the ability to return to their original length after being stretched

*Flashpoint*
Skeletal muscles account for approximately 45% of a man's body weight and 36% of a woman's body weight.

## Smooth Muscle

**Smooth muscle** is also called visceral muscle or involuntary muscle. It is called visceral because it is found in the walls of the internal organs. Because it is not consciously controlled, it is involuntary. These muscle cells are shorter than skeletal muscle cells and are spindle-shaped, which means they taper at the ends. Smooth muscle cells have a single nucleus and are not striated. This type of muscle stretches, but not as much as skeletal muscle.

Smooth muscles line the walls of hollow organs, such as the stomach, respiratory tract, and urinary bladder. The lining of this type of muscle is usually two layers thick with one layer running transversely and the other layer running sagittally. The difference in direction allows one layer to contract while the other relaxes. The result is a wavelike movement that propels substances along a pathway. For example, the simultaneous contraction and relaxation of the urinary bladder allows urine into and out of the organ. Contraction in smooth muscle is slower and more sustained than contraction of skeletal muscle to maintain the constant activity of the organs.

## Cardiac Muscle

Cardiac tissue is found only in the wall of the heart. **Cardiac muscle** has characteristics of skeletal and smooth muscle. Similar to smooth muscle, it is involuntarily controlled and has one nucleus per muscle fiber; similar to skeletal muscle, it is striated. The striations give the heart the ability to contract.

Cardiac tissue has four functions. Similar to skeletal muscle, cardiac muscle has the ability to contract, to become excitable by a stimulus, and to conduct that stimulus. Cardiac muscle has an internal mechanism, however, that can stimulate its own contraction without needing electrical stimulus from the nervous system. Cardiac tissue differs from skeletal muscle because it is automatic. Each cardiac cell can beat on its own. If a heart were divided into individual cells, each one would beat on its own. These muscle cells also have the unusual ability to synchronize. If the individual cells from different hearts are placed side by side, they slow down or speed up until all of them have the same beat.

## Muscle Structure

Muscle cells of skeletal and smooth muscle have an elongated, cylindrical shape and are referred to as **muscle fibers** (see Fig. 4–2). The fibers found in skeletal muscles are the longest, with some being 1 foot in length. A single muscle fiber is weak and easily broken, but groups of fibers can withstand great force and provide the strength and support the body needs to move and maintain posture.

Individual muscle fibers are wrapped in a sheath of connective tissue called an **endomysium** (within the muscle). Muscles are composed of bundles of individual muscle fibers. Each bundle or **fascicle** is surrounded by another sheath of loose connective tissue called a **perimysium** (around the muscle). Several

*Flashpoint*

Each muscle fiber is thinner than a single human hair and can support 1000 times its own weight.

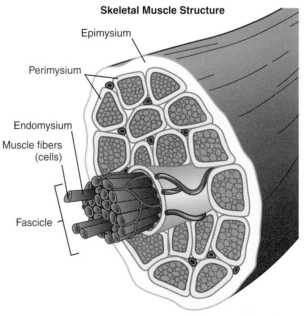

**Skeletal Muscle Structure**

Epimysium

Perimysium

Endomysium

Muscle fibers (cells)

Fascicle

FIGURE 4–2  General structure of skeletal muscle.

fascicles grouped together form a single muscle. Each muscle is surrounded by another sheath of connective tissue called the *epimysium* (on the muscle). The ends of the epimysium form tendons that connect the muscles to bone.

See Box 4–1 for a description of common diseases and disorders that affect the muscle.

## Action Potential

Similar to all cells, muscle cells have the ability to conduct electrical current and respond to an electrical stimulus. Muscle cells also have contractility, or the ability to contract in response to the electrical stimulus. For a muscle to contract, changes must occur inside and outside of the cell. This change is the *action potential* (see Fig. 4–3).

For a cell to respond to a stimulus, it must first be at rest. A muscle cell at rest is in a state of *polarization*. When a cell is polarized, it contains more

### Box 4-1 Common Diseases and Disorders of Muscles

Many problems and disorders can affect the muscles. These problems can be temporary or permanent and may occur for a variety of reasons, such as simply overstretching a muscle, dietary deficiencies, neurological disorders, or genetic mutations.

A cramp is a contraction that does not relax. It is usually a result of lactic acid retention because of strenuous exercise. Treatment is to cease activity, rest the muscle, and massage. Other cramps of the feet and legs are not due to exercise and seem to occur spontaneously. Commonly called a "charley horse," the cramp is most often due to an injury, hormone imbalance, dehydration, or dietary deficiency. Treatment is to stretch the muscles and massage the area.

A strain is an overuse or overextension of a muscle. It causes pain, weakness, swelling, redness, and an inability to use the muscle. Treatment for strain is rest, ice to relieve swelling, then heat, and medication to relieve pain.

Myasthenia gravis is a disease that occurs during adulthood and is a result of muscle cells not being stimulated properly. It results in drooping eyelids, difficulty swallowing and talking, and generalized muscle weakness and fatigue. Eventually death occurs as the muscles of the respiratory system fail. The cause is unknown, and there is no treatment at this time.

Duchenne muscular dystrophy is one of the most common forms of muscular dystrophy. This disease occurs most often in males, and the onset is age 2 to 6 years. The child appears normal, but becomes progressively clumsy as the muscles weaken. The extremities are the first to be affected followed by the muscles of the chest and head. Most victims of Duchenne muscular dystrophy are wheelchair bound by age 12 and do not live beyond the teenage years. The cause is a lack of a protein called dystrophin in the muscle fibers. Treatments and cures are still unavailable.

Restless legs syndrome (RLS) is characterized by an intense urge to move the legs because of sensations of crawling, itching, or pain. Movement is especially prevalent during sleep. There is no one cause of RLS, although anemia, hormone imbalances, and dietary deficiency are suspected. Treatment for RLS includes prescription medications if treatment of the suspected cause is ineffective.

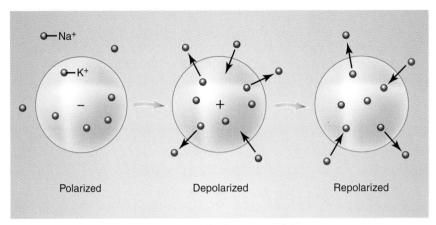

FIGURE 4–3 Action potential.

potassium ions (K$^+$) than sodium ions (Na$^+$) and has a negative charge. An electrical impulse stimulates the cell and causes it to change. The Na$^+$ ions flow into the cell and the K$^+$ ions flow out, changing the cell to a positive charge. This change is called ***depolarization***. When a cell is depolarized, it is able to perform an action. When a muscle cell depolarizes, it shortens or contracts, which causes contraction in the whole muscle.

A cell cannot remain stimulated and cannot be stimulated again without going back to a polarized state. A muscle cell must relax before it can contract again. To go back to its polarized state, the Na$^+$ ions flow out of the cell. The K$^+$ ions return to the inside, and the cell becomes negatively charged. The act of a cell returning to it resting state is ***repolarization***. This part of the action potential allows the muscle to relax.

## Muscle Movement

Muscles attach to bones by connective tissue called ***tendons***. Muscles and tendons work together to create the force that causes movement. ***Ligaments*** are similar to tendons, but they attach bone to bone at a joint. Movement of muscle depends on how the muscle is attached to the bone. Contraction causes muscles to change in length and is the basis for body movement. To maintain posture, muscles are always in a slight state of contraction. This slight contraction is called ***muscle tone***.

The point of ***origin*** is where a muscle attaches to a stationary bone, and the point of ***insertion*** is where a muscle attaches to a bone with more movement. For example, the sternocleidomastoid has its origin at the stationary sternum, or breast bone, and inserts behind the ear onto the temporal bone. The sternum, is a stationary bone, and the skull is a moving bone. This muscle causes the head to turn side to side.

All movement is created by the contraction of one set of muscles and the relaxation of the opposite muscles. Muscles move the body by working either with or against each other. ***Antagonist*** muscles are muscles that work against each other, meaning they have an opposite function. For example, the hamstrings and quadriceps of the thigh are antagonistic. These types of muscles either increase or decrease an angle at a joint. When the quadriceps on the ventral thigh contract, the leg extends or increases the angle of the joint, but the quadriceps cannot perform the opposite motion. The hamstrings on the dorsal thigh contract causing the muscle to flex or decrease the angle of the joint and bend the leg back.

*Synergistic* muscles are groups of muscles that work together to perform a function. The quadriceps are four individual muscles, but they work together to extend the leg. If one muscle in a group of synergistic muscles plays more of a role in the movement, it is called the *prime mover*. A *fixator* is a muscle that holds one bone in place while a more distal bone moves. A fixator muscle stabilizes a joint.

## Types of Body Movements

The different muscles of the body move the bones to which they are attached in specific ways (see Fig. 4–4). Muscles that move a body part away from the midline of the body are performing *abduction*. Moving the arm away from the torso is an example of abduction. Muscles that move a body part toward the midline of the body are performing adduction. Bringing that arm back to the torso is *adduction*.

*Circumduction* is a movement made when the proximal end of a limb is stationary, and the distal end moves in a circle. Moving the arm in a circle at the shoulder joint is circumduction. Moving a bone around a central point is *rotation*. The radius of the forearm moves over the ulna turning the forearm, but not in a complete circle. This is rotation.

When muscles increase the angle between joints, it is *extension*, and shortening the angle is *flexion*. When the quadriceps pulls the leg outward, this is an example of extension, and when the hamstrings bend the leg back, this is flexion. *Hyperextension* occurs when the joint is pushed past its normal range of extension.

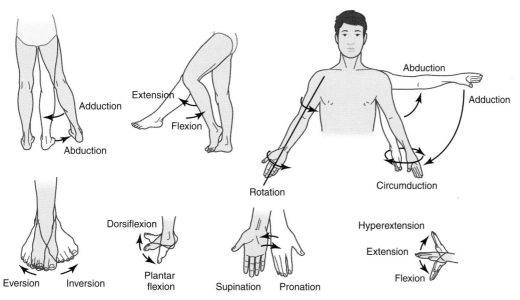

**FIGURE 4–4  Types of muscle movement.**

Some movements are done only in a specific body part, such as the foot, the thumb, and the forearm. The foot is capable of lifting so that the toes point toward the ankle; this is **dorsiflexion**. If the foot points downward so that a person is standing on the toes, this is **plantar flexion**. If the foot is turned so that the sole of the foot turns to the inner ankle, this is **eversion**, and turning the foot so the sole moves outward is **inversion**. The thumb can move so that it touches the tip of each finger. This is **opposition**. The forearm is capable of **pronation**, which is moving the radius and ulna so that the palm faces downward, and **supination**, which is turning the radius and ulna so that the palm faces upward.

See Table 4–1 for a summary of the different body movements.

## Energy Sources for Muscle Contraction

Muscle movement is made possible by the energy produced by the mitochondria of the cells. ATP is the preferred energy source for muscle fiber contraction, although the ATP supply is usually not enough to fuel the muscle fibers for more than a short time. When the stored ATP is used, muscles have a means to replenish it. **Cellular respiration** is the process of creating new ATP to power muscle contraction. This process can be done with or without oxygen.

The most abundant source of energy for muscle fibers to use is glucose. Glucose originally is stored in the body as glycogen, but through a process called **glycolysis** (sugar breaking), the glycogen is broken down into a form the cell can use.

All cells need oxygen to perform efficiently. Oxygen is also needed to break glucose down further into ATP. When oxygen and glucose are combined, they

| TABLE 4–1 | |
|---|---|
| **TERMS OF MOVEMENT** | |
| **Type of Movement** | **Description of Movement** |
| Abduction | Moving away from the midline of the body |
| Adduction | Moving toward the midline of the body |
| Circumduction | Proximal end of limb is stationary, and distal end moves in a circle |
| Dorsiflexion | Lifting the foot so that toes point toward the ankle |
| Eversion | Turning the sole of the foot laterally |
| Extension | Increasing the angle between two joints; straightening |
| Flexion | Decreasing the angle between two joints; bending |
| Hyperextension | Moving a joint past its normal range of motion |
| Inversion | Turning the sole of the foot medially |
| Opposition | Touching the tip of the fingers with the thumb |
| Plantar flexion | Pointing the toes |
| Pronation | Movement of radius and ulna so that the palm of the hand faces downward |
| Rotation | Moving a bone around a central point or axis |
| Supination | Movement of radius and ulna so that the palm faces upward |

produce 36 ATP molecules for every glucose molecule. This is like getting 36 miles to a gallon of gas. During cellular respiration, carbon dioxide, water, and heat are also produced as waste. Even though these substances are considered waste, they are not all excreted from the body. The heat produced is what maintains body temperature. Water is recycled and is absorbed by the body to maintain hydration. Carbon dioxide is not used by the body and is excreted by being exhaled through the lungs. This process of energy production is called ***aerobic respiration***. Aerobic means "in the presence of oxygen," and is the typical means of producing energy when the body is resting, or when there is low or moderate stress on the muscles.

During strenuous exercise, ATP production cannot always keep up with the demand, and oxygen is used faster than it can be delivered to the cells. Because the muscles still need to function even when all the oxygen stores are gone, glycolysis continues. When glycolysis occurs without oxygen present, it is called ***anaerobic respiration***. This is not the preferred or most efficient means of creating energy for the body. Less ATP is produced—only two ATP molecules for every glucose molecule. The waste products of anaerobic respiration are pyruvic acid and lactic acid. These wastes cannot be used in the body.

If anaerobic respiration continues for an extended time, the body enters ***oxygen debt***. This state is reached when all oxygen stores have been used by the muscle fibers, yet the fibers need to continue working. Lactic acid is stored in the muscle as anaerobic respiration continues. Eventually the lactic acid causes fatigue or cramping as the muscle continues to work without adequate energy. The lactic acid is responsible for the pain and stiffness you may feel during a strenuous workout. When the exercise has ended and the muscles return to resting, the body restores its normal oxygen levels, and the lactic acid breaks down and is excreted from the body.

## Exercise

Contraction is needed to provide muscles with good muscle tone. Toned muscles move faster and more efficiently than muscles that are soft and have poor tone. Muscle tone can be improved and increased by exercise or physical activity. Two types of contractions are produced by exercise: isotonic and isometric.

***Isotonic*** (same tone) ***contractions*** cause the muscles to shorten to create movement. Weight lifting, running, and swimming are examples of isotonic exercises. This type of exercise improves tone, size, strength, and endurance of the muscles. Size and strength of muscles improve because the force or extra weight on individual fibers causes them to thicken. The muscles fibers may even break and thicken as they heal. Pain that occurs a day or two after a workout can be blamed on breaks in the muscle fibers.

The cardiovascular system also improves with isotonic exercise. As more oxygen is needed to meet the skeletal muscle demand, the heart muscle must work harder to keep up. Because it is also working harder similar to the other muscles of the body, it strengthens and becomes more efficient.

***Isometric*** (same measurement) ***contractions*** do not shorten the muscle. Tension on the muscle increases, but the muscle does not move. Pushing against a wall or another stable object is using isometric contraction. This type of exercise increases tone and strength, but does not increase muscle mass because the individual fibers are not broken, and it does not improve cardiovascular function.

Flashpoint
Muscle mass starts to decline at about 1% per year after age 30.

# Muscles of the Body

There are hundreds of muscles in the body; only the more superficial and larger groups of muscles are discussed here. These muscles are the ones used for medical procedures, such as vaccine injections, and are most commonly injured (see Fig. 4–5).

## Head and Neck

The head and neck together use the most muscles of the whole body. These muscles not only allow movement, but also create facial expressions. The *frontalis* is a scalp muscle and controls movement of the ears and eyebrows. It gives us the ability to raise our eyebrows and furrow our brows. Some people can use this muscle to wiggle their ears.

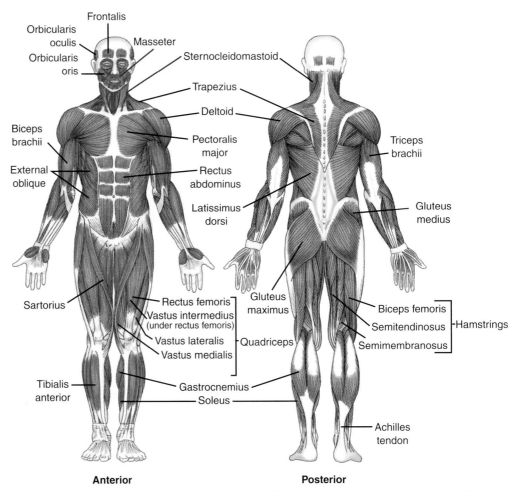

**Anterior**          **Posterior**

FIGURE 4–5 **Anterior and posterior views of superficial muscles of the human body.** (Adapted from Eagle S. *Medical Terminology in a Flash!* Philadelphia, PA: FA Davis; 2006:223.)

Surrounding the eye socket is the ***orbicularis oculi***, which controls movement of the upper eyelid. The ***orbicularis oris*** circles the mouth and allows us to move our lips to speak and pucker. A rounded mass of muscle called the ***masseter*** is located in front of the ear and moves the lower jaw from side to side. This movement allows us to chew. The ***temporalis*** located on the temporal bone aids in moving the lower jaw. It is responsible for opening the mouth and aids the ***pterygoid*** in closing the mouth. Located under the cheek, the ***buccinator*** muscle compresses the cheek against the teeth and allows us to blow.

The ***platysma*** covers the ventral surface of the neck and can pull the head forward. The ***sternocleidomastoid*** is the large muscle on the lateral neck that stops behind the ear. This muscle allows us to turn our heads (see Fig. 4–6). It is prominent when turning the face to the side. See Table 4–2 for a summary of the muscles of the head and neck.

Flashpoint

The masseter can close the mouth with a force of 55 lb on the incisors and 200 lb on the molars.

## Shoulder and Arm

The muscles of the shoulder are the ***deltoids***. These muscles cover the shoulder joints and are responsible for moving the arm away from the body. The deltoid is a muscle commonly used for vaccine injections. The upper arm has the ***biceps brachii*** on the inner side of the arm, which allow the arm to flex, and the ***triceps brachii*** on the outer side, which allow it to extend. Also part of the upper arm are the ***brachialis*** and the ***brachioradialis***, which attach on the upper arm and insert on the forearm. The brachialis flexes the elbow, and the brachioradialis is responsible for turning the forearm.

The muscles of the forearm are responsible for flexion and extension of the wrist and movement of the fingers. The ***flexor carpi*** flex the wrist, and the ***extensor carpi*** extend the wrist. Fingers are flexed by the ***flexor digitorum*** and extended by the ***extensor digitorum*** (see Fig. 4–7). Table 4–3 gives an overview of the muscles of the shoulders and arms.

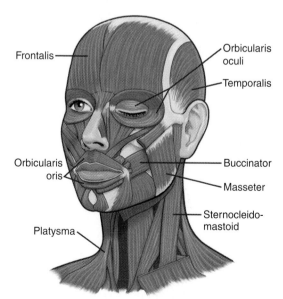

**FIGURE 4–6  Muscles of the head and neck.**

## TABLE 4–2
### MUSCLES OF THE HEAD AND NECK

| Muscle | Function | Location |
| --- | --- | --- |
| Frontalis | Moves the ears and eyebrows | Scalp |
| Masseter | Moves mandible up and down in chewing motion | In front of the ear |
| Orbicularis oculi | Moves upper eyelid | Around the eye socket |
| Orbicularis oris | Allows the lips to pucker | Around the mouth |
| Platysma | Allows head to bend forward | Ventral neck |
| Buccinator | Compresses cheek against the teeth | Under the cheek |
| Sternocleidomastoid | Turns head from side to side | Lateral neck to ear |
| Temporalis | Aids in moving mandible upward | Temporal bone |
| Pterygoid | Aids in moving mandible upward | Under the cheek |

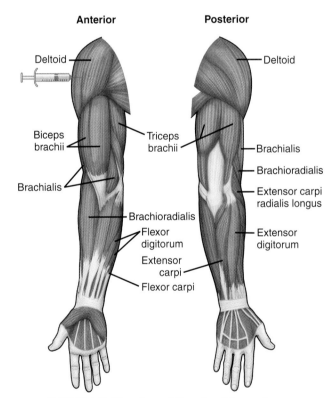

FIGURE 4–7  Muscles of the shoulder and arm.

## Torso and Back

The torso consists of the chest and abdomen. The ***pectoralis major*** and ***pectoralis minor*** muscles form the chest. The pectoralis major is the larger of the two muscles and is responsible for moving the arm across the chest. The

### TABLE 4-3
### MUSCLES OF THE ARM AND SHOULDER

| Muscle | Function | Location |
| --- | --- | --- |
| Biceps brachii | Flexes lower arm | Inner upper arm |
| Brachialis | Flexes elbow | Upper arm and forearm |
| Brachioradialis | Turns lower arm | Upper arm and forearm |
| Deltoid | Turns and abducts arm | Shoulder |
| Extensor carpi | Extends wrist | Forearm |
| Extensor digitorum | Extends fingers | Forearm |
| Flexor carpi | Flexes wrist | Forearm |
| Flexor digitorum | Flexes fingers | Forearm |
| Triceps brachii | Extends lower arm | Outer upper arm |

pectoralis minor located under the pectoralis major helps to stabilize the shoulder. The abdomen is covered by the **rectus abdominis** and the **external obliques**. The rectus abdominis muscles create the abdominal wall and are joined at the medial abdomen by the **linea alba**, a thin band of tissue. These muscles flex and allow the body to bend forward. The external obliques allow the torso to turn.

On the posterior body, the diamond-shaped muscle called the **trapezius** covers the back of the neck, partially covers the deltoids, and attaches to the spine. This muscle allows the shoulders to shrug by moving up and back. Below the trapezius are the **latissimus dorsi**, which move the arm downward and back. The buttocks are composed of two muscles: the **gluteus medius**, which covers the hips, and the **gluteus maximus**, which makes up the bulk of the buttocks (see Fig. 4–8). The gluteus medius abducts the leg, and the gluteus maximus adducts the leg. Vaccines and other injectable medications can be given in the gluteus medius. Table 4–4 summarizes the muscles of the torso and back.

*Flashpoint*
The gluteus maximus is the largest muscle in the human body.

## Legs

The upper leg or thigh comprises four muscles: the vastus lateralis, rectus femoris, vastus intermedius, and vastus medialis. Collectively, these four muscles are called the **quadriceps femoris**. Crossing the quadriceps is a long, thin muscle that originates at the pelvis and attaches to the tibia. This muscle is the **sartorius**, and it aids in turning the leg laterally to achieve a cross-legged position. The muscles of the posterior thigh are the semitendinosus, biceps femoris, and semimembranosus. Together these are the **hamstrings**. The quadriceps extend the leg, and the hamstrings flex the leg.

The largest muscle of the calf is the **gastrocnemius**. This muscle raises the heel so that you can stand on your toes. The gastrocnemius attaches to the heel by the **Achilles tendon**. Under the Achilles tendon is the **soleus** muscle, which covers the lower leg and inserts into the foot (see Fig. 4–9).

*Flashpoint*
The sartorius is the longest muscle in the body.

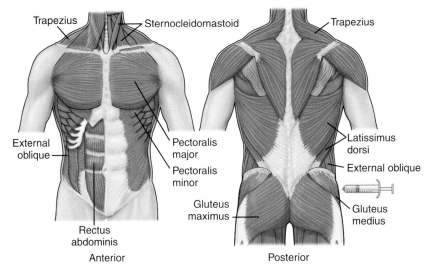

FIGURE 4–8  **Muscles of the torso and back.**

This muscle lowers the heel. On the front of the anterior of the lower leg is the extensor digitorum longus, which extends the toes, and the extensor hallucis longus, which extends just the big toe. The *intrinsic foot muscles* flex, extend, abduct, and adduct the toes. See Table 4–5 for an overview of the leg muscles.

For information about diseases and disorders of the muscular system, see Table 4–6.

### TABLE 4–4

### MUSCLES OF THE TORSO AND BACK

| Muscle | Function | Location |
|---|---|---|
| External obliques | Allow torso to turn | Lateral abdomen |
| Gluteus maximus | Extend leg to the rear | Buttocks |
| Gluteus medius | Move leg to the side | Hip |
| Latissimus dorsi | Pull arms downward and stabilize torso | Lateral back |
| Pectoralis major | Pulls arm across the chest | Chest |
| Pectoralis minor | Causes shoulder to move forward | Chest |
| Rectus abdominis | Movement of body between ribs and pelvis | Medial abdomen |
| Trapezius | Movement of scapula | Covers neck, shoulders, and spine |

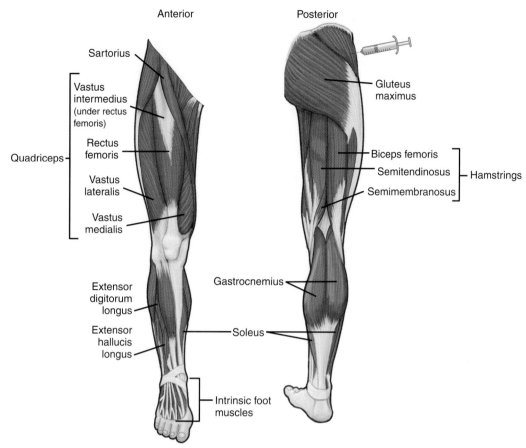

Anterior

Posterior

Sartorius

Vastus
intermedius
(under rectus
femoris)

Rectus
femoris

Quadriceps

Vastus
lateralis

Vastus
medialis

Extensor
digitorum
longus

Extensor
hallucis
longus

Gluteus
maximus

Biceps femoris

Semitendinosus

Hamstrings

Semimembranosus

Gastrocnemius

Soleus

Intrinsic foot
muscles

**FIGURE 4–9  Muscles of the anterior leg and posterior leg.**

TABLE 4–5

## MUSCLES OF THE LEGS

| Muscle | Function | Location |
|---|---|---|
| Gastrocnemius | Elevates heel | Calf muscle |
| Extensor digitorum longus | Extends toes | Lower leg |
| Extensor hallucis longus | Extends big toe | Lower leg |
| Hamstrings | Flexes lower leg | Back of thigh |
| Intrinsic foot muscles | Flex, extend, abduct, and adduct toes | Foot |
| Quadriceps femoris | Extends lower leg | Front of thigh |
| Sartorius | Turns leg laterally | Front of thigh |
| Soleus | Elevates heel when the knee is bent | Lower leg |

## TABLE 4–6
### PATHOLOGY TERMS FOR THE MUSCULAR SYSTEM

| | |
|---|---|
| Atrophy | Deterioration of muscle because of disease, injury, or disuse |
| Hypertrophy | Abnormal increase in growth of a muscle, organ, or body part |
| Hypotrophy | Abnormal decrease in growth of a muscle, organ, or body part |
| Muscular dystrophy | General term for many inherited disorders in which the muscle fibers degenerate resulting in muscle weakness |
| Myalgia | Muscle pain |
| Myoclonia | Irregular muscle twitching because of a nervous system disorder |
| Myotonia | General term for muscle spasm or temporary rigidity of a muscle |
| Sprain | Twisting or tearing of a ligament |
| Strain | Overuse or overextension of a muscle |
| Tetanus | Bacterial infection that causes the muscles to contract until they spasm resulting in paralysis; the jaw is the first to be affected (sometimes called lockjaw); also a general term for paralysis of a muscle because of overcontraction |

# Practice Exercises

## Multiple Choice

1. The muscle that allows the jaw to make a chewing motion is the
   _____.

   a. mandible

   b. masseter

   c. platysma

   d. temporalis

2. The _____ muscle of the shoulder is used for intramuscular injection.

   a. frontalis

   b. temporal

   c. deltoid

   d. soleus

3. The muscle that causes the leg to adduct is the _____.

   a. gluteus maximus

   b. gluteus medius

   c. gastrocnemius

   d. gratis

4. The upper thigh is composed of the _____ muscle.

   a. biceps

   b. triceps

   c. quadriceps

   d. quintceps

5. The muscle that turns the forearm is the _____.

   a. biceps

   b. brachioradialis

   c. gluteus medius

   d. soleus

6. Oxygen and glucose make energy in the process of _____ respiration.

   a. anaerobic

   b. anabolic

   c. aerobic

   d. antagonistic

7. The muscle that allows the lips to pucker is the _____.

   a. orbicularis oris

   b. orbicularis oculi

   c. platysma

   d. pterygoid

8. The muscle that moves the arm across the chest is the _____.

   a. gluteus maximus

   b. pectoralis major

   c. gluteus medius

   d. pectoralis minor

9. Anaerobic respiration causes _____ to build up in the muscle.

   a. citric acid

   b. acetic acid

   c. salicylic acid

   d. lactic acid

10. The muscle that flexes the arm is the _____.

    a. biceps brachii

    b. triceps brachii

    c. brachioradialis

    d. temporal

## Fill in the Blank

1. A muscle attaches to a stable bone at its point of _____.

2. An increase in muscle mass is called _____.

3. The quadriceps is an antagonist to the _____.

4. _____ is the shortening of the angle of two joints.

5. A _____ attaches muscle to bone.

6. Voluntary muscle is also called _____ muscle.

7. The type of exercise that causes an increase in muscle mass is _____.

8. Muscles that work together to create movement are called _____.

9. _____ is moving away from the midline of the body.

10. The _____ tendon holds the gastrocnemius muscle to the heel.

## Matching

1. _____ The thumb touching the tip of each finger.

2. _____ Moving a bone around a central point.

3. _____ Decreasing the angle between joints.

4. _____ Movement of the radius and ulna so that the palm faces upward.

5. _____ Increasing the angle between joints.

a. extension

b. circumduction

c. opposition

d. inversion

e. eversion

f. pronation

g. rotation

h. flexion

i. supination

j. plantar flexion

6. _____ The proximal
         end of a limb is
         stable, and the
         distal end
         moves in a
         circle.

7. _____ Turning the
         sole of the foot
         laterally.

8. _____ Movement of
         the ulna and
         radius so that
         the palm faces
         downward.

9. _____ Pointing the
         toes downward.

10. _____ Turning the
          sole of the foot
          medially.

## Short Answer

1. **Describe the three types of muscle.**

2. **What are the antagonistic muscles of the upper arm and thigh?**

3. **Describe the muscle structure.**

## Labeling

*Fill in the blanks with the appropriate anatomical terms.*

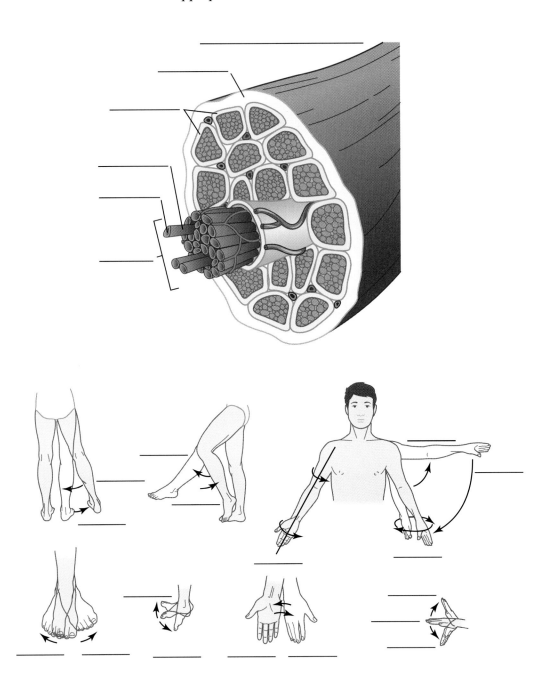

# THE SKELETAL SYSTEM 5

The skeletal system consists of the bones, the **cartilage** that connects the bones to form joints, and the ligaments that cover the joints where the bones join. The skeleton has several functions: It forms the body, supports the body, it aids in movement, acts as protection, stores minerals, and is the site of blood cell formation.

The bones create the framework that gives the body its shape. Because the human body is upright, the bones are needed to support the weight of the upper body. Leg bones are sturdier and larger than the other bones to bear the weight of the body. The ribs also act as support to the chest wall and create the thoracic cavity. Bones are the places of muscle attachment. As the muscles contract, or shorten, they pull on the bones, which produces movement. Bones provide protection to the internal organs by enclosing them. The skull encases and protects the brain, and the ribs protect the heart and lungs. The skeleton is the storage area for minerals. Bones store calcium and phosphorus, which are needed for bone growth, muscle contraction, and nerve conduction. The marrow found inside the bones is responsible for blood cell formation.

This chapter discusses the types of bone and their classifications and structure. It also discusses the fetal and adult skeletons, and gives an overview of the names and location of bones in the adult skeleton. In addition, bone healing and the different joints are described.

## Bones

Bones are made of a connective tissue called **osseous tissue**, which is one of the strongest tissues in the body. When the bones of the skeleton are shown in their proper location, the skeleton is said to be **articulated** or joined (see Fig. 5–1). Each bone of the skeleton can be identified based on bone type, shape, and function.

### Types of Bone

There are two types of bone in the body. One type is **compact bone**, which is dense and heavy. It can be found in the bones that need strength for lifting, carrying, and holding the body upright. Compact bone can be found in the bones of the arms and legs.

The other type of bone is **spongy bone**, also called cancellous bone, which looks like its name. This bone is much lighter and more porous than compact

## Key Terms

amphiarthroses

appendicular skeleton

articulated

axial skeleton

callus

cartilage

compact bone

diaphysis

diarthroses

epiphysis

fontanel

joint

ligament

osseous tissue

ossification

osteoblast

osteoclast

osteocytes

periosteum

process

*Continued*

### Flashpoint

The skeletal system maintains homeostasis by providing blood cells and storage for calcium so that blood calcium levels remain constant.

## Key Terms—cont'd

red marrow

spongy bone

sutures

synarthroses

yellow marrow

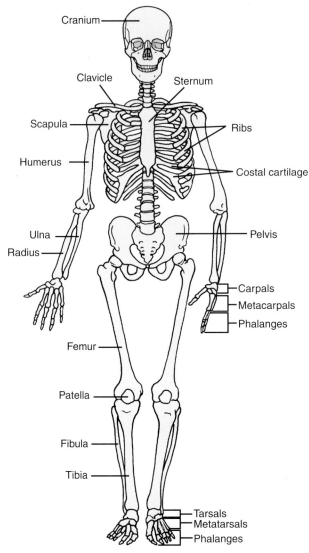

FIGURE 5–1  **Articulated skeleton.** (Adapted from Eagle S. *Medical Terminology in a Flash!* Philadelphia, PA: FA Davis; 2006:219.)

Flashpoint

Bone marrow transplant can be used to treat or cure anemia, leukemia, and other immune deficiency diseases. There is only a 35% chance of having a sibling who is a perfect match for donation.

bone. It is found in bones that do not need to be as strong or heavy, such as the skull and ribs. These two different types of bone not only give the bones their weight and strength, but they also act as storage areas for bone marrow.

Bone marrow can be either red or yellow. Compact bone is the storage site for **yellow marrow**, which is made mostly of adipose tissue or fat. Spongy bone stores the **red marrow**, which is site of blood cell production.

## Classification of Bones

Bones of the adult skeleton can be classified into four categories based on their shape: long, short, flat, or irregular. **Long bones** are much longer than they are wide and have a sticklike appearance. These bones are found in the arms and legs. The bones of the wrist and ankle are cube-shaped and are classified as **short bones**. **Flat bones** are thin, have a smooth appearance, and usually curve. Examples of these bones include the skull, ribs, shoulder blades, and sternum. **Irregular bones** are ones that do not have a similar shape. Some examples are the vertebrae of the spine and the facial bones.

## Structure of Long Bones

Long bones have a different structure and function than the other bones (see Fig. 5–2). These bones are stronger, are heavier, and provide support to the body. All long bones are wrapped in a protective tissue called the **periosteum** (around the bone). The shaft of a long bone is called the **diaphysis**. The diaphysis is made of compact bone. It contains an inner cavity called a medulla that stores the yellow bone marrow. Each end of a long bone has a rounded shape and is called an **epiphysis**. A band of hyaline cartilage spans the epiphysis and is called the **epiphyseal plate**. The epiphyseal plate is the place of growth in the long bones. When the body has reached its point of maximal growth, the epiphyseal plate hardens. The epiphyses are made of spongy bone and store red bone marrow.

*Flashpoint*
Growth of the epiphyseal plates stops around age 18 for women and around age 20 for men.

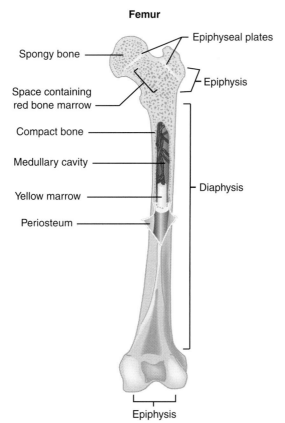

**Femur**

Spongy bone

Epiphyseal plates

Epiphysis

Space containing red bone marrow

Compact bone

Medullary cavity

Yellow marrow

Diaphysis

Periosteum

Epiphysis

FIGURE 5–2 **Parts of a long bone.**

# Skeleton

We begin life with cartilage making up the framework of our developing bodies. As hard bone replaces the cartilage, we are able to grow, stand, and walk as the bones become strong enough to support the weight of the body.

## Fetal Skeleton

*Flashpoint*

Ossification of all bones is complete by age 25.

The fetal skeleton comprises mostly cartilage and other fibrous connective tissue. About the third month of fetal development, bone-forming cells called **osteoblasts** (bone-producing) change the cartilage to bone in a process called **ossification**. The production of bone occurs from the inside of the bone outward as osteoblasts lay down calcium salts in the collagen that makes up the skeletal cartilage. When cartilage changes to bone, it is said to be ossified. At birth, the body has around 300 soft or cartilaginous bones.

Because the fetus needs to pass through the birth canal, its body needs to be flexible. The skull, especially, needs to be able to compress to move through the birth canal. For this reason, the skull bones are not completely joined at birth and are surrounded by fibrous cartilage called a **fontanel**, or "the soft spot" (see Fig. 5–3). The sites of bone growth in the long bones are also still fully cartilaginous. These sites are called epiphyseal plates; they are a disc of cartilage found on both ends of a long bone. Here the osteoblasts lay down bone vertically to increase the length of the bones. Growth in the human body continues until about age 16 to 25 depending on gender and hormone levels. When a bone is ossified, the osteoblasts mature to **osteocytes** (bone cells), which live in the bone and maintain the bone structure.

*Flashpoint*

The fontanel fully closes by 18 months of age. The posterior fontanel closes by 2 months, and the anterior fontanel closes by 9 to 18 months.

Another bone cell in the fetal bone is called an **osteoclast** (bone breaker), which is responsible for breaking down and reabsorbing the minerals of the bone matrix. In the fetal skeleton, these cells reabsorb the minerals in the centers of the long bones to carve out a hollow space for the storage of bone marrow and to allow blood vessels into the bone. After birth, the osteoclasts continue to shape the bone as it grows.

See Box 5–1 for a discussion of some common diseases and disorders of the skeletal system that affect children.

## Divisions of the Skeleton

The adult human skeleton has 206 bones. These bones have two divisions: the axial skeleton and the appendicular skeleton (see Fig. 5–4). The **axial skeleton** is the axis of the body or the main point to which the limbs are attached. The **appendicular skeleton** refers to the bones of the appendages or limbs.

### Axial Skeleton

The axial skeleton is formed by 80 individual bones. It consists of the skull, spine, and rib cage.

The **skull** is the superior portion of the axial skeleton, which is composed of cranial and facial bones. The skull is formed from 22 individual bones.

The cranium is the part of the skull that houses the brain. The **cranial bones** are eight bones that fuse together after the fontanel has ossified:

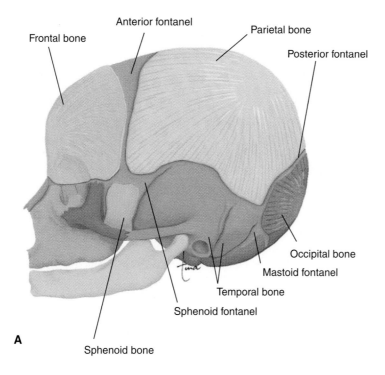

Anterior fontanel

Frontal bone

Parietal bone

Posterior fontanel

Occipital bone

Mastoid fontanel

Temporal bone

Sphenoid fontanel

**A**

Sphenoid bone

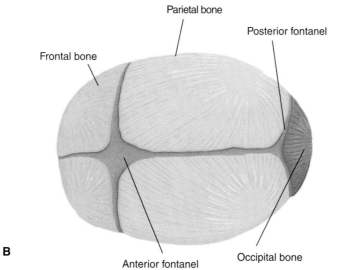

Parietal bone

Posterior fontanel

Frontal bone

**B**

Anterior fontanel

Occipital bone

FIGURE 5–3  **Fetal skull** *(A)* **Lateral view.** *(B)* **Superior view.** (From Scanlon VC. *Essentials of Anatomy and Physiology.* 5th ed. Philadelphia, PA: FA Davis; 2007:109.)

one frontal bone that forms the forehead, two parietal bones that are the sides of the skull, one occipital bone that is the base of the skull, two temporal bones on which the ears are located, one sphenoid bone that makes a portion of the interior eye socket, and one ethmoid bone located behind the lacrimal bones that completes the eye socket (see Fig. 5–5). When ossified, the grooves showing where the cranial bones fused are called **sutures**.

*(text continues on page 84)*

## Box 5-1 Childhood Diseases and Disorders of the Skeletal System

Skeletal defects are common disorders and diseases of the human body. Some are minor, but others can be life-threatening. Many skeletal disorders affect children and young adults.

Rickets occurs from a lack of dietary vitamin D and calcium during childhood when bones are growing. The result is bowed legs, a curved spine, and an enlarged skull. Prevention is the best treatment by having a diet high in calcium and vitamin D.

Scoliosis is a lateral curvature of the spine so that it bends in an "S" shape. The curvature can be a result of abnormal fetal development, or there can be a problem with another part of the body that causes the spine to curve. In most cases, the cause is unknown. Although scoliosis can occur at almost any age, adolescence (13 to 18 years old) is the most common time for scoliosis to develop. Treatment includes bracing and, if needed, surgery to fuse the spine in a more normal curvature.

Talipes, or clubfoot, is a congenital deformity in which the foot is twisted. Affected children appear to be walking on their ankles or the outside of the foot. Boys are affected more often than girls, and 50% of cases are bilateral, or occurring in both feet. Treatment is surgery to place the foot in the correct position. The child wears a series of casts, braces, and custom shoes until the deformity is corrected.

Osteosarcoma is a cancer that develops in growing bone; individuals 10 to 25 years old are most often affected. The tumor appears on the ends of the long bones; 50% of cases are located near the knee. Symptoms are pain and swelling around the tumor site. Treatment includes surgery to remove the tumor or the limb if the tumor is extensive, chemotherapy, and radiation. Survival rate with treatment is very low with only 60% surviving 5 years after treatment.

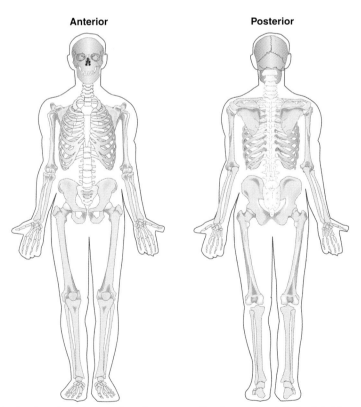

**Anterior**          **Posterior**

FIGURE 5-4  **Articulated skeleton showing appendicular and axial skeletal bones.**

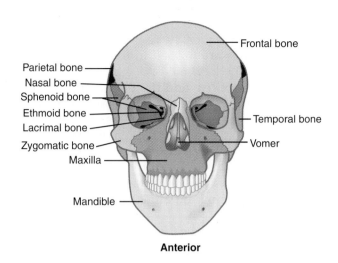

**Anterior**

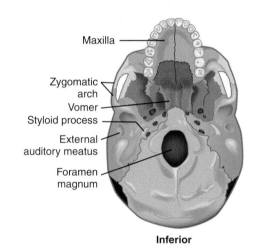

**Inferior**

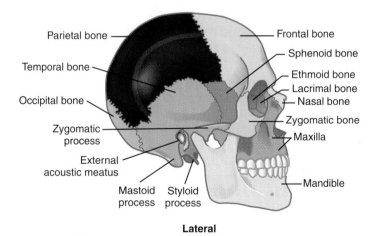

**Lateral**

FIGURE 5–5  Bones of the skull.

Flashpoint

Because of the location of the hyoid, fracture of this bone is rare. Trauma to this bone is indicative of hanging or strangulation.

Flashpoint

When it was fashionable for women to wear corsets to create the appearance of a small waist, the floating ribs became deformed by the constant tightening of the laces. Some women had the floating ribs surgically removed so they could pull the corset even tighter.

The *facial bones* include the nasal bone that forms the bridge of the nose and the vomer located within the nasal cavity that creates the nasal septum. Hollow spaces created by the nasal cavity are called *sinuses* and allow for the passage of air. The cheek bones are formed from the curved zygomatic bones. Just inside the eye orbit are the lacrimal bones, where the tear ducts are found. The upper jaw is called the *maxilla*, and the hard palate or the roof of the mouth is formed by the palatine bone. The lower jaw is the *mandible*.

Also in the skull are three small bones called ossicles located inside the ear. The ossicles are the smallest bones in the body and are not articulated to any other bone of the skull. These bones vibrate to carry sound to the brain.

A small bone called the *hyoid* is located under the mandible near the throat. Its job is to hold up the tongue. This bone is the only bone not articulated to the skeleton and is held in place by the muscles that aid in movement of the tongue.

Each of us, unless we are an identical twin, has an individual face. The face is the primary way of recognizing another person. We associate the skin with the individuality of the face. Skin and tissue are really just wrappings of the face, and the thickness of these tissues differs only slightly between gender and ethnicity. The structure of the bones beneath the tissue creates the shape of the face and makes it unique.

The skull has an opening on the inferior portion of the occipital bone called the *foramen magnum* (great hole), which allows the spinal cord to attach to the brain. The spinal cord is protected by the spinal column, also called the vertebral column.

The *spinal column* (see Fig. 5–6) is composed of 24 individual bones called vertebrae. There are three sections of spinal vertebrae. The first seven bones are called the *cervical*, or neck, vertebrae. The first two cervical vertebrae do a special job, so they also have special names. The first vertebra that the skull sits on is called the *atlas*. The second vertebra has a specialized piece of bone that allows the skull to pivot. This bone is called the *axis*. The next section of the vertebral column comprises 12 thoracic, or chest, vertebrae. The last five vertebrae are called *lumbar*, and they are the largest vertebrae and hold the weight of the other vertebrae. Between the vertebrae are discs or *intervertebral discs* made of cartilage that join the vertebrae together. Below the lumbar vertebrae is a bone called the *sacrum*. The sacrum is actually a fusion of five bones. Inferior to the sacrum is the *coccyx* bone, also called the tailbone. This bone is formed by three to five small bones fused together.

The shape of the chest is formed by 24 bones called *ribs* (see Fig. 5–7). The ribs join to the thoracic vertebrae. There are 12 pairs of ribs—one pair for each thoracic vertebra. The first seven pairs of ribs are called "true ribs." One side of a true rib joins to the thoracic vertebrae, and the other end joins to the sternum, or breast bone. The next three pairs of ribs are called "false ribs." These ribs have one side that joins to the thoracic vertebrae, and the other side joins to cartilage attached to the true ribs. The last two pairs of ribs are called "floating ribs." They get their name because they have one side that joins to the thoracic vertebrae, and the other side remains unattached.

The *sternum* (see Fig. 5–7), sometimes referred to as the breast bone, is the place of rib attachment. It is actually composed of three different bones. The uppermost bone is shaped like a shield and is called the *manubrium*. The middle bone is rectangular and the largest bone of the sternum. This bone is called the *body*. Attached to the inferior portion of the body is a small piece of bone called the *xiphoid process*.

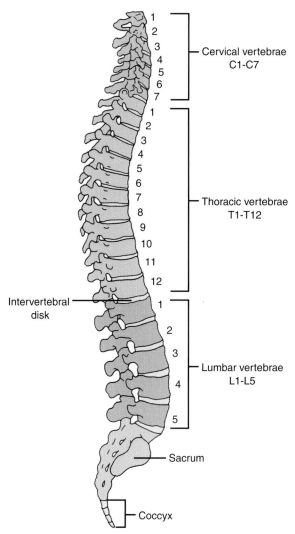

1
2
3
4
5
6
7
— Cervical vertebrae
C1-C7

1
2
3
4
5
6
7
8
9
10
11
12
— Thoracic vertebrae
T1-T12

Intervertebral — 1
disk
2
3
— Lumbar vertebrae
4　　L1-L5
5

— Sacrum

— Coccyx

**FIGURE 5-6** **Lateral view of the spinal column.** (Adapted from Eagle S. *Medical Terminology in a Flash!* Philadelphia, PA: FA Davis; 2006:220.)

## Appendicular Skeleton

The appendicular skeleton is formed by 126 individual bones. It consists of the bones of the arms, legs, shoulder girdle, and pelvis.

The superior appendicular skeleton begins with the two shoulder blades. Each is called a *scapula*, and they are located on the dorsal body below the cervical vertebrae. On the posterior surface of each scapula is an outcropping of bone, or **process**, called the spine, which broadens as it curves toward the shoulder. This broad piece of bone is the acromion process.

The collar bones are the *clavicles*. They are located on the ventral body below the cervical vertebrae. The clavicles are an elongated "S" shape, and the lateral portion of the clavicle meets the acromion process. These two bones form the shoulder girdle, which is the place of attachment for the arms. See Figure 5–8 for the bones of the shoulder girdle.

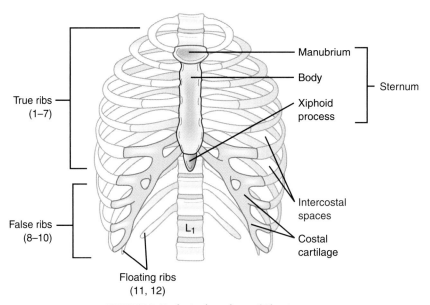

FIGURE 5-7  Anterior view of the torso.

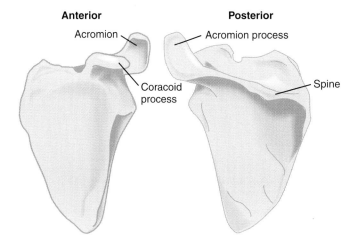

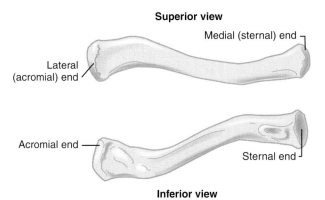

FIGURE 5-8  Scapula and clavicle.

The upper arm bone is the *humerus*, and it attaches at the shoulder girdle. The proximal humerus has a rounded head that fits into the shoulder girdle. Distally the humerus has two rounded portions called epicondyles. Between the epicondyles is a flattened depression called the olecranon.

Two bones are found in the *forearm*. They are the *ulna*, which is located on the little finger side of the palm, and the *radius*, which is on the thumb side of the palm. The proximal end of the ulna has a hook-shaped notch called the trochlea that attaches to the humerus. The distal ulna ends in a rounded knob called the head. The proximal radius is a wheel-shaped knob called the head and ends distally with a curved process called the styloid. These two bones are actually parallel to each other, but movement of the forearm is created by the radius crossing over the ulna. See Figure 5–9 for bones of the arm.

Flashpoint

The "funny bone" is not really a bone. The tingly, numb feeling that comes from hitting the inside of the elbow is actually the ulnar nerve being pushed against the humerus.

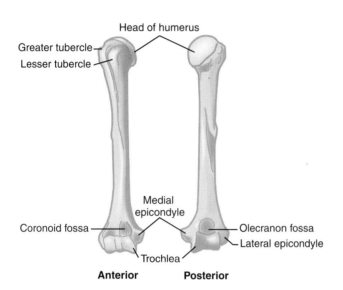

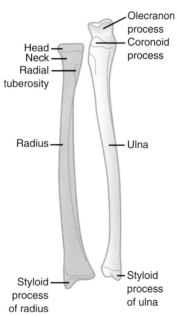

FIGURE 5-9 **Bones of the arm.**

The wrist is composed of eight cube-shaped bones that form two rows of four bones called *carpals*; the five bones of the palm are the *metacarpals*. Fingers are called *phalanges*, and each finger is composed of three small bones called phalanx bones. The thumb is made of two phalanx bones.

The *pelvis* (see Fig. 5–10) surrounds the lower spine and consists of two hip bones. Each hip bone, or coxa, has three sections. The flared upper portion of the hip bone is called the *ilium*. At the superior ilium of each hip bone is a ridge referred to as the iliac crest. The lower portion of the hip bone curves posteriorly and anteriorly. The *ischium* is the rounded posterior section. These bones are often called the "sit bones" because they can be felt when sitting on a firm surface. The anterior curve of the hip bone is the *pubis*. Where the ilium curves above the ischium, a bony socket or acetabulum forms the hip joint. The fibrous cartilage that holds the hip bones together at the pubis is called the *pubic symphysis*. The angle that the pubis forms is the pubic arch. See Box 5–2 for a description of the differences between the male and female pelvis. When the hip bones are articulated anteriorly at the pubis and posteriorly to the sacrum, a ring of bone is formed, which is referred to as the pelvic girdle.

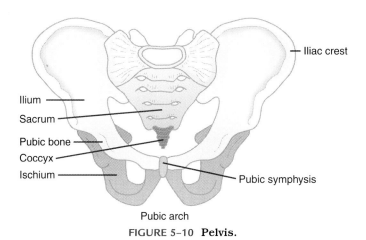

FIGURE 5–10 **Pelvis.**

## Box 5–2 Gender Differences in the Pelvis

The bones of the pelvis are the same in men and women; however, the shape of the pelvis differs between the genders.

The female pelvis is wider and lower than the male pelvis, which has a higher ilium and a more narrow width. The angle of the female pubic arch is wide and round, and the angle of the male pubic arch is narrow. A pubic arch of a female is greater than a 90-degree angle, and a pubic arch of a male is less than a 90-degree angle. The inside of the pelvis is more round or oval in the female, whereas the male pelvis is more heart-shaped.

The female sacrum is wider and more triangular in shape than the sacrum of the male. It also curves back away from the pelvic opening, whereas the male sacrum curves inward.

The female pelvis differs from the male pelvis to create space for a fetus to pass through the birth canal.

The legs join the axial skeleton at the pelvic girdle (see Fig. 5–11). The *femur*, the largest and heaviest bone in the body, is found in the upper leg or thigh. At the proximal end of the femur is a large rounded knob of bone called the head. The head is the portion of the femur that inserts into the hip socket. The distal end of the femur has two rounded processes called condyles. This is the place of attachment to the lower leg.

The lower leg has two bones. The larger bone of the ventral lower leg is the shin bone, or *tibia*. The proximal end of the tibia also has rounded ends called condyles that join with the condyles of the femur. The other bone is a thin bone located under the calf muscle called the *fibula*. It is not weight-bearing, but acts as a site of muscle attachment. Between the upper and lower leg is the knee joint. A small bone called the *patella*, or kneecap, covers and protects this joint.

The bones of the feet are similar to the bones of the hand. Each ankle is formed by seven small bones called *tarsals*. The largest tarsal is the heel or *calcaneus* bone. *Metatarsals* are the bones of the instep of the foot. The toes, similar to the fingers, are phalanges; the big toe, or *hallux*, has two phalanx bones, and the other toes have three (see Fig. 5–12).

# Bone Repair

Although bone is one of the hardest substances in the body, it can still be fractured or broken secondary to stress, trauma, or disease. Healing of the bone occurs in three phases: inflammatory response, repair, and remodeling.

When a bone is broken, the tissue surrounding the break is damaged, the injured blood vessels bleed, and white blood cells come to the area. The

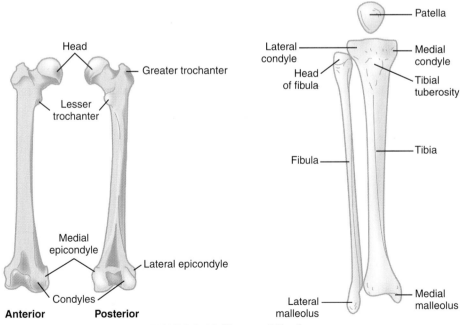

FIGURE 5–11  **Bones of the leg.**

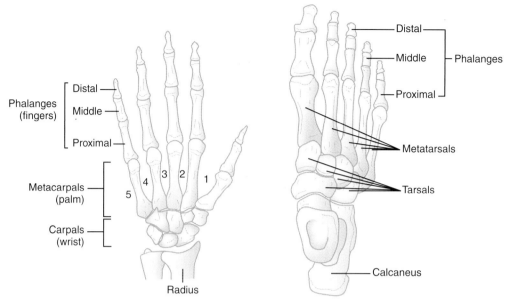

FIGURE 5-12 Bones of the hand and foot.

presence of these cells causes inflammation, which is the pain and swelling at the fracture site. As the vessels stop bleeding and the cells begin to die, a *hematoma* or clot forms at the break.

Cells in the blood called *fibroblasts* (fiber-producing) begin repair of the break by producing collagen fibers that form a structure similar to scaffolding on a building over the clot. Osteoblasts stored in the periosteum migrate to the area. These cells add calcium to the collagen to turn it to bone. A raised area called a **callus** is left around the fracture. The callus ossifies, completely repairing the break.

As the bone continues to strengthen, osteoclasts remodel the bone and remove any excess osseous tissue. During this stage, the bone should return to its original shape and strength (see Fig. 5-13).

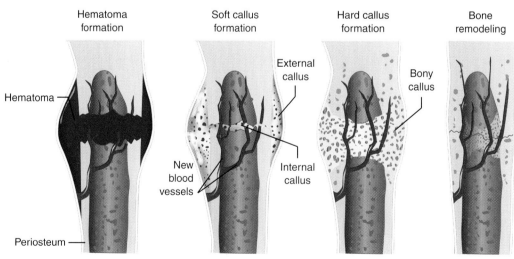

FIGURE 5-13 Bone repair.

Bone healing takes 3 to 6 weeks depending on the age of the person, the bone that is broken, and the type of fracture (see Fig. 15–14). To heal adequately, the injured bone needs to be reduced or immobilized to allow the ossification process to occur. If a bone is not reduced, or if the bone is not aligned properly during ossification, the result is a malformed bone or one that does not heal. Table 5–1 describes the different types of bone fractures.

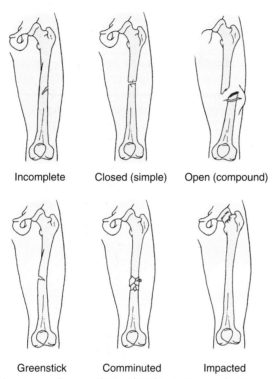

Incomplete    Closed (simple)    Open (compound)

Greenstick    Comminuted    Impacted

FIGURE 5-14 **Types of fractures: incomplete, simple, compound, greenstick, comminuted, impacted.** (Adapted from Eagle S. *Medical Terminology in a Flash!* Philadelphia, PA: FA Davis; 2006:231.)

Flashpoint
Bone mineral density (BMD) is measured with a dual-energy X-ray absorptiometry test (DEXA scan). This test can predict future fracture risk as bone ages.

## TABLE 5–1
### TYPES OF FRACTURES

| | |
|---|---|
| Comminuted | Two or more intersecting breaks result in bone fragments |
| Compound (open) | Ends of the broken bones have pierced the skin |
| Greenstick | Occurs in children who still have more collagen than solid bone, and the bone breaks longitudinally |
| Incomplete | Occurs when the bone breaks, but is not completely separated across the width of the bone |
| Impacted | Occurs when two bones are forced against each other, and the bone ends fragment |
| Pathological | Bone breaks because of weakness secondary to a disorder of the bone |
| Simple (closed) | Bones are broken, but do not move, and there is little trauma to surrounding tissue |

# Types of Joints

The place where two bones come together is called a *joint*, or articulation. A type of fibrous connective tissue called a *ligament* stabilizes the joint by joining the bones. There are three types of joints in the body: synarthroses, amphiarthroses, and diarthroses. They can be classified by function and by structure.

*Synarthroses* are joints that are incapable of movement. Structurally, these joints are composed of fibrous tissue. The best example of this type of joint is the sutures of the skull. *Amphiarthroses* are slightly movable. This joint can be found in the discs between the spinal vertebrae. The slight movement is created by cartilage that has limited flexibility, so it does not stretch very far. *Diarthroses* are freely movable joints. Sacs of cartilage filled with fluid occur between the bones at these joints. These are synovial joints, and the sacs are filled with synovial fluid. These sacs act as a cushion between the bones and allow a greater range of movement. There are several different types of diarthroses in the body: ball-and-socket, hinge, condyloid, plane, pivot, and saddle (see Fig. 5–15). Table 5–2 gives examples of these types of joints.

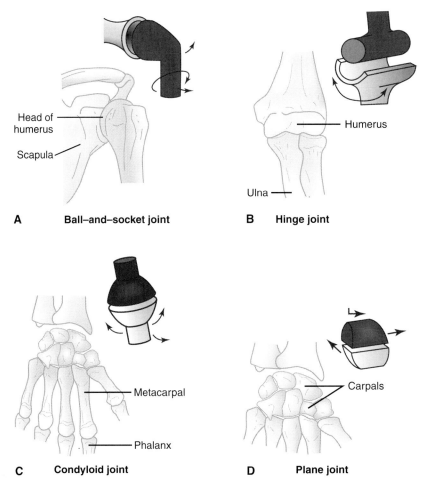

**A**   **Ball–and–socket joint**

Head of humerus

Scapula

**B**   **Hinge joint**

Humerus

Ulna

**C**   **Condyloid joint**

Metacarpal

Phalanx

**D**   **Plane joint**

Carpals

FIGURE 5–15  **Types of diarthroses.** *(A)* Ball-and-socket. *(B)* Hinge. *(C)* Condyloid. *(D)* Plane. *(E)* Pivot. *(F)* Saddle.

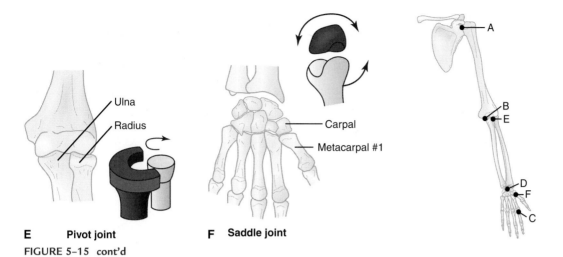

**E** **Pivot joint** **F** **Saddle joint**

FIGURE 5–15 cont'd

## TABLE 5–2

### TYPES OF DIARTHROSES

| Term | Definition | Example |
|------|-----------|---------|
| Ball-and-socket joint | Round head of one bone fits into socket of another and allows rotating movement | Shoulder and hip |
| Condyloid joint | Oval shape of one bone fits to another concave bone; this joint can move side to side | Finger and toes |
| Hinge joint | One cylindrical-shaped bone fits into the trough-shaped surface of another and allows movement one way | Elbow and knee |
| Pivot joint | Rounded end of one bone fits into a ring of bone and allows rotation | Atlas and axis |
| Plane joint | Articulating bone ends are flat, and one glides against another | Wrist and ankle |
| Saddle joint | One bone is convex, and the articulating bone is concave forming a "saddle"; allows circumduction movement | Thumb |

A ***ball-and-socket*** joint allows a rotating movement because the rounded end of one bone fits into a socket of another bone. The shoulder and hip joints are examples of this type of joint. A ***hinge*** joint allows one-way movement, such as at the knee and elbow. This joint is created by a ***cylindrical***-shaped bone attaching to a trough-shaped groove in another bone. When a rounded end of one bone fits into a concave end of another bone, it forms a ***condyloid*** joint. This joint has a side-to-side movement and can be found in the fingers and toes. A ***plane*** joint is found in the wrists and ankles, and is created where two flat bones slide against one another. When a rounded end of bone fits into a ring-shaped opening in another bone, a ***pivot*** joint is formed. The axis fitting in the atlas to give a turning movement to the head is an example of this type of joint. The thumb is the only example of a ***saddle*** joint in the body; a convex-shaped bone fits into the concave shape of another creating a joint capable of circumduction or circular movement.

For information about common diseases and disorders of the skeletal system, see Table 5–3.

Flashpoint
The knee is the most common surgically replaced joint.

## TABLE 5–3
## PATHOLOGY TERMS FOR THE SKELETAL SYSTEM

| | |
|---|---|
| Achondroplasia | Genetic disease of the connective tissue that results in a normal-sized torso but shortened limbs |
| Dislocation | Displacement of a bone from the joint |
| Kyphosis | An exaggerated thoracic curve called hunchback |
| Lordosis | An exaggerated lumbar curve called swayback |
| Osteoarthritis | Progressive wearing away of joints because of age or injury; symptoms include pain and stiffness, which increase during cold, damp weather |
| Osteoporosis | Loss of bone density caused by decreased mineral retention in the bones secondary to a lack of estrogen so that bones weaken and break easily; commonly affects postmenopausal women |
| Paget disease | Abnormal bone destruction and repair, which creates bone irregularities and deformities; affects middle-aged and elderly adults |
| Scoliosis | Lateral curvature of the spine; occurs more often during adolescence |
| Talipes | Congenital deformity of the foot where the foot is in a fixed twisted position; also called clubfoot |

# Practice Exercises

## Multiple Choice

1. Red bone marrow is found in the _____ of a long bone.

   a.  diaphysis

   b.  epiphysis

   c.  periosteum

   d.  endomysium

2. An example of a synarthrosis joint is _____.

   a.  ball-and-socket

   b.  hinge

   c.  suture

   d.  pubis symphysis

3. The shin bone is the _____.

   a.  ulna

   b.  radius

   c.  tibia

   d.  fibula

4. The ribs are connected to the _____ vertebrae.

   a.  cervical

   b.  thoracic

   c.  lumbar

   d.  coccyx

5. The only bone not connected to the skeleton is the _____.

   a.  thyroid

   b.  sacrum

   c.  hyoid

   d.  hilus

6. The _____ is the lower portion of the pelvis.

   a.  ilium

   b.  ischium

   c.  ileum

   d.  idiom

7. A _____ joins bone to bone.

   a.  joint

   b.  ligament

   c.  tendon

   d.  muscle

8. The _____ skeleton is the main point to which the limbs are attached.

   a.  atlas

   b.  appendicular

   c.  anterior

   d.  axial

9. The spinal cord is found in the _____ column.

   a.  vertical

   b.  ventral

   c.  vertebral

   d.  vernal

10. The calcaneus bone is commonly called the _____.

    a. foot

    b. knee

    c. heel

    d. toe

## True or False

1. True   False    A fibrous joint and a synarthrosis are the same.

2. True   False    The femur is found in the upper arm.

3. True   False    Phalanges are both fingers and toes.

4. True   False    The false ribs are connected to the sternum

5. True   False    There are 206 bones in the adult skeleton.

## Fill in the Blank

1. _____ bone marrow is the site of blood cell production.

2. The _____ is the protective covering of a long bone.

3. The cartilage in the fetal skull is known as a _____.

4. The _____ turns over the _____ to produce movement in the arm.

5. The largest bone in the human body is the _____.

6. The site of growth in a long bone is the _____.

7. There are _____ pairs of ribs.

8. Another name for the breast bone is the _____.

9. _____ is the process of making bone.

10. The flared portion of the hip bone is the _____.

11. The _____ bone is made of a fusion of three to five small bones.

12. The _____ of a long bone stores yellow marrow.

13. The mandible is the _____ jaw bone.

14. An example of a _____ joint is the bend of the elbow.

15. The _____ protects the knee joint.

16. A _____ fracture is found most often in children.

17. A slightly movable joint is called a(n) _____.

18. The bones of the palm are the _____.

19. Mature bone cells are _____.

20. The scapula is commonly called the _____ bone.

## Short Answer

1. **Name and describe the three types of joints in the body.**

2. **Name and define the different fractures.**

3. **List the types of diarthroses and give an example of each.**

## Labeling

*Fill in the blanks with the appropriate anatomical terms.*

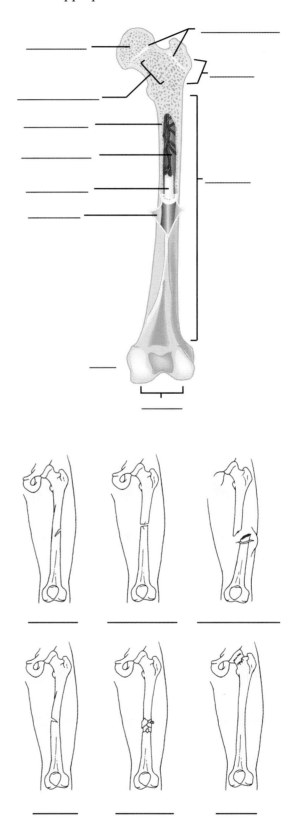

_____

_____

_____

_____

_____

_____

_____

_____

_____

_____

_____

_____

_____     _____     _____

_____     _____     _____

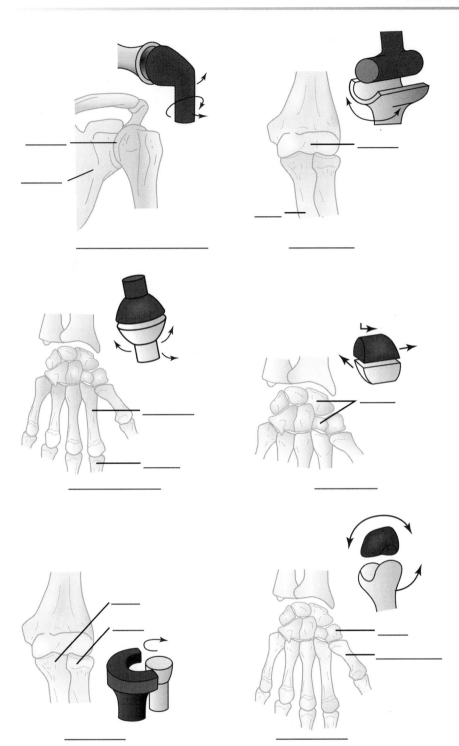

# 6

# BLOOD

## Key Terms

agglutination

colony-stimulating factors

erythrocyte

erythropoietin

hematopoiesis

hemolytic disease of the newborn

hemostasis

leukocyte

plasma

thrombocyte

thrombopoietin

Blood is a specialized body fluid because it is actually a fluid tissue. Blood circulates throughout the body and performs the functions of transportation, protection, and regulation.

Blood transports oxygen and other nutrients to the tissues, and transports wastes from the tissues to be removed from the body. Some cells in the blood can detect and destroy foreign substances that may harm the body. Blood also regulates fluid and electrolyte balance and maintains body temperature.

This chapter discusses and describes the components of blood. The human blood groups and the importance of blood typing are also discussed.

## Blood Components

Blood accounts for about 8% of our body weight, which equals about 5 or 6 liters. It is thicker and heavier than water because blood is part fluid and part solid (see Fig. 6–1). The fluid portion is a clear, yellowish liquid called plasma, and the solid portion is composed of formed elements or cells.

### Plasma

The fluid portion of blood is **plasma**; it makes up 55% of the total blood volume. The main component of plasma is water, which makes up about 90% of the fluid. The other substances in plasma are soluble, or able to be dissolved in water. Because plasma is a solvent, which means it is capable of dissolving substances, it is able to transport many different substances. Nutrients such as oxygen and electrolytes are carried to all body cells. The fluid waste products created from the use of nutrients are transported to the kidneys to be excreted. Another waste product called carbon dioxide is actually a gas, but it is transported in the plasma as bicarbonate ions. When the bicarbonate ions reach the lungs, the carbon dioxide is re-formed and is exhaled as a gas. Hormones are water-soluble and travel in the plasma to their target organs.

Plasma proteins are another substance in the plasma. These proteins are responsible for blood clotting, maintaining pressure in the blood, and providing immunity. The clotting proteins are prothrombin and fibrinogen. They are made in the liver and circulate in the plasma until they are needed to form a clot to plug a damaged vessel. Albumin is another protein made by the liver. This is the most abundant of the plasma proteins and maintains the osmotic pressure within the blood. Osmotic pressure occurs when two different solutions of

Flashpoint
Blood maintains homeostasis by delivering oxygen to the cells and removing carbon dioxide, fighting infection, and maintaining fluid volume.

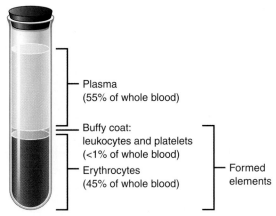

FIGURE 6–1 **Blood components.**

- Plasma
  (55% of whole blood)
- Buffy coat:
  leukocytes and platelets
  (<1% of whole blood)
- Erythrocytes
  (45% of whole blood)
- Formed elements

different concentrations are separated by a membrane. In higher osmotic pressure, blood pulls tissue fluid into the capillaries to maintain blood volume and blood pressure. The globulins are another type of plasma protein. Some globulins are made by the liver and act as carriers for other molecules. The lymphocytes make others globulin called immunoglobulins or antibodies, which provide protection from foreign substances and provide immunity.

## Formed Elements

The formed elements constitute about 45% of the total volume of whole blood. There are three types of *formed elements*, or blood cells: erythrocytes, leukocytes, and thrombocytes (see Fig. 6–2). All three blood cells are created in the red bone marrow found in the ends of the long bones and in the flat and irregular bones such as the skull, ribs, and vertebrae.

### Red Blood Cells

**Erythrocytes**, or red blood cells (RBCs), are the most common formed elements (see Fig. 6–3). They are anucleate, meaning they have no nucleus, so they appear hollow in the middle. Because of this feature, RBCs are sometimes

*Flashpoint*

Serum is the clear fluid that is separated from blood that has clotted, so it lacks the clotting proteins that would still be present in the plasma.

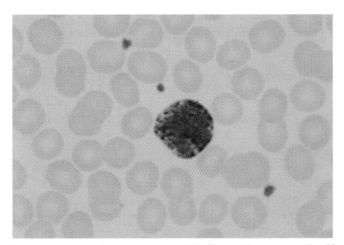

FIGURE 6–2 **Red blood cells, platelets, and basophil.** (From Harmening D. *Clinical Hematology and Fundamentals of Hemostasis*, 5th ed. Philadelphia, PA: FA Davis; 2009:5.)

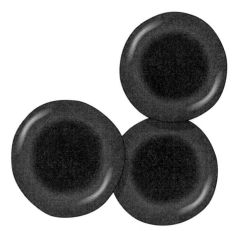

FIGURE 6–3  Red blood cell.

referred to as biconcave discs because the centers are thinner than the edges and the middle looks caved in on both sides. These cells are the only cells in the human body that contain no nucleus. The nucleus is not needed because these cells do not go through mitosis to reproduce.

Erythrocytes live for approximately 120 days, and the old cells become part of the debris that is removed by another cell called a macrophage (big eater). Because these cells do not replicate, they are constantly being produced in the bone marrow to maintain the 4 to 6 million cells found in each blood droplet. It is estimated that 2 to 3 million new RBCs are made each second.

The purpose of RBCs is to carry oxygen to all cells of the body. Erythrocytes contain an iron protein called **hemoglobin** (Hb), which binds to oxygen and releases it in the capillaries to be used by the other cells. By not having a nucleus, the RBCs have more space to carry hemoglobin. The heme, or iron, in the hemoglobin gives RBCs their color. When RBCs are digested by macrophages, the breakdown of the cells releases several color pigments that are excreted from the body. Bilirubin is a pigment that is removed from the blood by the liver. It is secreted from the liver into the bile, giving the bile its yellowish green color. Bile is removed with the waste from the digestive system and gives feces its brown color. Another pigment called urochrome is removed by the kidneys and is excreted in the fluid waste, giving urine its distinctive yellow color.

Iron is also released into the blood after the RBCs are broken down. Instead of being excreted, iron returns to the red bone marrow where it is used for new RBC production. This iron is recycled over and over. Any excess iron not used immediately for new RBCs is stored in the liver for future use.

## White Blood Cells

**Leukocytes**, or white blood cells (WBCs), are part of the body's defense system (see Fig. 6–4). These cells are larger than RBCs, but are far less numerous. The average number of WBCs is 5000 to 10,000 per drop of blood. Leukocytes are able to move in and out of blood vessels and circulate throughout the body to defend it against bacteria, viruses, parasites, and tumor cells.

There are five different types of leukocytes, and each differs in size, shape of the nucleus, and features of the cytoplasm (see Fig. 6–5). Leukocytes can be classified as granulocytes or agranulocytes. Leukocytes that have granules in the cytoplasm are called **granulocytes**, and cells without granules are **agranulocytes**.

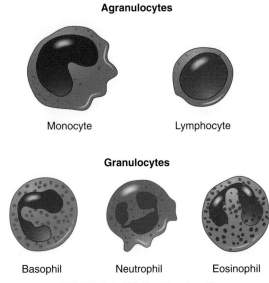

**Agranulocytes**

Monocyte          Lymphocyte

**Granulocytes**

Basophil     Neutrophil     Eosinophil

FIGURE 6–4  **White blood cells.**

Of the five different WBCs, three are granulocytes. They are neutrophils, eosinophils, and basophils.

- *Neutrophils* are the most numerous of the leukocytes. These cells act as phagocytes, cleaning up small debris throughout the body. An immature neutrophil is called a band cell.
- *Eosinophils* are present in small numbers in the blood, but increase in response to a parasitic infection or allergic reaction.
- *Basophils* are present in small amounts. They secrete heparin and histamine. Heparin is an anticoagulant that prevents abnormal clotting. Histamine makes vessels leak tissue fluid as part of the inflammatory response secondary to injury or allergic reaction.

The other two types of WBCs are agranulocytes. They are monocytes and lymphocytes.

- *Monocytes* are the largest of the WBCs. They change into a large phagocyte called a macrophage to clear large particles and clean debris from the site of an immune response. Macrophages also aid in tissue repair by phagocytizing dead or damaged tissue at an injury site.
- *Lymphocytes* are the smallest WBCs. They increase in response to the presence of foreign substances and provide two different types of immunity to the body.

## Platelets

**Thrombocytes** are also called platelets. They aid in stopping blood flow because of tissue trauma. Platelets are actually not cells, but fragments of another larger cell called a *megakaryocyte* (see Fig. 6–6). In response to trauma, the megakaryocyte breaks open, and the platelets spill out. The platelets travel to the injured site and form a plug causing the blood to clot. The average number of platelets is about 150,000 to 400,000 in each drop of blood.

Flashpoint
Whole blood can be donated, but so can the plasma or the platelets. The process of removing the plasma or platelets is called apheresis.

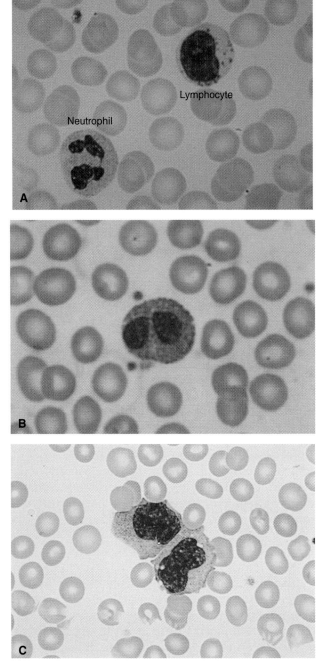

FIGURE 6–5  *(A)* **Lymphocyte and neutrophil.** *(B)* **Eosinophils.** *(C)* **Monocytes.** (From Harmening D. *Clinical Hematology and Fundamentals of Hemostasis*, 5th ed. Philadelphia, PA: FA Davis; 2009:5, 6, 7.)

## Hematopoiesis

**Hematopoiesis** (blood creation), also called hemopoiesis, is the process of making blood cells. All three of the formed elements are made in the red bone marrow found in the ends of the long bones and in the ribs, skull, sternum, and pelvis.

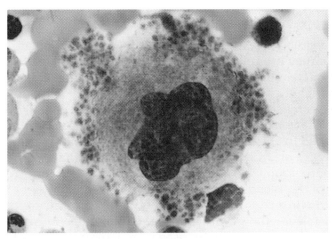

**FIGURE 6–6 Megakaryocyte.** (From Harmening D. *Clinical Hematology and Fundamentals of Hemostasis*, 5th ed. Philadelphia, PA: FA Davis; 2009:30.)

Each cell comes from the same stem cell, called a **hemocytoblast**. The hemocytoblast (embryonic blood cell) is described as pluripotent, meaning it has the ability to change into several different cells. Production of blood cells depends on which of the three types is needed. A wound that causes blood loss would stimulate the production of RBCs to replace the cells that were lost. The presence of a microorganism would signal the manufacture of WBCs to fight that microorganism.

A hemocytoblast can become one of two types of cell lines. One is lymphoid, and the other is myeloid. The lymphoid cell line produces only lymphocytes. The myeloid cell line produces the other formed elements. Which formed element the myeloid cell becomes depends on the hormone that stimulates the myeloid cell (see Fig. 6–7).

The rate of RBC production is controlled by a hormone called **erythropoietin**. This hormone is produced by the kidneys at a constant rate. If **hypoxia** occurs,

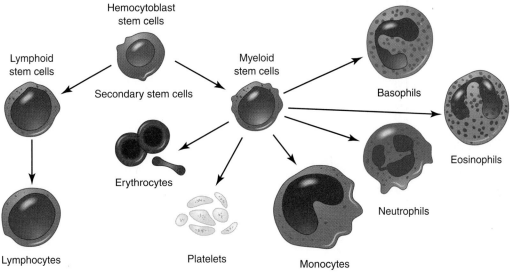

**FIGURE 6–7 Hematopoiesis.**

which means the oxygen level of the blood decreases, the kidneys increase the manufacture of erythropoietin. This stimulates the myeloid cells to change to reticulocytes. Reticulocytes are immature RBCs, and they remain in the marrow for 4 days before they are released into the bloodstream. After entering the bloodstream, the reticulocytes circulate for another day before becoming fully mature erythrocytes.

An abnormal increase in the number of erythrocytes, usually resulting from an abnormality of the bone marrow, is *polycythemia. Anemia* is a general term for a decrease in the number of RBCs, an abnormality in the shape of the RBCs, or a decrease or an abnormality of the hemoglobin so that it cannot transport adequate supplies of oxygen. See Box 6–1 for a summary of hemorrhagic diseases of the blood.

*Colony-stimulating factors* (CSFs) are produced by several tissues, and they are responsible for the production of the different WBCs. CSFs are also responsible for enhancing the ability of mature leukocytes to detect foreign substances.

A high level of leukocytes is called *leukocytosis* and is often an indication of infection. A low level of leukocytes is *leukopenia* and may be an indication of chemical or radiation exposure or the early stages of tuberculosis.

*Thrombopoietin* is the hormone that controls the manufacture of megakaryocytes. This hormone is produced in the liver and the kidneys. *Thrombocytosis* is an abnormal increase in the number of platelets in the blood. A decrease in platelets is *thrombocytopenia*, and it may be due to a virus or medications or have no known cause.

## Box 6–1 Hemorrhagic Blood Disorders

Many blood-borne pathogens that infect humans are transmitted from insects and other mammals. Some commonly transmitted diseases are those that cause hemorrhagic reactions or severe blood loss in the victims.

Malaria is one of the most common blood-borne illnesses. It is spread by mosquitoes that can live in the tropical and subtropical climates of the United States, Asia, and Africa. Symptoms begin with a fever and chills and progress to anemia owing to hemolysis of the red blood cells. Malaria can cause seizures, coma, and death if untreated. Treatment includes supportive measures of fluids, rest, and administration of antimalarial drugs. Full recovery can by achieved by early treatment.

Dengue fever is carried by mosquitoes in tropical climates. Symptoms include sudden onset of fever, headache, joint, and muscle aches. A rash then develops that starts on the limbs and spreads to the rest of the body. The fever progresses to spontaneous bleeding from the mucous membranes. Symptoms of the fever last 6 to 8 days. Many infected individuals survive, but some go into shock from blood loss, which can lead to death. Treatment includes fluid regulation and rest. Blood transfusions may be given to patients with significant blood loss. Currently there is no vaccine.

Ebola virus is a deadly virus transmitted from the fruit bat. Most outbreaks have been in Africa; infected individuals have only a 20% survival rate. Symptoms begin with fever, vomiting, and diarrhea, then progress to internal and then external bleeding. Death occurs from shock because of blood loss and organ failure. Currently there is no treatment or vaccine.

# Hemostasis

The clotting of blood to stop blood flow is called **hemostasis** (blood stoppage). Hemostasis involves several steps. If a blood vessel is damaged, vasoconstriction of that vessel occurs first to slow the flow of blood. Next, the megakaryocytes burst and release platelets that go to the damaged site and bind to the collagen on the broken vessel and form a plug. A protein in the blood called fibrinogen binds to the platelet plug and causes a clot. This clot stimulates fibroblasts to repair the broken vessel and to dissolve the clot after the vessel is healed.

# Human Blood Groups

Identification of human blood, or blood typing, is based on the presence or absence of markers, or **antigens**, on the surface of the RBCs. Antigens provide a means of identification for all cells because each has a unique shape.

Having the correct blood type is so important that antibodies against foreign blood types are present without having to come in contact first with the foreign blood type. An **antibody** is a defense against foreign substances. Human blood is most commonly identified by the ABO blood system (see Table 6–1) and the Rh blood system.

## ABO Blood System

In the **ABO blood system**, people have Type A, Type B, Type AB, or Type O blood. Individuals with Type A have A antigen on the cell surface, individuals with Type B have B antigen on the cell surface, individuals with Type AB have both A antigen and B antigen, and individuals with Type O have neither A antigen nor B antigen.

Antibodies are made whenever the body comes in contact with a new antigen. The purpose of an antibody is to destroy a foreign antigen. If an antibody comes in contact with the antigen it was made for, it attaches itself to the antigen like a jigsaw puzzle piece. The antibody then destroys the antigen.

In the ABO system, people with A antigen would see the B antigen as foreign, so they would make the antibody anti-B. People with B antigen would see the

*Flashpoint*

There are more than 600 known possible blood antigens. Many of them are rare or found only in certain ethnic groups.

*Flashpoint*

Karl Landsteiner discovered the four basic human blood types in 1900.

| TABLE 6-1 | | | | |
| --- | --- | --- | --- | --- |
| **ABO BLOOD TYPES** | | | | |
| Blood Type | Antigen | Antibody | Percentage of Population | Who Can Donate |
| A | A | Anti-B | 41 | A, O |
| B | B | Anti-A | 10 | B, O |
| AB | A and B | None | 4 | A, B, AB, O |
| O | None | Anti-A and anti-B | 45 | O |

A antigen as foreign, so they would make the anti-A antibody. People with the Type AB blood would not make either antibody because they have both antigens. People with Type O would make both anti-A and anti-B because both antigens would be foreign to them.

Because Type O blood has no antigens, it is not seen as foreign by the other blood types and can be mixed with any of those blood types. It is often referred to as the universal donor. All blood types can mix with Type AB, so this type is called the universal recipient. See Figure 6–8 for the antigens and antibodies of the ABO blood system.

Blood antibodies differ from other antibodies because we naturally make antibodies against other blood antigens so we do not need to come in contact with a foreign blood antigen before antibodies are produced. Blood antibodies also differ from other antibodies because instead of destroying the foreign blood, they cause clumping of the blood cells. This clumping of blood cells is called **_agglutination_**. Agglutination occurs if different blood types are mixed, such as in a transfusion of the incorrect blood type. The clumping of the blood cells can cause organ damage or failure and even death. The amount of agglutination depends on how much foreign blood was introduced, and how strongly the blood antibodies react to the foreign antigens.

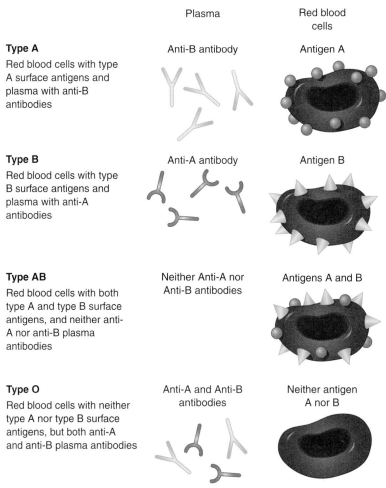

|  | Plasma | Red blood cells |
|---|---|---|
| **Type A** Red blood cells with type A surface antigens and plasma with anti-B antibodies | Anti-B antibody | Antigen A |
| **Type B** Red blood cells with type B surface antigens and plasma with anti-A antibodies | Anti-A antibody | Antigen B |
| **Type AB** Red blood cells with both type A and type B surface antigens, and neither anti-A nor anti-B plasma antibodies | Neither Anti-A nor Anti-B antibodies | Antigens A and B |
| **Type O** Red blood cells with neither type A nor type B surface antigens, but both anti-A and anti-B plasma antibodies | Anti-A and Anti-B antibodies | Neither antigen A nor B |

FIGURE 6–8  ABO antigens and antibodies.

# Rh Blood Group

The other commonly typed blood antigen is Rh, also called D antigen. Rh is named for the Rhesus monkeys that were used to identify this blood antigen. In the **Rh blood system**, a person either has the Rh antigen on the blood cells or does not have it. People with the antigen are Rh⁺, and people without it are Rh⁻.

It is important that ABO and Rh are typed together. Even if the ABO system matches, if the Rh does not, agglutination would still occur. With Rh factored in, the true universal donor is O⁻, and the true universal recipient is AB⁺.

## Hemolytic Disease of the Newborn

The importance of correct blood typing is important not only for blood transfusions, but also for identifying women who are at risk for infants with **hemolytic disease of the newborn** (HDN). HDN, also called erythroblastosis fetalis, occurs when an Rh⁻ woman is pregnant with an Rh⁺ fetus (see Fig. 6–9).

*Flashpoint*
Type O⁻ blood is found in about 7% and Type AB⁺ blood is found in about 4% of the population worldwide.

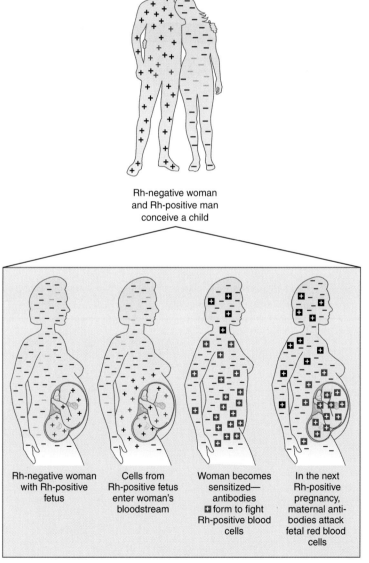

Rh-negative woman and Rh-positive man conceive a child

| Rh-negative woman with Rh-positive fetus | Cells from Rh-positive fetus enter woman's bloodstream | Woman becomes sensitized— antibodies ⊞ form to fight Rh-positive blood cells | In the next Rh-positive pregnancy, maternal anti-bodies attack fetal red blood cells |

**FIGURE 6–9  Rh⁻ mother and Rh⁺ father resulting in hemolytic disease of the newborn.**

Because fetal blood and maternal blood mix, the woman comes in contact with a foreign blood type. Antibodies to Rh do not occur naturally in the body the way antibodies for antigen A and antigen B do. The woman has to make antibodies against the Rh antigen. The first child is usually not affected because not enough antibodies have been made against the Rh antigen. The next Rh⁺ fetus would have its RBCs attacked, however, by the anti-Rh antibodies produced by the mother. The lack of blood cells can cause the fetus to be stillborn or to die shortly after birth. An infant born with this condition has been commonly called a "blue baby" because of *cyanosis*, or blueness, of the skin caused by the lack of RBCs.

Because the fetus cannot be blood-typed (even after birth it is difficult to type blood until about 6 months of age), precautions must be taken to prevent HDN. A woman who is Rh⁻ is given an injection of a substance called RhoGAM just before and just after birth. This prevents her body from producing antibodies if the fetus has Rh⁺ blood.

For other diseases and disorders of the blood, see Table 6–2.

## TABLE 6–2
### PATHOLOGY TERMS FOR BLOOD

| | |
|---|---|
| Anemia | General name for several different conditions; can be a result of decrease in number of RBCs, deficiency in hemoglobin, or lack of iron in the diet |
| Hemophilia | Inherited disorder; defect is found on the X chromosome, so it is more common in males; patient is missing certain clotting proteins so the blood does not clot |
| Hematoma | Collection of blood under the skin; also called a bruise |
| Leukemia | Cancer of WBCs; caused by abnormality in the myeloid cells so that WBCs cannot function normally; treatment includes chemotherapy, radiation, or bone marrow transplant |
| Sickle cell anemia | Inherited from both parents; RBCs are sickle-shaped or C-shaped and cannot deliver oxygen efficiently; more common in those of African ancestry |
| Thalassemia | Inherited disorder from both parents; type of anemia where RBCs are smaller than normal and have reduced amount of hemoglobin; more common in those of Mediterranean ancestry |
| Thrombocytopenia | Decrease in number of platelets because of virus, trauma, blood transfusion, medications, or unknown cause |

# Practice Exercises

## Multiple Choice

1. Formed elements are _____.
   a. cells
   b. plasma
   c. salts
   d. hormones

2. Erythropoietin is responsible for the production of _____.
   a. platelets
   b. white blood cells
   c. red blood cells
   d. megakaryocytes

3. The smallest formed elements are _____.
   a. red blood cells
   b. white blood cells
   c. granulocytes
   d. platelets

4. The clumping of incompatible RBCs is _____.
   a. clotting
   b. hemostasis
   c. agglutination
   d. hemopoiesis

5. All of the following are granulocytes except _____.
   a. neutrophil
   b. basophil
   c. lymphocyte
   d. eosinophil

## True or False

1. True    False      White blood cells aid in fighting infection.

2. True    False      Megakaryocytes break and release platelets.

3. True    False      Someone with Type A blood can receive Type O blood.

4. True    False      Red blood cells have a nucleus.

5. True    False      The Rh antigen is also called D.

## Fill in the Blank

1. Someone with AB⁺ blood is called the universal _____.

2. _____ is the main component of plasma.

3. Red blood cells are also called _____.

4. An Rh⁺ fetus born to an Rh⁻ mother can develop a disease called

   _____.

5. _____ or _____ is the production of

   blood cells.

6. White blood cells are classified as _____ and

   _____.

7. The stem cells for blood production are called _____.

8. Someone with O⁻ blood is called the universal _____.

9. A cell surface marker is also called a(n) _____.

10. Blood cells are made in the _____ marrow.

## Short Answer

1. **Describe the components of whole blood.**

2. **Discuss the differences between each white blood cell.**

3.  **Describe how hemolytic disease of the newborn occurs.**

## Labeling

*Fill in the blanks with the appropriate anatomical terms.*

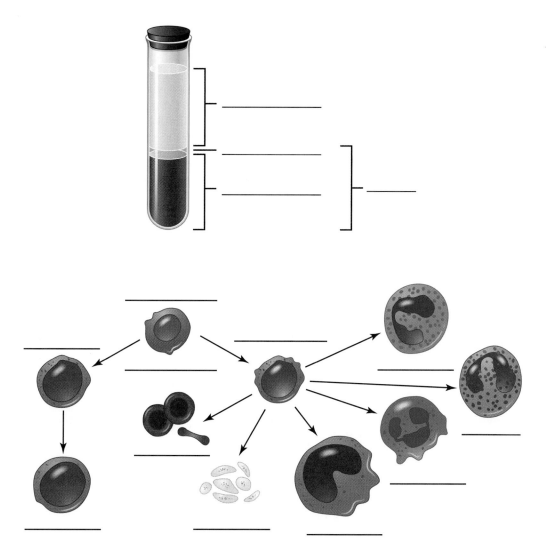

# 7

# THE LYMPHATIC SYSTEM

*Flashpoint*

The lymphatic system maintains homeostasis in the body by providing immunity.

The lymphatic system, sometimes called the immune system, is a collection of vessels, tissues, and organs. This system is a functional system, rather than a true organ system, because the parts of the lymphatic system are not totally dependent on each other. The vessels, tissues, and organs are scattered throughout the body, and the vessels can work independently of the organs. The organs do not need the vessels to perform their duties. The functions of the lymphatic system are fluid transportation and removal, protection, and resistance to disease.

Fluid transportation is done by the lymphatic vessels. These vessels collect *interstitial fluid* or cellular fluid from the tissues. Interstitial fluid is actually blood plasma that brought nutrients to the tissues, but did not get fully reabsorbed into the blood capillaries. Collection of this fluid prevents edema, or swelling, by draining the excess fluid from the tissues.

Protection of the body is provided by the lymph nodes and the lymphocytes. The lymph nodes are structures that filter and remove foreign substances and microorganisms from the fluid in the lymph vessels. The lymphocytes are cells that travel the body to detect and destroy foreign substances. Collectively, the structures of the lymphatic system protect the body by creating either a non-specific or a specific defensive response to foreign substances. The protection of the body against foreign substances is called *immunity*.

This chapter discusses the structure of the vessels, tissues, and organs of the lymphatic system. The defenses of the body and the different types of immunity and antibodies and their role in immunity are described.

## Structures of the Lymphatic System

All the vessels, tissues, and organs of the lymphatic system have a role in protecting the body from outside threats and aiding in resistance to disease. The lymph vessels and lymph nodes filter microorganisms from the blood. The other tissues and organs are the bone marrow, thymus gland, spleen, tonsils, and Peyer patches. Each structure aids in protection by playing a role in creating and maintaining the body's defense systems.

### Lymph Vessels and Nodes

The *lymphatic vessels* begin as lymph capillaries in the tissues of the body. The capillaries enlarge to vessels as they leave the tissues. Lymph vessels are located beside the blood vessels and are found in a similar path throughout the body. These vessels are responsible for draining excess interstitial fluid from the tissues to prevent edema. When this fluid enters the lymphatic vessels, it is called *lymph*. Carried along in the lymph are large proteins that cannot enter the capillaries, and viruses, bacteria, and cell debris. The lymph vessels do not have a pump the way the blood vessels have the heart to push the lymph along, so movement of lymph is done by constriction and relaxation of the surrounding tissues. To cleanse the lymph and to prevent microorganisms from using the lymphatic vessels as transportation around the body, the lymph gets filtered through the lymph nodes.

*Lymph nodes* are a mass of tissue that can range in size from a small pea to a marble and are found clustered around the lymph vessels (see Fig. 7–1). They are most prevalent in the neck, armpits, umbilicus, and groin. The lymph nodes act as filters for any foreign substances, tumor cells, or microorganisms in the lymph fluid.

*Flashpoint*

There are 500 to 700 lymph nodes in the body.

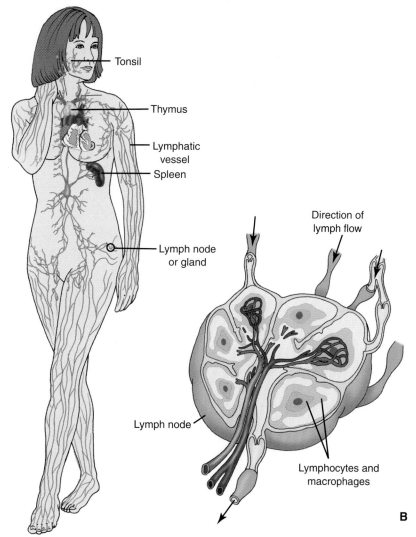

FIGURE 7-1  *(A)* Locations of lymph nodes in the body. *(B)* Individual node. (From Eagle S. *Medical Terminology in a Flash!* Philadelphia, PA: FA Davis; 2006:71.)

When lymph enters a node, it flows into sinuses within the node. Cells in the sinuses detect and destroy foreign substances. ***Macrophages*** are cells that engulf foreign substances and cell debris. ***Lymphocytes*** are cells that are also present in the nodes to assist the macrophages in detecting foreign substances. When the lymph flows out of the node, it should be cleansed of debris and microorganisms. The filtered lymph returns to the bloodstream free of any potentially harmful substances.

## Tissues and Organs

The tissues and organs of the lymphatic system are divided into primary and secondary lymphoid tissues. ***Primary lymphoid tissues*** produce the cells responsible for immunity. These tissues are the bone marrow and thymus gland. ***Secondary lymphoid tissues*** aid the immune system, and they are the spleen, tonsils, and Peyer's patches (see Fig. 7–2).

### Primary Lymphoid Tissues

The primary lymphoid tissues are the bone marrow and the thymus gland. These tissues produce and control the cells of the lymphatic system. The ***bone marrow***—specifically, the red bone marrow—makes all blood cells. The red bone marrow is found in the ends of long bones and in flat bones such as the ribs and sternum.

One type of cell produced in the bone marrow is the leukocytes, or white blood cells (WBCs). The WBCs are responsible for protecting the body from harmful substances. There are five different types of leukocytes. The smallest are the lymphocytes, and they control the immune system. There are two types of lymphocytes: B and T. The B lymphocytes, or B cells, are created in and

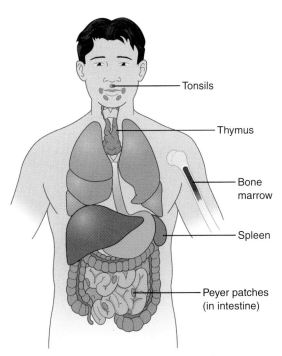

FIGURE 7–2  **Lymphoid tissues and organs.**

mature in the bone marrow before being released into the bloodstream. The T lymphocytes, or T cells, leave the bone marrow when produced and travel to another primary lymphoid organ called the thymus gland.

The **thymus gland** is located in the chest inferior to the thyroid gland and anterior to the heart. This gland stores the immature lymphocytes and produces hormones that cause the T lymphocytes to mature before being released into the bloodstream. T lymphocytes aid in creating immunity, so the thymus gland is most active during childhood. As children come in contact with new substances, more cells are created in response. The immune system of a child is fully functioning by about 2 years of age. As we age and come in contact with fewer new substances, the thymus decreases in size and use.

### Secondary Lymphoid Tissues

The secondary lymphoid tissues are the spleen, tonsils, and Peyer patches. Secondary lymphoid tissues do not produce or control cells. These tissues and organs aid the lymphocytes produced by the primary lymphoid tissues.

The **spleen** is located in the upper left quadrant of the abdominal cavity. It sits just behind the lower rib cage, and it curves around the anterior portion of the stomach. The spleen has many varied functions. It is responsible for filtering blood and cleansing it of bacteria, viruses, and other debris. The spleen also breaks down old red blood cells and transports the by-products to the liver. Platelets, which are clotting cells, are stored in the spleen. This organ also acts as a blood reservoir so that if the body loses blood for any reason, the spleen can release its extra supply to maintain blood volume. In a fetus, the spleen produces red blood cells because the bone marrow is not functional until after birth.

The spleen is not considered a vital organ, so it may be removed. Its functions can be compensated for by other organs. For example, the liver can remove and break down old red blood cells if the spleen is unavailable.

The **tonsils** are small masses of tissue located in the soft palate at the entrance to the throat. Tonsils trap and destroy any foreign substances entering through the mouth. Because tonsils filter so much bacteria, they can become clogged. When this happens, the tonsils swell and become red and sore. This condition is called **tonsillitis**. Someone who has repeated swelling and redness of the tonsils has them removed. Removal of the tonsils does not interfere with the body's ability to protect itself because of the other lymph nodes near the mouth.

**Peyer patches** are masses of tissue that resemble tonsils and are located in the small intestines. These tissues capture and destroy harmful microorganisms that enter into the intestines. These microorganisms can enter from the stomach after being swallowed or from the large intestine, which opens to the external environment.

## Body Defenses

The body is under constant attack from microorganisms, such as viruses, bacteria, and mold. The cells of our bodies can also change so that they become a threat to our health. There are many ways the body defends itself against these foreign and domestic invaders. These defenses are known collectively as immunity, and they can be nonspecific or specific (see Table 7–1).

| TABLE 7-1 | | |
|---|---|---|
| **TYPES OF BODY DEFENSES** | | |
| Nonspecific Defenses | | Specific Defenses |
| First Line of Defense | Second Line of Defense | Third Line of Defense |
| • Skin<br>• Mucous membrane<br>• Natural flora | • Physiological changes<br>• Phagocytes<br>• Natural killer cells<br>• Inflammatory response | • Lymphocytes<br>• Antibodies |

## Nonspecific Immunity

First the body protects itself by **nonspecific immunity**, which is also called natural or innate immunity. These are the defenses humans are born with. Nonspecific immunity has four types of defense: anatomical, physiological, phagocytic, and inflammatory.

An *anatomical defense* or barrier is the first line of defense against harmful substances. These barriers meet the external environment and include the skin and mucous membranes. The body's greatest natural defense is the skin. As long as it remains intact, it keeps substances out. Sweat and oil produced by the glands of the skin also help to prevent microorganisms from entering the body.

The mucous membranes are another natural defense; they trap particles and microorganisms that enter through the nose and mouth. Trapped particles are swallowed with the mucus and are destroyed in the stomach.

Additionally, the body has **natural flora**, also called normal flora, which are the microorganisms that normally live both on the surface of the body and within the body to aid in resistance to foreign substances. Some examples of natural flora are the bacteria *Escherichia coli* in the large intestine, *Lactobacillus acidophilus* in the digestive tract, and the yeast *Candida albicans* in the mouth and female reproductive tract.

*Physiological defenses* are defenses that change the chemical makeup of the body. This can include changes in temperature and pH. When a microorganism has made its way inside the body, leukocytes detect them. Leukocytes then produce chemicals to signal the brain to increase body temperature. This occurs because most microorganisms prefer to live at normal body temperature, which is 98.6°F. Any increase in temperature causes death of the microorganism.

The pH of the stomach is low, so it is highly acidic. If a harmful substance enters the mouth or nose, it is swallowed along with food, drink, or mucus. The acids in the stomach aid in digestion. Very few microorganisms can live in a highly acidic environment, so they are destroyed.

Another innate defense mechanism is the *phagocytic response. Phagocytes* (cell eaters) are cells that patrol the body looking for debris and microorganisms. When a phagocyte finds a foreign particle, it wraps its cell membrane around the particle and brings it inside the cell. The particle is destroyed by the enzymes within the phagocyte.

Another protective cell is the natural killer (NK) cell. NK cells are specialized WBCs that constantly patrol the body. NK cells look for virus-infected cells and tumor cells. These cells do not kill by digestion of the foreign antigen. When the NK cell finds a foreign particle, it produces a chemical that breaks apart the cell membrane of the foreign substance.

The inflammatory response is a natural defense to any substance that has penetrated the skin. If the skin is damaged, the body must react to stop any natural flora that should remain outside or any foreign substance from entering. The reaction of the body to damage or trauma is the ***inflammatory response***. There are four cardinal signs or major symptoms of the inflammatory response: redness, heat, swelling, and pain.

In the first step in the inflammatory response, the damaged tissue leaks interstitial fluid causing swelling. Then blood capillaries constrict causing redness, also called ***erythema***, and heat. The damage to the skin causes pain receptors to be activated. Finally, WBCs and phagocytes swarm to the area to fight any invaders that may have entered.

Sometimes an area may be too small to feel the heat of the blood and increased cell activity, but even a paper cut shows the swelling, pain, and redness of the an inflammatory response (see Fig. 7–3). The purpose of this response is to protect the body from invading microorganisms and provide means for the body to clean the debris from the area. Inflammation also begins the healing process.

## Specific Immunity

The other type of immunity that protects the body is **specific immunity**, also called acquired immunity. This type of immunity is not innate. The body must first come in contact with a foreign substance before defenses can be made against it. Specific immunity is responsible for:

- ***Recognition***, which is the ability of the immune system to recognize differences in antigens and to know which antigens belong to the body and which ones do not.
- ***Specificity***, which gives the immune system the ability to direct a response to a specific antigen while leaving similar antigens alone.
- ***Memory***, which is the ability of the immune system to remember an antigen after the initial exposure to it.

Specific immunity is controlled by the type of leukocytes called lymphocytes. The two types of lymphocytes are B lymphocytes and T lymphocytes, also referred to as B cells and T cells. These cells are responsible for two different types of specific immunity: humoral and cell-mediated.

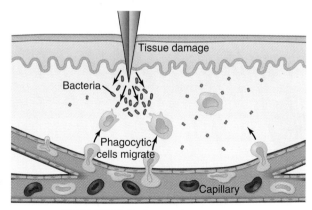

FIGURE 7–3  Inflammatory response.

## Humoral Immunity

B lymphocytes control **humoral immunity**. *B lymphocytes*, similar to all blood cells, are created in the red bone marrow. After B lymphocytes mature, they circulate freely in the blood searching for foreign antigens, such as bacteria and mold. An **antigen** is the identification of a cell located on the cell's surface. When a B lymphocyte comes in contact with a foreign antigen, it changes into a cell called a plasma cell. Plasma cells have the ability to make **antibodies** (see Fig. 7–4). These are the weapons the immune system uses to defend the body. Antibodies are created so that they can fit onto the antigen of the foreign substance, similar to a jigsaw puzzle piece. When an antibody binds to the antigen it was made for,

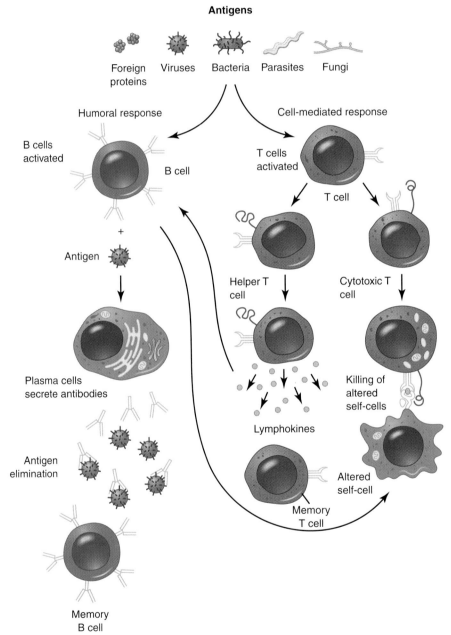

FIGURE 7–4 **Summary of humoral immunity.**

the antigen is destroyed. Another cell called a memory B cell is also made after the antibodies. Memory B cells remember the foreign antigen so that if it is found again, the antibodies already created can be used to fight the antigen.

Antibodies are also called ***immunoglobulins***. There are five classes of immunoglobulins: IgG, IgM, IgA, IgD, and IgE (see Table 7–2). Each antibody has a different size, shape, and function in the immune response.

* ***IgM*** is the antibody made first when the body comes in contact with a foreign antigen.
* ***IgG*** is the second antibody made when a foreign antigen is detected. It is the most abundant in the body because it stays for weeks or even years after contact with a foreign antigen. IgG also has the ability to cross the placenta and give immunity to the fetus.
* ***IgA*** is found in the mucous membranes and body secretions such as breast milk, saliva, and tears.
* ***IgE*** increases in response to a parasitic infection and when the body is having an allergic reaction to a substance.
* ***IgD*** is found only in very small amounts in the body. The function of this antibody is unknown at this time.

Figure 7–5 shows the structures of the different immunoglobulins.

## Cell-mediated Immunity

***T lymphocytes*** are responsible for **cell-mediated immunity**. These lymphocytes are made in the bone marrow, but leave soon after and travel to the thymus gland where they mature. After maturity, T lymphocytes leave the thymus and circulate throughout the body in the blood. These lymphocytes are responsible for recognizing the body's own antigens as being different from foreign antigens. This is called recognizing self from nonself. T lymphocytes also have the ability to identify body cells that have been changed by a virus or mutation.

T lymphocytes do not make antibodies. If a changed cell is detected, T lymphocytes need assistance from B lymphocytes to make antibodies and destroy the antigen.

There are five types of T lymphocytes, and each has a role in recognizing self from nonself (see Fig. 7–6). Because T lymphocytes do not make antibodies, if an unusual cell is found, they cannot destroy it. The T lymphocyte holds onto the foreign cell or changed body cell. Helper T cells interact with B lymphocytes by sending out chemicals called lymphokines to signal the B lymphocytes that a foreign antigen has been found. B lymphocytes come to the captured cell and

### TABLE 7–2

### IMMUNOGLOBULINS

| Type | Function |
| --- | --- |
| IgG | Second responder to foreign antigens and can cross the placenta to give immunity to the fetus |
| IgM | First responder to foreign antigens |
| IgD | Found in small amounts; role is unknown |
| IgE | Responsible for allergic reactions and increases in response to parasitic infections |
| IgA | Found in body secretions such as breast milk, saliva, and tears |

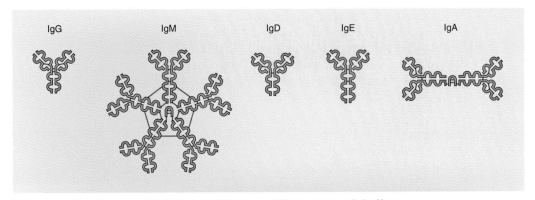

IgG          IgM          IgD          IgE          IgA

FIGURE 7–5  Structures of the immunoglobulins.

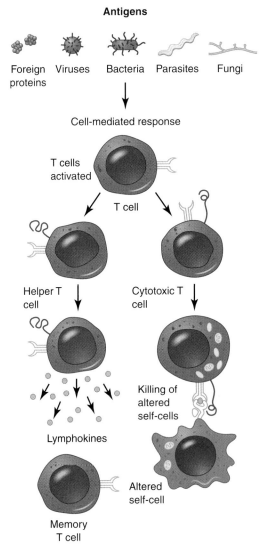

**Antigens**

Foreign    Viruses    Bacteria    Parasites    Fungi
proteins

Cell-mediated response

T cells
activated

T cell

Helper T
cell

Cytotoxic T
cell

Lymphokines

Killing of
altered
self-cells

Altered
self-cell

Memory
T cell

FIGURE 7–6  Summary of cell-mediated immunity.

create antibodies to destroy it. Suppressor T cells stop the immune response when enough antibodies have been produced. Cytotoxic T cells find and destroy cancer cells and foreign tissue grafts. The final type of T lymphocytes are memory T cells. Similar to memory B cells, these cells remember each new antigen in case it returns.

*Flashpoint*

Major histocompatibility complex (MHC) is the medical term for the ability of T lymphocytes to recognize self from nonself.

# Immune Response

The body's reaction to a foreign antigen is called an immune response. There are two types of responses: primary and secondary. Both responses are controlled by B lymphocytes as part of humoral immunity.

## Primary Response

When the body first comes in contact with a foreign antigen, it triggers the **primary response**. The B lymphocyte must recognize that the antigen is foreign to start the immune response. When this happens, B lymphocytes change to plasma cells and begin to make antibodies. It can take several days for enough antibodies to be made by the plasma cells to fight the antigen. IgM is the first antibody to be made. This antibody lasts only a few days after it is produced, so another antibody then takes over. The second antibody is IgG. This antibody is made several days after IgM, but continues to fight the foreign antigen after IgM cells die. IgG lasts several weeks to several months after the initial contact. Memory B cells are made after the initial response, and they remain in the bloodstream to recognize the foreign antigen if it returns.

## Second Response

If the foreign antigen returns, the memory B cells recognize it and organize a faster response. In the **secondary response**, antibodies have already been made for this antigen, so the IgM reacts within 1 or 2 days. IgM remains active for a few weeks fighting the returning antigen. IgG also reacts faster in the second response and is ready within 3 or 4 days. IgM and IgG not only react sooner, but also in greater numbers than with the primary response. IgG can remain in the blood for months or years after the second response. Figure 7–7 shows the difference in the primary and secondary immune response.

*Flashpoint*

The anamnestic response, or the memory response, is the principle behind immunizations. A dead or changed antigen can be injected into the body, and memory cells can be created without a patient being exposed to a possible pathogen. The memory cells then respond should the actual antigen be encountered.

# Types of Immunity

There are two types of immunity: passive and active (see Fig. 7–8). In **passive immunity**, the body does not have to detect a foreign antigen and make an antibody before immunity can occur. One type of passive immunity is called *naturally passive immunity*. This type of immunity occurs when IgG passes

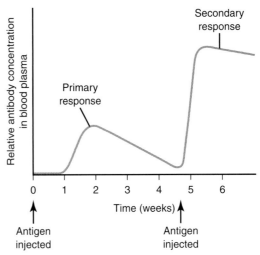

FIGURE 7-7  **Primary and secondary immune responses.**

the placenta and gives immunity to the fetus and when IgA passes from breast milk to the newborn. The immune system of the newborn is not functional, and so it uses the antibodies of the mother for protection.

*Artificially passive immunity* is obtained by injection of immunoglobulins. Someone born lacking lymphocytes or who has a suppressed immune system may receive donated immunoglobulins. Because the cells only live a short time, the injections have to be repeated.

*Active immunity* is when the body must find and recognize a foreign antigen and then create an antibody against it. *Naturally active immunity* comes when antibodies and memory cells are made by the body in response to a foreign antigen.

*Artificially active immunity* comes from the injection of a vaccine containing a dead or altered pathogen. The pathogen does not make the recipient ill, but because the antigen is foreign, the body makes antibodies and memory cells.

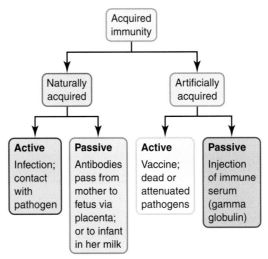

FIGURE 7-8  **Types of immunity.**

# Organ and Tissue Rejection

Organ and tissue transplantation is done for people whose organs have failed because of disease or trauma. Almost any organ or tissue can be transplanted; the kidney and heart are the most commonly transplanted organs. Because the tissues of the implanted organ contain foreign antigens, T lymphocytes in the recipient's body recognize it as foreign. T lymphocytes begin an immune response to attack the tissue.

There are four types of grafts that can be performed: autografts, isografts, allografts, and xenografts.

- ***Autograft*** is moving tissue from one area to another in the same person. This transplant may be for someone with a third-degree burn who would need skin removed from an undamaged area of the body to replace the burned skin. Because the tissue antigens are the recipient's own, there is no rejection.
- ***Isografts*** are grafts done between identical twins. Tissue types are the same in identical twins, so antigens on the tissues are identical. The chances of rejection are slight.
- ***Allografts*** are grafts taken from an unrelated person. Because the tissues have different antigens, this type of graft causes an immune response and death of the donated tissue. Recipients of an allograft take immunosuppressant drugs for the rest of their lives to protect the donated tissue.
- ***Xenografts*** are grafts from a different animal species. Pig heart valves are commonly used to replace human ones. These grafts also result in an immune response so that as with an allograft the recipient needs immunosuppressant drugs.

Even with the use of immunosuppressant drugs, the immune system cannot be totally turned off. The body slowly attacks the tissue without creating an active immune response. Over time, the tissue fails, and rejection occurs. Donated organs have an average of 8 to 12 years before failure, depending on the organ. Kidneys tend to function the longest of the donated organs. When rejection of the donated organ occurs, the recipient needs another transplant.

# Autoimmune Disease

Sometimes a T lymphocyte loses the ability to recognize the body's own antigens. T lymphocytes then attack those cells. This failure to recognize self from nonself is called an ***autoimmune disease***. Any cell or tissue of the body can come under attack if T lymphocytes mistakenly identify it as foreign. In ***rheumatoid arthritis***, T lymphocytes no longer recognize the antigens found on the joints and begin an attack. The result is pain, swelling, and deformity of the joints of the hands and feet (see Fig. 7–9). Another common autoimmune disease is ***systemic lupus erythematosus*** (SLE). T lymphocytes create a generalized response against the body's connective tissue. Patients with SLE have joint pain, weakness, skin rashes, and fatigue.

There are no cures for any autoimmune disease; only treatment of the symptoms can be offered. Because the effects of autoimmune disease can differ from patient to patient and even differ in the same patient, treatment is variable.

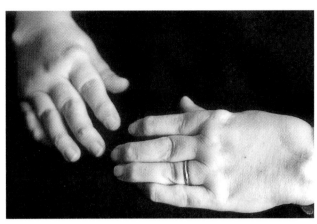

**FIGURE 7–9  Rheumatoid arthritis.** (From Williams, Hopper. *Understanding Medical Surgical Nursing.* 3rd ed. Philadelphia, PA: FA Davis; 2007:1021.)

Commonly, hormone treatments, anti-inflammatory drugs, corticosteroids, and antimalarial drugs are used.

Why autoimmune diseases occur is unknown. Women tend to have a higher incidence of autoimmune diseases. For this reason, a genetic link is suspected, although environmental factors, such as parasitic infections and certain drugs, have also been linked to autoimmune disease.

## Allergy

*Flashpoint*

More than 50 million Americans have allergies. Allergies are the sixth most common chronic condition in the United States.

An **allergy**, also called hypersensitivity, is an overreaction of the immune system to a substance that is perceived as a threat, but actually is harmless. When an allergic reaction to a substance occurs, the body increases the immunoglobulin IgE and increases the number of WBCs called eosinophils. IgE and eosinophils stimulate the release of histamine. The histamine causes vessels to become leaky, resulting in a runny nose, watery eyes, and itching reddened skin. In the respiratory system, an allergic response can cause constriction of the muscles of the lungs, restricting air flow.

Most allergies can be controlled by taking a medication called antihistamines to block the production of histamine and prevent symptoms. Any substance can cause an allergic reaction; pollen, animal dander or hair, dust, certain fabrics, and foods such as peanuts and strawberries are common allergens (see Box 7–1).

*Flashpoint*

An estimated 150 people die each year from anaphylaxis because of food allergies. Peanuts cause the most severe food allergies. Penicillin is the most common cause of drug allergies. An estimated 400 patients die each year from penicillin-induced anaphylaxis.

Some allergens can cause an extreme systemic response called anaphylactic shock. This response occurs when the allergen enters the bloodstream and causes rapid response. **Anaphylaxis** includes constriction of the airway and dilation of the blood vessels resulting in rapid collapse of circulation and a sudden decrease in blood pressure. Death can occur quickly, often within minutes. To reverse these effects, epinephrine is injected to open the vessels and increase heart rate and blood flow. Common allergens that cause anaphylaxis are venoms from spiders and bees, medicines such as penicillin, and food such as peanuts or shellfish.

See Table 7–3 for more information about diseases and disorders of the immune system.

## Box 7–1 Allergies

About 20% of Americans are afflicted with the same disorder—allergies. An allergy is an overreaction of the immune system to an antigen that is not truly harmful. In response to the antigen, the lymphatic system produces an inflammatory response that increases the level of white blood cells, IgE, and histamine.

Almost anything can trigger an allergic reaction. Common allergens are pollen, animal hair, peanuts, shellfish, bee venom, milk, latex, penicillin, and dust. People who have allergies have a long-term sensitivity, but a one-time allergic reaction can occur from any new substance the body comes in contact with, such as a perfume, soap, medication, or vaccine.

The most common symptoms of an allergy are itching, sneezing, red and watery eyes, runny nose, and cough. More severe reactions are rash, hives, and breathing problems. The most severe form of allergic reaction is anaphylaxis.

Anaphylaxis is a life-threatening condition in which the airway constricts, and blood pressure decreases. People with anaphylactic reactions can go into a coma and die.

Treatment for allergies includes antihistamines, oral and topical steroids, and immunotherapy that results in desensitivity to the allergen.

## TABLE 7–3
### PATHOLOGY TERMS FOR LYMPHATIC SYSTEM

| | |
|---|---|
| Acquired immunodeficiency syndrome (AIDS) | Destruction of the cell-mediated immune system by HIV; patients die of opportunistic infections |
| Allergy | Overresponse of immune system to antigens that would be harmless to the body; common reactions are sneezing, watery eyes, itching skin, or hives |
| Hodgkin disease | Tumor of the lymph nodes, spleen, or bone marrow; occurs more often in people 15-35 years old; 90% survival with treatment |
| Human immunodeficiency virus (HIV) | Virus that targets and destroys T lymphocytes causing AIDS; it is found in semen, blood, vaginal secretions, and breast milk; HIV is spread through contact with contaminated body fluids that have entered the body through a needle stick, broken skin, or sexual intercourse |
| Lymphedema | Accumulation of lymph fluid in the tissues where the lymph nodes have been surgically removed |
| Multiple sclerosis | Autoimmune disease that targets the myelin sheath surrounding motor neurons; this slow degeneration causes various symptoms, such as loss of balance and coordination, muscle weakness and pain, visual problems, and speech impairment |
| Non-Hodgkin lymphoma | General name for >30 types of lymphoma that are a malignancy of the B or T lymphocytes that have spread to the body tissues; occurs more often in people 40-70 years old; depending on the type, there is a 70% survival rate after the first year of diagnosis |
| Rheumatoid arthritis | Autoimmune disease where immune system attacks the joints mostly of the hands and feet causing deformities of the joints; occurs more often in women 40-60 years old |
| Severe combined immunodeficiency virus (SCID) | Deficiency of cell-mediated and humoral immunities. Death occurs within first few months of life from infection |
| Systemic lupus erythematosus (SLE) | Autoimmune disease where immune system attacks the connective tissue, usually affecting women of childbearing age |

## Practice Exercises

### Multiple Choice

1. B lymphocytes are responsible for _____ immunity.

   a.  cell-mediated

   b.  humoral

   c.  innate

   d.  natural

2. The function of _____ is unknown.

   a.  IgA

   b.  IgG

   c.  IgM

   d.  IgD

3. When a B lymphocyte comes in contact with a foreign substance, it changes to a _____.

   a.  T cell

   b.  platelet

   c.  plasma cell

   d.  leukocyte

4. _____ is found in body secretions such as saliva and breast milk.

   a.  IgA

   b.  IgG

   c.  IgM

   d.  IgD

5. Peyer's patches are located in the _____.

   a.  throat

   b.  spleen

   c.  small intestine

   d.  thymus

### True or False

1. True    False     B lymphocytes mature in the thyroid gland.

2. True    False     All immunoglobulins can cross the placenta.

3. True  False    Cell-mediated immunity is responsible for recognizing self from nonself.

4. True  False    Lymph nodes filter blood.

5. True  False    T lymphocytes are made in the bone marrow.

6. True  False    Tonsils are found in the small intestines.

7. True  False    An autoimmune disease occurs because of a malfunction of B lymphocytes.

8. True  False    Cell-mediated immunity is a nonspecific immunity.

9. True  False    IgD is found in secretions.

10. True  False    Natural immunity is the type of immunity you are born with.

## Fill in the Blank

1. The immunoglobulin that is the first responder is _____.

2. The _____ lymphocytes control cell-mediated immunity.

3. _____ is the first natural defense against foreign antigens.

4. _____ protect against substances entering through the mouth.

5. Pain, redness, heat, and swelling are part of the _____ response.

6. B lymphocytes are responsible for _____ immunity.

7. Antibodies are made by _____ cells.

8. The spleen filters foreign material from the _____.

9. Excess tissue fluid is called _____ when it enters the lymphatic vessels.

10. The _____ response is faster and stronger when a foreign antigen returns.

## Short Answer

1. **List and describe the different immunoglobulins.**

2. **List and describe the different T lymphocytes.**

## Labeling

*Fill in the blanks with the appropriate anatomical terms.*

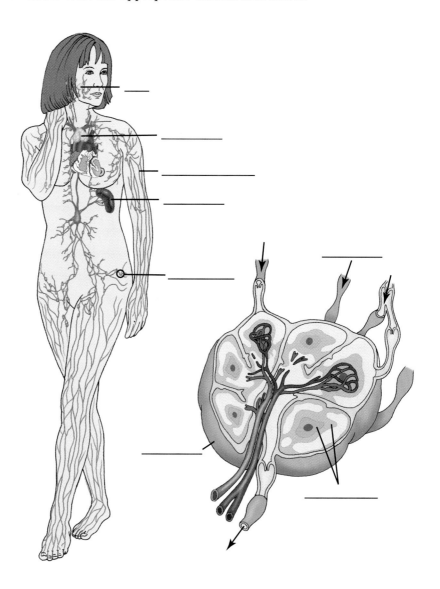

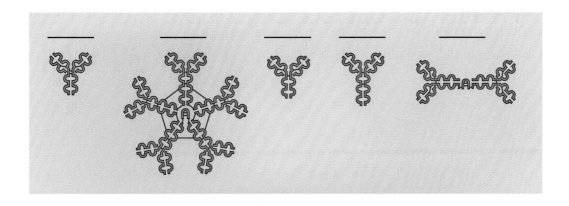

# THE CARDIOVASCULAR SYSTEM

The cardiovascular system includes the heart, blood, and all the vessels that circulate blood throughout the body. The vessels alone are often referred to as the circulatory system or vascular system. Transportation is the main function of the cardiovascular system.

This system uses the heart as a pump to keep blood moving through the blood vessels to provide oxygen, glucose, minerals, hormones, and other nutrients to the cells. The same blood vessels take wastes away from the cells so that they can be removed from the body.

This chapter outlines the structures of the heart and other vessels of the cardiovascular system. How the heart conducts electricity and the difference between adult and fetal circulation are also discussed.

## Structures of the Cardiovascular System

The cardiovascular system consists of the heart and vessels, called veins and arteries, that transport blood throughout the body. The heart is responsible for keeping the blood flowing through the vessels. Blood is carried from the cells and tissues to the heart by the veins, and the arteries carry blood away from the heart back to the tissues and cells.

### Heart

The main organ of the cardiovascular system is the heart. It is the muscular pump that forces blood though the vessels to keep it circulating around the body. The heart is located in the thoracic cavity above the diaphragm and between the lungs in a space called the *mediastinum* (see Fig. 8–1). The heart is protected anteriorly by the sternum and ribs.

The heart is oval in shape and about the size of a man's fist. It sits at a slight diagonal in the chest. The flattened top of the heart is the *base*. It points toward the right shoulder and is the site of attachment for the large vessels. The pointed bottom of the heart is the *apex*, which sits on the diaphragm and is angled toward the left side.

The heart is composed of three layers of tissue. The outer layer is the *epicardium* (on the heart), and it is a protective layer of connective tissue. The middle layer is the *myocardium* (heart muscle). This tissue is thought of as the actual heart because it is a thick layer of cardiac muscle tissue that

## Flashpoint

The cardiovascular system maintains homeostasis in the body by providing oxygen to the cells and removing carbon dioxide.

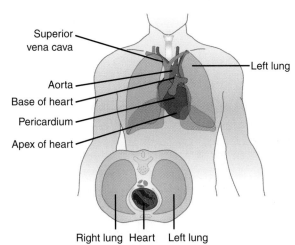

Superior vena cava

Left lung

Aorta

Base of heart

Pericardium

Apex of heart

Right lung  Heart  Left lung

**FIGURE 8–1  The heart in the mediastinum.**

Key Terms—cont'd

tricuspid valve

vein

vena cava

ventricles

causes the pumping action that circulates blood. The inside of the heart is called the **endocardium** (within the heart), and it is made of smooth epithelial tissue.

On the outside of the heart is a serous membrane that surrounds it like a sac. This membrane is called the **pericardium** (around the heart). Between the pericardium and the epicardium is serous fluid called pericardial fluid that acts as lubricant to prevent friction between the heart and the membrane when the heart beats.

The adult heart beats an average of 60 to 80 times a minute, which equates to more than 100,000 times a day. In a fetus, the heartbeat is more rapid pumping at about 120 to 160 bpm. After birth, the heart rate slows to about 130 bpm, and it continues to slow with age. At age 4, the average heart rate is 100 bpm. During adolescence, the heart rate settles into the normal adult rate.

## Chambers and Valves

There are four chambers within the heart (see Fig. 8–2). The interior of the heart chambers are lined with epithelial tissue called the endocardium. The heart is divided into a right and left side. A thick wall of tissue called the **septum** (wall) separates the two sides. Each side of the heart contains an upper and a lower chamber. The two upper chambers of both sides are the **atria**, and the two lower chambers of both sides are the **ventricles**.

There are four valves in the heart, and they are named for the shape or number of cusps or flaps in each valve. These valves act as doorways between the chambers. Between the right atrium and right ventricle is the **tricuspid** (three flaps) **valve**. The valve between the left atrium and left ventricle is the **bicuspid** (two flaps) **valve** or mitral valve. These valves open with each contraction of the heart allowing blood into the ventricles and close when the ventricles are full. Because blood flow is one way, these valves also prevent blood from flowing back into the atria.

At the entrance to the pulmonary artery is the **pulmonary semilunar** (half moon) **valve**, which keeps blood in the pulmonary artery and prevents it from flowing backward into the right ventricle. The **aortic semilunar** (half moon) **valve** is located at the entrance of the aorta. This valve keeps blood in the aorta and prevents backflow into the left ventricle. Similar to the other valves, the semilunar valves open with each contraction and close when the vessels are full.

Flashpoint

The "lub-dub" sound heard when listening to the heart is made by the heart valves opening and closing.

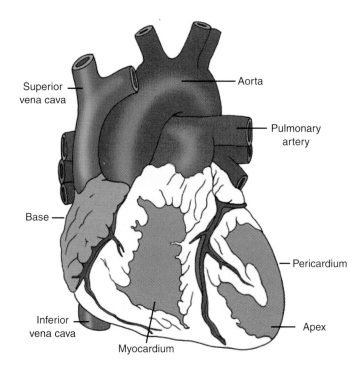

**A**

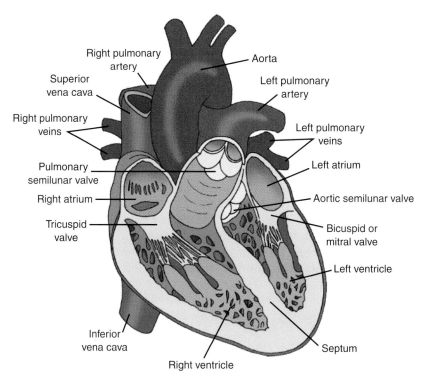

**B**

FIGURE 8–2 *(A)* **Exterior view of the heart.** *(B)* **Interior view of the heart.** (Adapted from Eagle S. *Medical Terminology in a Flash!* Philadelphia, PA: FA Davis; 2006:81 *(A)*, 69 *(B)*.)

## Blood Vessels

The vessels of the cardiovascular system are the means of transportation for the blood. It is estimated that if all the vessels in an adult body were put in a line they would reach a length close to 100,000 miles. The two main types of vessels are veins and arteries. Veins and arteries travel the same route and are like opposite lanes of traffic on a highway (see Fig. 8–3). Both vessels are used for transportation, but they differ in structure and in the composition of the blood they carry.

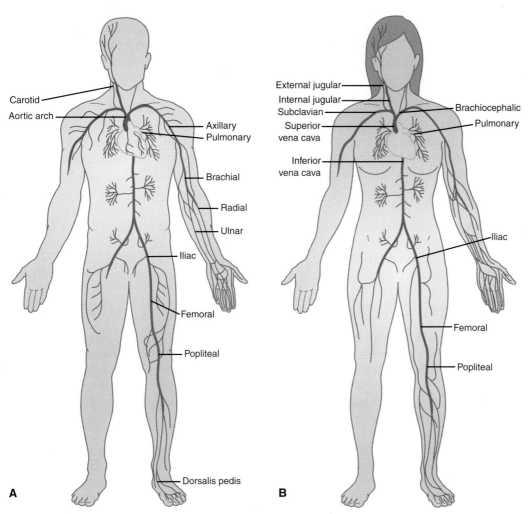

**FIGURE 8–3** *(A)* **Arteries of the body.** *(B)* **Veins of the body.**

### Veins

**Veins** are thin vessels that are part of the blood transportation system throughout the body. The purpose of veins is to carry deoxygenated blood from the tissues back to the heart. Most veins have flaplike valves called venous valves that prevent blood from flowing backward because of the pull of gravity. Blood in the veins is full of the waste product carbon dioxide, which is left over after oxygen is converted to energy by the cells. Veins are shown as blue because that color is associated with a lack of oxygen. When blood is drawn from a vein, it is actually a deep red or even brownish color depending on the amount of carbon dioxide in the blood.

Veins begin in the tissues as capillaries. Capillaries are the smallest vessels and can be seen only with a microscope. They are so small that an estimated 40 billion of them are found in an adult body. These vessels are only one cell thick and are able to let oxygen and carbon dioxide, which are both gases, diffuse or flow freely through the vessel wall. Many capillaries form a mesh called a capillary bed. These capillary beds are found throughout the tissues of the body. Here oxygen is able to be picked up by the cells at the same time carbon dioxide is being pushed out. When carbon dioxide diffuses into a capillary, it has to find its way to the lungs to leave the body. To get to the lungs, the blood must first go to the heart. Veins are responsible for getting that deoxygenated blood to the heart.

After leaving the tissues, the capillaries enlarge to vessels called venules (little veins); these vessels enlarge to bigger vessels called veins. The superior and inferior **venae cava** are the largest veins in the body. The superior vena cava drains blood from the upper body, and the inferior vena cava drains blood from the lower body. Both venae cava connect to the heart at the right atrium.

*Flashpoint*

Capillaries are so thin that it takes 10 of them to equal the width of a single hair.

## Arteries

**Arteries** are thicker and stronger than veins and carry oxygenated blood. These vessels are also part of the blood transportation system. Arteries are shown as red because they appear red owing to the oxygen being carried by the red blood cells. Blood taken from an artery is bright red and, if compared, is clearly different from the darker venous blood.

The purpose of arteries is to take the oxygenated blood that comes into the heart from the lungs to the tissues of the body. The largest artery of the body is the **aorta**. This artery is attached to the left ventricle and is responsible for bringing oxygenated blood into the body from the heart. From the aorta blood flows into smaller vessels called arteries. Arteries act like small pumps that push blood into smaller vessels called arterioles (little arteries), which lead to the capillary beds. Here oxygen is exchanged with carbon dioxide, and blood begins its journey back to the heart.

Because arteries are small pumps, they have a pulse and beat in time with the heart. If an artery is severed, blood spurts from the opening because of the force created by the heartbeat. How often the heart beats is called the heart rate, and the force of the beat is the blood pressure. Heart rate and blood pressure can be measured by palpating or pressing the different arteries (see Fig. 8–4). Heart rate is most often taken with the radial artery on the thumb side of the wrist. Blood pressure is commonly measured using the brachial artery on the little finger side of the upper arm. When doing cardiopulmonary resuscitation (CPR), the carotid artery in the neck is preferred for counting heart rate.

## Pulmonary Vessels

There is an exception to the rule of veins carrying deoxygenated blood and arteries carrying oxygenated blood. This exception is found in the pulmonary veins and pulmonary artery that attach the heart to the lungs.

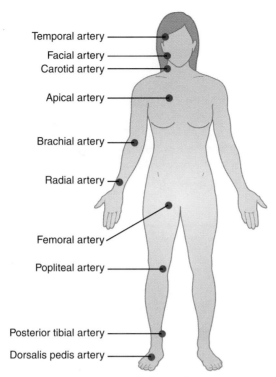

Temporal artery

Facial artery

Carotid artery

Apical artery

Brachial artery

Radial artery

Femoral artery

Popliteal artery

Posterior tibial artery

Dorsalis pedis artery

**FIGURE 8–4  Pulse points.**

The ***pulmonary veins*** bring oxygenated, not deoxygenated, blood back from the lungs to the left atrium. The ***pulmonary artery*** carries deoxygenated instead of oxygenated blood from the right ventricle to the lungs. These vessels differ from the other vessels of the body because of structure. Arteries are thick and elastic, whereas veins are thinner and weaker. The pulmonary artery could not be a vein because the strong contraction of the heart forcing the blood upward would burst a thin vessel. Likewise, the pulmonary veins are not arteries because the oxygenated blood flows by gravity from the lungs to the heart, so it does not need to be a thick-walled vessel.

## Cardiac Vessels

The heart provides blood to the tissues so that they receive the nutrients needed to live. These same nutrients are needed by the tissues of the heart. The heart has its own veins, called coronary veins, to remove wastes and arteries to supply it with nutrients (see Fig. 8–5). The arteries are as follows:

- ***Left anterior descending*** (LAD) feeds the anterior wall of the left ventricle.
- ***Circumflex*** feeds the lateral wall of the left ventricle.
- ***Right coronary artery*** (RCA) feeds the right ventricle and the inferior wall of the left ventricle.

In contrast to the other tissues that receive their blood supply when the heart contracts, the heart has its blood supply pushed out during the contraction. When the heart relaxes, blood flows into the heart tissues. If blood flow to the tissues is decreased for any reason, it is called ***ischemia***. Lack of blood flow means a lack of oxygen to the heart and other tissues, which can result in death of the tissue. Tissue death is called an ***infarction***. If too much tissue death occurs in the heart, a ***myocardial infarction*** or heart attack occurs (see Box 8–1).

*(text continues on page 140)*

Flashpoint

Coronary artery disease (CAD) occurs when atheroma, or plaque, builds up on the walls of the arteries. Plaque is formed from cholesterol, fat, cells, and calcium, and slows the flow of blood through the heart.

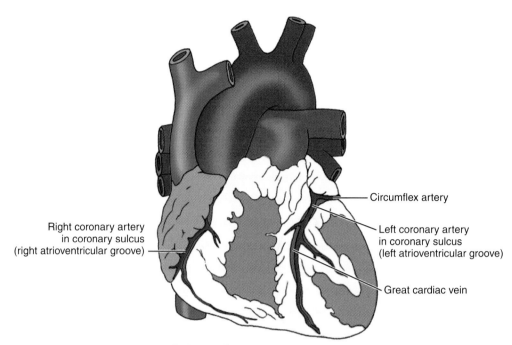

**FIGURE 8-5  Coronary arteries.** (Adapted from Eagle S. *Medical Terminology in a Flash!* Philadelphia, PA: FA Davis; 2006:81.)

## Box 8-1 Myocardial Infarction

Heart disease is a leading cause of death for men and women in the United States. Almost 14 million people have a history of heart disease.

Poor diet and lack of exercise lead to high blood pressure and high cholesterol, both of which lead to heart disease. Fatty deposits and cholesterol called plaque can collect in the arteries and build up over time. This is atherosclerosis. As the plaque builds, it eventually closes the artery, stopping all blood flow. Calcium can also deposit in the arteries making them rigid and thickened. This is arteriosclerosis, and this hardening of the arteries has the same results as atherosclerosis.

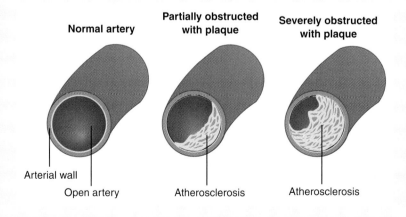

## Box 8-1 Myocardial Infarction—cont'd

Lack of blood flow is ischemia. As blood flow decreases, so does the oxygen to the tissues. Because of the lack of oxygen, the heart slowly suffocates. As the heart struggles for more blood and oxygen, it causes chest pain called angina. Angina is a warning that the heart is not getting what it needs to survive. Eventually, ischemia leads to death of the tissues, called an infarction. If too much blood flow ceases to the heart, a myocardial infarction or heart attack occurs.

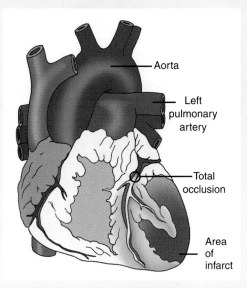

Myocardial infarction. (From Eagle S. *Medical Terminology in a Flash!* Philadelphia, PA: FA Davis; 2006:81.)

Symptoms of a heart attack are crushing chest pain, pain radiating down the left arm or into the left jaw, shortness of breath, nausea, indigestion, pallor (paleness of the skin), diaphoresis (cold sweat), and feeling as though one may die. These are the classic symptoms of a heart attack. Someone may have all or just a few of these symptoms. Women tend not to have the crushing pain in the chest and arm. Usually women have nausea and difficulty breathing that gets worse when they lie down. Because these are not the symptoms that one thinks of for a heart attack, many women do not realize they are having a heart attack. They may also be ignored by medical personnel because they are not showing classic symptoms.

If symptoms of a heart attack occur, the person must seek emergency aid immediately. If conscious, the person may take an aspirin and chew it so that it reaches the bloodstream faster. Aspirin is an anticoagulant (blood thinner) and helps the blood move around a clogged area. If someone has had angina in the past, he or she may have nitroglycerin tablets. These pills open the blood vessels to allow more blood flow. Nitroglycerin pills are placed sublingually (under the tongue) and absorb into the mucous membranes. These pills should be stored only in a glass container and with a metal lid. They should not be touched with the bare hands. If administering nitroglycerin, one should wear gloves to prevent the nitroglycerin from penetrating the skin. If gloves are unavailable, one should shake a pill into the cap and let the patient place the pill under the tongue. If the patient is unable to do this for himself or herself, one should not try to place anything in the patient's mouth.

An ECG is performed to see if there is any damage to the heart. The patient may be placed on a telemetry monitor. The clogged artery needs to be opened. This is done by

*Continued*

## Box 8-1 Myocardial Infarction—cont'd

heart catheterization, which consists of taking small tubes and passing them through the arteries around the heart. Angioplasty, which is the repair of the artery, is done, and the clot is enlarged or removed. A piece of wire may be left at the site of the blockage to strengthen the wall; this is called a stent.

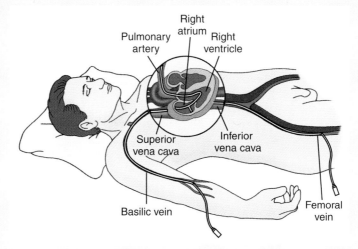

Cardiac catheterization. (From Eagle S. *Medical Terminology in a Flash!* Philadelphia, PA: FA Davis; 2006:83.)

After cardiac surgery, patients continue to take anticoagulants and cholesterol-lowering medicines most likely for the rest of their lives. The patient also is advised to exercise and maintain a healthy diet.

If the myocardial infarction is too severe, death occurs. A heart attack occurs about every 20 seconds, and 50% of individuals having a heart attack die within 1 hour of the attack without medical treatment. With medical treatment, 8% to 10% still die from the irreversible damage to the heart.

# Types of Circulation

There are two types of circulation in the adult body: systemic and pulmonary. *Systemic circulation* occurs when blood travels throughout the whole body. The pathway of systemic circulation is a continuous flow from the heart to the tissues to the cells and then back through the tissues to the heart.

If the process is started at the capillary beds, systemic circulation begins when blood exchanges oxygen for carbon dioxide. Blood leaves the tissues by venules, which become veins. All veins connect to either the superior vena cava or the inferior vena cava. The vena cavae connect to the right atrium. Blood then flows through the tricuspid valve into the right ventricle. From the right ventricle, blood flows through the pulmonary semilunar valve into the trunk of the pulmonary artery. At this point, blood flows into either the right or the left branch of the pulmonary artery and enters the lungs. In the lungs, carbon dioxide is exhaled, and oxygen is inhaled. After becoming oxygenated, blood leaves the lungs by the pulmonary veins, which connect to the left atrium.

The blood flow from the heart to the lungs and back to the heart is called *pulmonary circulation*. When in the left atrium, systemic circulation continues, and blood flows through the bicuspid valve into the left ventricle. From the left ventricle, blood passes the aortic semilunar valve and enters the aorta. Oxygenated blood leaves the aorta and enters the arteries and then the smaller arterioles. Finally, blood enters the capillary beds where oxygen and carbon dioxide are again exchanged, and the process begins again.

Circulation is a continuous loop, and blood is always present in all the chambers of the heart and all the vessels. Blood leaves both atria at the same time, and both ventricles fill at the same time. Blood moves into the pulmonary artery and the aorta at the same time without a gap in the flow. Figure 8–6 is a flowchart of all the steps in systemic circulation and pulmonary circulation.

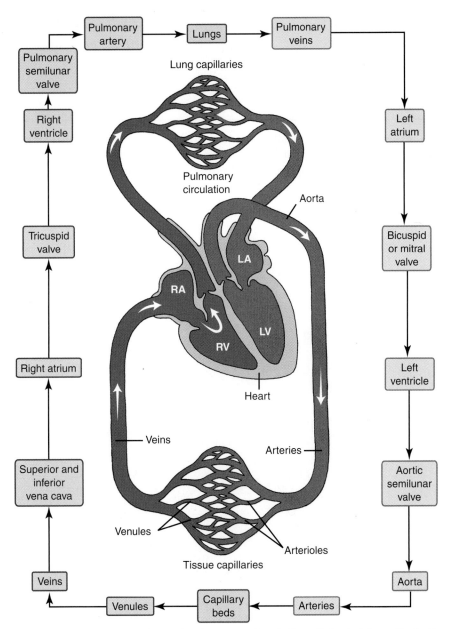

**FIGURE 8–6 Flowchart of systemic and pulmonary circulation.** (Adapted from Eagle S. *Medical Terminology in a Flash!* Philadelphia, PA: FA Davis, 2006:70.)

# Characteristics of Cardiac Cells

Cardiac cells have four characteristics: contractility, conductivity, excitability, and automaticity. Similar to skeletal muscle, cardiac muscle has the ability to contract or shorten. Cardiac cells like skeletal tissue cells also have the ability to become excitable or stimulated by an electrical impulse. These cells can conduct that stimulus to another cell. Cardiac cells differ from skeletal muscle cells because they are automatic. Cardiac muscle has an internal mechanism that can stimulate its own contraction without needing electrical stimulus from the nervous system.

Each cardiac cell is also automatic because it can beat on its own. If a heart was divided into individual cells, each one would beat or pulse. These cardiac cells also have the unusual ability to synchronize. If the individual cells from different hearts are placed side by side, they slow down or speed up until all of them have the same beat.

## Intrinsic Conduction System

Electrical impulses are responsible for the workings of all cells. In the heart, the electrical impulses control contraction by a built-in conduction system called the *intrinsic conduction system*, also called the cardiac conduction system (see Fig. 8–7).

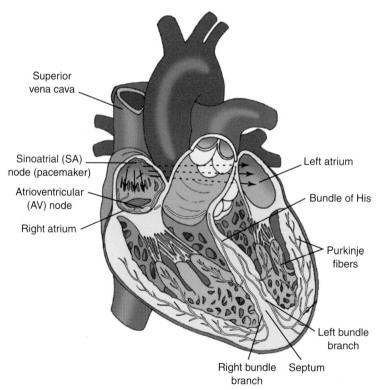

FIGURE 8–7  Intrinsic conduction system of the heart.

Conduction begins with the ***sinoatrial (SA) node***, also called the sinus node, located in the upper right atrium near the attachment of the superior vena cava. It is a small specialized piece of tissue that acts like a trigger. This node controls heart rate, so it is referred to as the "natural pacemaker." When blood flows into the right atrium, the SA node sends an electrical impulse to the left atrium and the ***atrioventricular (AV) node***. This node is located near the bottom of the right atrium at the entrance to the right ventricle. The signal from the SA node causes a small contraction that pushes blood from both atria into the ventricles. As blood flows past the AV node, it sends the impulse into the septum.

Located in the septum is a mass of conductive tissue connected to the AV node called the ***bundle of His***. The bundle of His has a right and left bundle branch that attaches to the right and left sides of the heart. When the bundle branches receive the stimulus from the AV node, they conduct the impulse to the ***Purkinje fibers***. These fibers surround the ventricles like a net. When the impulse gets to the Purkinje fibers, they are stimulated and pull upward causing a strong contraction in the ventricles. This strong contraction pushes blood against gravity into the aorta and the pulmonary artery. This strong contraction, called ***systole***, is measured when taking blood pressure and is also felt when counting heart rate. After stimulation, the cells of the Purkinje fibers must return to a resting state. The resting or relaxation phase of the heart is called ***diastole***.

*Flashpoint*

Any change in cardiac conduction causes an abnormal heartbeat, also called an arrhythmia.

### Action Potential

The electrical impulse that triggers the cardiac conduction system is controlled by the action potential, which is the process of a cell going from a relaxed to an active state. For a cell to be active, changes need to occur on the inside of the cell. The cell goes through three changes or phases: polarization, depolarization, and repolarization (see Fig. 8–8).

The exterior environment of a cell is positively charged because it contains more sodium ions ($Na^+$). The inside of a cell is negatively charged and contains more potassium ions ($K^+$). In this state, the cell is ***polarized*** or at rest. When an electrical current stimulates the cell, the state of the cell changes so that $K^+$ flows out and $Na^+$ flows in. The inside of the cell becomes positively charged, and it is now stimulated and capable of producing an action. The cell is called ***depolarized***. When a cell is stimulated, it cannot be stimulated again until it goes back to a resting state. The $Na^+$ inside the cell must flow out, and the $K^+$ must flow back

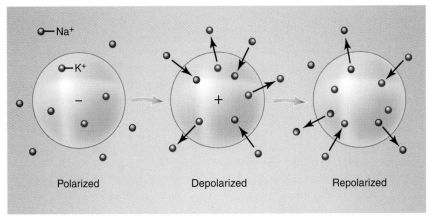

FIGURE 8–8 Action potential.

in, changing the inside again to a negative charge and the outside to a positive charge. The act of the cell changing back to resting is called *repolarization*.

The electrical activity of the action potential can be seen with a device called an electrocardiogram (ECG or EKG). It converts the electrical charge into a graph (see Fig. 8–9). This graph can be used to detect any abnormalities or changes in the rhythm of the heart called arrhythmias or dysrhythmias (see Box 8–2).

## Cardiac Cycle

The intrinsic conduction system is responsible for the ability of the heart to beat. Each heartbeat has two phases: contraction and relaxation. One contraction and one relaxation are considered to be one *cardiac cycle*, or one heartbeat. The contraction phase of the heart is systole, and the relaxation phase is diastole. The average number of cardiac cycles is 60 to 80 bpm. Each cardiac cycle lasts about 0.8 second.

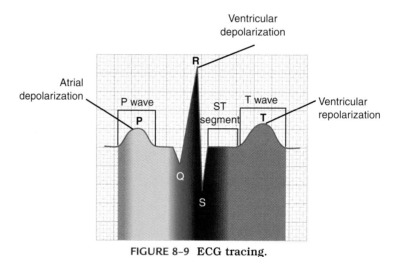

**FIGURE 8–9  ECG tracing.**

## Box 8–2 Heart Monitors

Cardiovascular disease (CVD) is one of the leading causes of death in the United States. Individuals who are at risk of CVD or individuals who have known cardiac disease can be monitored.

The ECG is the most common device for predicting people at risk for heart disease and detecting any damage caused by a myocardial infarction. The ECG was invented in 1903 by Wilhelm Einthoven; this device converts the electrical activity of the intrinsic conduction system into a graph. Any abnormality in the rhythm of the heart shows on the graph.

A patient who needs constant monitoring can be attached to a continuous ECG called a telemetry monitor. Medical personnel view the recordings as they are made and look for any abnormalities in the pattern.

Another device is a Holter monitor, which is a small box attached to the patient's waist for 24 to 48 hours to record the heart during normal activity. After the monitoring period, the device is returned to the physician's office where the recording is analyzed.

Changes in heart rate depend on such factors as age, gender, weight, emotions, and medications. As the heart rate changes, so does the strength of the beat, which changes the blood pressure. The rate of the heartbeat also changes how much blood is being pumped through the body. Increased rate results in blood moving faster than normal.

Determining how much blood is pumped out of the heart in 1 minute is the *cardiac output*. Cardiac output can be determined by the heart rate multiplied by the stroke volume. Stroke volume is the amount of blood pumped out of the ventricles with each contraction. For example, a heart rate of 75 bpm and a stroke volume of 70 mL per beat would equal 5250 mL per minute. Resting cardiac output is about 5 liters, or 5000 mL per minute, which is the average total amount of blood in the adult body.

### Regulation of the Cardiac Cycle

Heart rate and respiration are controlled by the autonomic nervous system, which controls all involuntary body functions. The autonomic nervous system is further divided into the sympathetic and parasympathetic nervous systems. When startled, afraid, or if a quick response is needed, the sympathetic nervous system produces a chemical called epinephrine, or adrenaline, to speed up the cardiovascular system.

The *vagus nerve* is one of the cranial nerves and is connected to several organs and tissues, including the SA node of the heart, the lungs, and the stomach. In response to epinephrine, the vagus nerve increases heart rate and blood pressure, causes the pupils to dilate, and slows digestion. The vagus nerve also quickens respiration to keep up with the increased oxygen demand. The sympathetic response is only short-term and is slowed down by the parasympathetic nervous system. This part of the autonomic nervous system produces a chemical called acetylcholine, which counteracts epinephrine. Acetylcholine is also responsible for controlling the heart rate and respiration when the body is at rest.

It is possible for the heart rate to be slowed too much, such as with breath-holding or straining, such as during a bowel movement or childbirth. Straining causes the vagus nerve to be stimulated, and acetylcholine is produced to counter the vagus nerve. If the acetylcholine slows the heart too much in response, syncope or fainting occurs. Usually when the straining has ceased, the acetylcholine stops being produced, and normal heartbeat and respiration return. In an extreme case of **syncope**, the heart may stop, and medical intervention is needed to start the heart again.

## Blood Pressure

The volume of blood in the body remains constant unless there is blood loss secondary to trauma. The blood pressure and heart rate are variable. When blood pressure and heart rate change, the blood may move faster or slower through the circulatory system, but the volume remains the same.

Blood pressure is the measurement of the systolic and diastolic pressure. A normal systolic range is 90 to 120 mm Hg (millimeters of mercury), and a normal diastolic range is 60 to 80 mm Hg. A rate greater than 140/90 mm Hg is called **hypertension**, and a rate less than 90/60 mm Hg is **hypotension**.

*Flashpoint*
In the United States, one out of three adults has hypertension. This condition can lead to coronary artery disease, stroke, kidney failure, and heart failure.

Many physiological factors affect blood pressure:

- *Heart rate*: If heart rate increases, so does the force of the blood, so blood pressure increases. If the heart rate is extremely rapid, the ventricles do not fill completely before the blood is forced out. This lessens the volume of blood leaving the heart and lowers the blood pressure.
- *Peripheral resistance*: The arteries and veins always maintain a slight constriction to maintain the force of the vessels. If the vessels become smaller than normal, the blood pressure increases because the same volume of blood is trying to move through a smaller space, so more force is needed to push the blood through.
- *Elasticity of the arteries*: The arteries are small pumps, and when blood enters them, the vessels stretch to accommodate the blood. This elasticity also absorbs some of the force of the blood. If the artery is unable to stretch because of a condition called **arteriosclerosis**, or hardening of the arteries, the pressure increases to push the same amount of blood into the artery.
- *Loss of blood*: If blood is lost because of trauma, a decrease in blood pressure occurs. The body compensates by increasing heart rate and vasoconstriction, which is constriction of the blood vessels to create more pressure. After severe blood loss, the body may be unable to compensate, and blood pressure and blood flow decrease. The result is a decrease in blood flow to the brain. A long-term decrease in blood flow to the brain may result in brain damage.
- *Blood viscosity*: Viscosity, or thickness, of the blood depends on the amount of blood cells and proteins present. If the red blood cells are increased, such as with the condition **polycythemia** (increased ROCs), the blood is more difficult to move through the cells. This increases the pressure to keep it moving. If the red blood cells are decreased, as with some types of **anemia**, blood loses viscosity, and blood pressure decreases. To prevent the decrease in pressure, the vessels constrict to maintain pressure.
- *Hormones*: Several hormones change blood pressure. Epinephrine produced during the sympathetic response increases blood pressure and heart rate by causing vasoconstriction. Antidiuretic hormone (ADH) secreted by the pituitary gland in the brain increases when the body becomes dehydrated. ADH causes the kidneys to absorb more water to increase hydration and stop the decrease of blood pressure. Aldosterone is secreted from the adrenal glands. This hormone also prevents pressure loss secondary to dehydration. It stimulates the reabsorption of sodium by the kidneys. Water flows with the sodium and goes back to the vessels to maintain blood pressure.

## Fetal Circulation

In a fetus, the heart of the mother is needed to bring blood carrying oxygen and nutrients into the developing body. The fetus cannot inspire oxygen, so fetal circulation bypasses the lungs. Because the lungs are not used in the fetus, they are the last organ to develop, usually around the sixth month of gestation.

The fetus is attached to the mother's cardiovascular system by the umbilical cord. Veins and arteries pass from the body of the mother through the placenta, which is attached to the uterine wall through the umbilical cord.

The fetal heart has a different structure than that of the adult heart (see Fig. 8–10). Blood entering the right atrium gets pushed through an opening called the *foramen ovale* at the same time blood enters the right ventricle. Blood enters the left atrium through the foramen ovale, bypassing the lungs and giving the left side the oxygen it needs. Blood from the right atrium, which in an adult would go the lungs, gets routed to the *ductus arteriosus*, which connects the pulmonary artery to the aorta. Oxygen is received from maternal blood, and carbon dioxide collected from fetal cells enters back into the maternal blood for disposal. After birth, the foramen ovale closes, and blood begins its normal path through the heart.

See Table 8–1 for common diseases and disorders of the cardiovascular system.

Flashpoint
The heart is the first organ to develop in a fetus and starts beating about 22 days after conception.

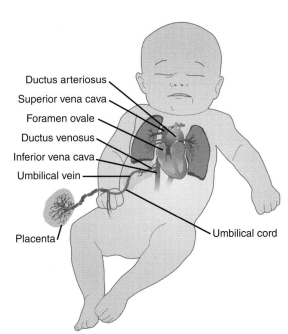

Ductus arteriosus
Superior vena cava
Foramen ovale
Ductus venosus
Inferior vena cava
Umbilical vein
Placenta
Umbilical cord

FIGURE 8–10  **Blood flow in the fetal heart.**

### TABLE 8–1
### PATHOLOGY TERMS FOR THE CARDIOVASCULAR SYSTEM

| | |
|---|---|
| Angina pectoris | Chest pain and discomfort that occurs when the heart is not receiving enough blood usually because of arteriosclerosis or atherosclerosis |
| Arrhythmia | Abnormal or irregular heartbeat, may be called dysrhythmias |
| Arteriosclerosis | Thickening of the arteries that slows blood flow |
| Atherosclerosis | Plaque called atheroma builds up in the arteries and slows blood flow |
| Bradycardia | Slow heartbeat <60 bpm |
| Coronary artery disease | Generalized term for decreased blood supply to the heart caused by either arteriosclerosis or atherosclerosis |
| Fibrillation | Type of arrhythmia where the heart is in spasm so that it is unable to pump blood |
| Flutter | Lesser form of fibrillation |
| Hypertension | Elevated blood pressure >140/90 mm Hg |
| Myocardial infarction | Death of the heart muscle because of loss of blood flow; heart attack |
| Phlebitis | Inflammation of the veins |
| Tachycardia | Rapid heartbeat >100 bpm |
| Varicose veins | Swollen and twisted veins most often formed in the legs because of defective valves in the veins; occurs often in elderly people |

## Practice Exercises

## Multiple Choice

1. The _____ nerve controls heart rate, blood pressure, and respiration.
   a. cardiac
   b. vagus
   c. renal
   d. carotid

2. The foramen ovale is part of the _____ circulation.
   a. pulmonary
   b. cardiac
   c. fetal
   d. systemic

3. The ability of a cardiac cell to work independently is _____.

    a. contractility

    b. conductivity

    c. excitability

    d. automaticity

4. One systole and one diastole are equal to one _____ cycle.

    a. cardiac

    b. heart

    c. pulmonary

    d. blood

5. The superior and inferior venae cava are the largest _____ in the body.

    a. arteries

    b. veins

    c. capillaries

    d. venules

## True or False

1. True    False    The bicuspid valve and mitral valve are the same.

2. True    False    Veins carry deoxygenated blood.

3. True    False    Systemic circulation goes from the heart to the lungs and back to the heart.

4. True    False    The aorta is the largest vein in the body.

5. True    False    The right side of the heart holds deoxygenated blood.

## Fill in the Blank

1. The _____ divides the heart into right and left halves.

2. The right atrium and right ventricle are separated by the _____ valve.

3. _____ is the relaxation phase of the heart.

4. Arteries have a _____, which can be felt.

5. Blood carries the waste product _____ back to the lungs.

6. The heart is located in the thoracic cavity in a space called the

   _____.

7. The _____ is the smooth epithelial tissue lining the heart.

8. The opening in the fetal heat that bypasses the lungs is the

   _____.

9. The largest veins in the body are the _____ and the

   _____.

10. The pacemaker of the heart is the _____.

## Short Answer

1. **Describe the path of blood flow through the body.**

2. **Name and describe the three layers of the heart.**

## Labeling

*Fill in the blanks with the appropriate anatomical terms.*

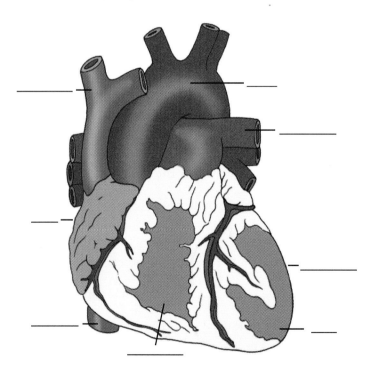

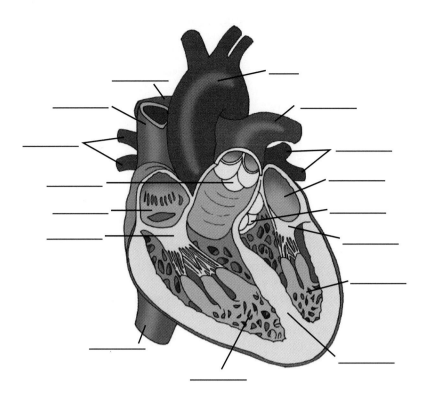

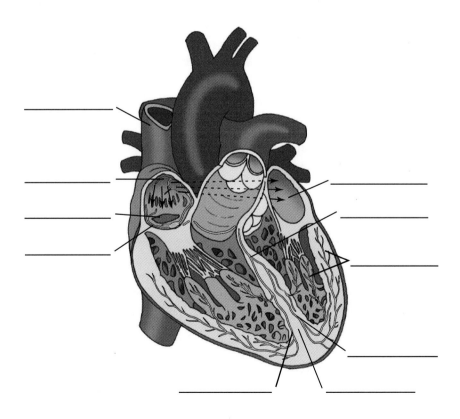

# THE RESPIRATORY SYSTEM

## Key Terms

expiration

expiratory reserve volume

external respiration

inspiration

inspiratory reserve volume

internal respiration

pulmonary ventilation

residual volume

respiratory cycle

surfactant

total capacity

tidal volume

vital capacity

The respiratory system provides the body with a means of gas exchange. It brings oxygen into the body and allows carbon dioxide to leave. Oxygen is vital for life. It is needed by all of the body's cells to live and make energy, or ATP. The body can live 3 or 4 days with no water and a few weeks without food, but can survive only a few minutes without oxygen.

The respiratory system and cardiovascular system are linked. Oxygen comes into the body by the respiratory system and is transported throughout the body by the cardiovascular system. Carbon dioxide is the waste product of making ATP and is transported back to the lungs where the respiratory system expels it from the body.

This chapter discusses the structures of the respiratory system. It also discusses the different types of respiration, how breathing occurs, and variations in respiration.

## Structures of the Respiratory System

The respiratory system moves air into and out of the lungs. This movement of air allows oxygen into the body and lets carbon dioxide leave. This action is called gas exchange. The organs and structures of the respiratory system include the nose, pharynx, larynx, trachea, and lungs (see Fig. 9–1). Gas exchange occurs in the lungs and the capillaries. The other structures of the respiratory system are a passageway for air to enter and leave the lungs.

### Nose

The nose is the only external structure of the respiratory system. Air enters the nose through the *nares*, or nostrils. Just within the nostrils are hairs that trap debris. Inside the nose is the nasal cavity, and it is divided by bone and cartilage called the nasal septum (wall). Within the cavity are small, scroll-like bones called the conchae. These bones create more space in the cavity. The nose is separated from the oral cavity by bone called the hard palate and by tissue called the soft palate.

The nasal cavity is lined with a mucous membrane called the respiratory mucosa. This membrane not only secretes mucus, but also has a network of capillaries just under the surface. Heat from the passing blood warms the air as it enters the nose. The mucus moistens the air and traps any particles or debris entering with the air. The cells of the mucosa are ciliated, and the cilia

*Flashpoint*

The respiratory system maintains homeostasis in the body by maintaining oxygen and carbon dioxide levels.

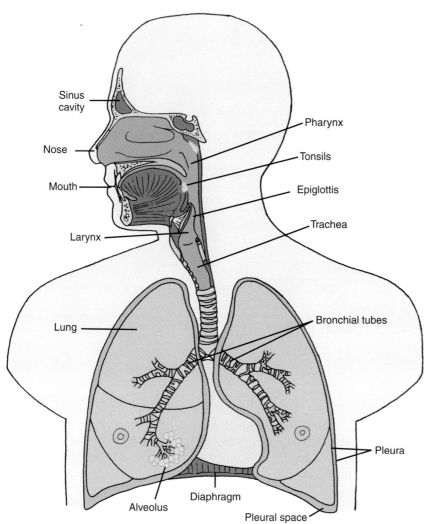

**FIGURE 9–1 Respiratory system.** (From Eagle S. *Medical Terminology in a Flash!* Philadelphia, PA: FA Davis; 2006:98.)

move the mucus into the throat, where it is swallowed and all the trapped debris is broken down by the stomach acids.

Also within the nose are the olfactory receptors located within the mucosa of the upper nasal cavity. These receptors detect odor. Above the nasal cavity are the nasal sinuses located within the skull bones. The sinuses are lined with ciliated epithelium, and the mucus they produce drains into the nasal cavities.

## Pharynx

From the nasal cavity, air enters the ***pharynx***, or throat (see Fig. 9–2). Air can also enter through the mouth or oral cavity and travel to the pharynx.

The pharynx is a muscular tube about 5 inches long and is a passageway for food and air. Because food passes through these structures, the pharynx and oral cavity are also part of the digestive system.

The pharynx is divided into three sections: the ***nasopharynx*** behind the nasal cavity, the ***oropharynx*** behind the oral cavity, and the ***laryngopharynx***

Flashpoint
The vertical groove on the upper lip located between the nose and mouth is called the philtrum.

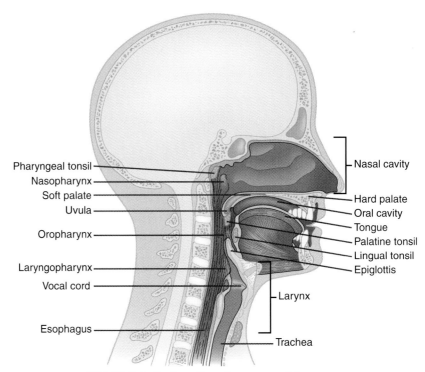

FIGURE 9-2 Oral cavity, pharynx, and larynx.

located in the neck. Located just behind the oral cavity is a punching bag–shaped piece of tissue that hangs from the soft palate. This is the *uvula*, and it blocks the entrance to the nasopharynx when swallowing to prevent food or liquid from entering the nasal cavity.

Also behind the oral cavity at the entrance to the oropharynx are the *tonsils*. These structures are clusters of lymphatic tissue that help prevent microorganisms from entering the pharynx. Tonsils are located at several places in the pharynx. Tonsils in the nasopharynx are called pharyngeal tonsils or adenoids. Palatine tonsils are located at the end of the soft palate, and lingual tonsils are located at the base of the tongue.

The third section of the pharynx is the laryngopharynx, and it is continuous with the trachea. Air and food both travel to this point. Food gets routed from the pharynx to another tube called the esophagus. Air continues to the larynx.

## Larynx

Air travels from the pharynx into the *larynx*, or voice box. The larynx not only is a passage for air, but it also gives us the ability to form speech. The larynx is a tube formed from eight rings of rigid hyaline cartilage called thyroid cartilage. It is located posterior to the pharynx and anterior to the esophagus. Within the larynx are two folds of tissue called *vocal cords* (see Fig. 9–3). As air passes these folds of tissue, they vibrate, and sounds are produced. Men have thicker cartilage in the larynx than women. This area is commonly called the Adam's apple, and the thicker cartilage causes deepening of the voice.

At the entrance to the larynx is a flap of cartilage called the *epiglottis*. This structure closes off the larynx when swallowing so that food and liquid continue

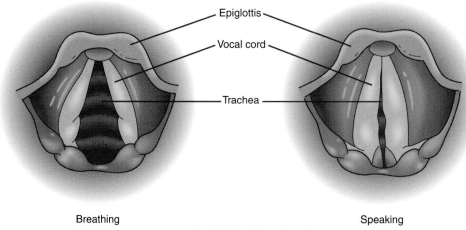

Breathing                              Speaking

**FIGURE 9–3  Vocal cords.**

into the esophagus instead of entering the larynx. If the flap fails to close
properly when swallowing and something enters the larynx, coughing occurs to
expel the substance before it enters the lungs. Air continues through the larynx
into another tube called the trachea.

## Trachea

The *trachea* or windpipe is a rigid tube about 4 inches in length. The trachea
is surrounded by rings of hyaline cartilage that support the trachea and keep it
open when breathing. The trachea is lined with a mucosa that contains cilia.
These cilia create waves to move the mucus filled with particles and debris
upward away from the lungs to the pharynx to be swallowed.

   The trachea bifurcates, or divides, into a right and left branch. Each branch
is called a *bronchus* and enters into a lung.

## Lungs

The *lungs* (see Fig. 9–4) sit in the central thoracic cavity in a space called the
mediastinum. The right lung comprises three sections called lobes. The left lung
has two lobes; the heart sits inside a curved section of the left lung called the
*cardiac notch* and uses the space that a third lobe would inhabit.

   Each lung is covered in a serous membrane called the pulmonary or visceral
pleura. Between the membrane and the lungs is serous fluid called parietal
fluid to prevent friction when the lungs rub against the pleura during breathing. The thoracic cavity is also lined in serous membrane called parietal pleura.
Parietal fluid also prevents the two membranes from rubbing when the lungs
expand against the chest cavity.

   Within the lungs, each bronchus divides into smaller branches called *bronchioles*. At the ends of the bronchioles are clusters of round, saclike structures called
*alveoli* (see Fig. 9–5). The bronchi and bronchioles resemble an upside-down tree
with the alveoli covering the ends of the bronchioles like leaves. The alveoli are the
place of gas exchange where oxygen is brought into the lungs and carbon dioxide
is pushed out. The alveoli are coated in a substance called *surfactant*, which
stops the alveoli from sticking together after exhalation. Surfactant is needed

*Flashpoint*
A tracheotomy is a surgical
procedure in which an inci-
sion is made in a blocked
trachea to open an airway.

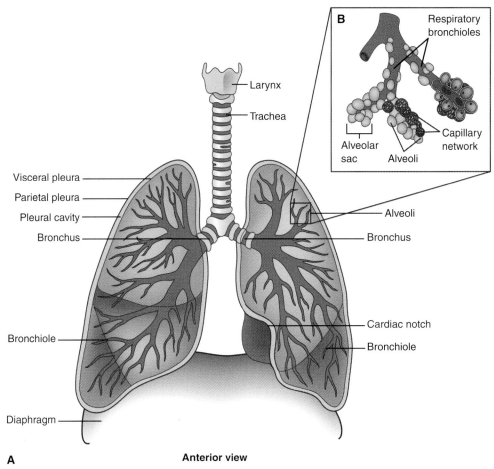

**FIGURE 9-4  Bronchial tree within the lungs.**

because, similar to a wet balloon that when deflated sticks together and is difficult, if not impossible, to inflate again, the alveoli deflate as air is breathed out. Without surfactant, the membrane of the alveoli would stick together and not inflate again.

In a fetus, the lungs are among the last organs to develop. A premature infant has poor or even no lung development. If the lungs are not fully developed, surfactant may not be present. Lack of surfactant prevents a newborn

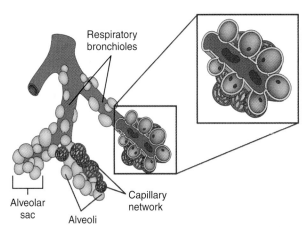

**FIGURE 9-5  Structure of the alveoli.**

from being able to breathe on his or her own. A synthetic surfactant is available that can be administered to premature infants until their lungs develop and make their own surfactant.

See Figure 9–6 for a flowchart showing the pathway of air through the respiratory system.

# Respiratory Cycle

Bringing oxygen into the body is called an **inspiration**, or inhalation. Releasing air out of the body is an **expiration**, or exhalation. Together, one inspiration and one expiration is equal to one breath or one **respiratory cycle**. The average respiration for an adult is 12 to 20 breaths per minute.

## Types of Respiration

To bring oxygen into the body and remove carbon dioxide, four different phases occur during the respiratory cycle. First, air must move into and out of the lungs so that the alveoli are constantly exposed to air for gas exchange to occur. This process is called **pulmonary ventilation**, or breathing.

The second phase is **external respiration**, which takes place only in the lungs. External respiration occurs when expiration releases the carbon dioxide

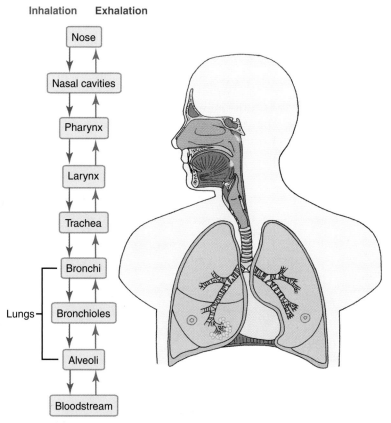

FIGURE 9–6  **Flow chart of air through the lungs.**

from the body and an inspiration brings oxygen in. Air is brought in from the external environment and returned to the external environment.

After gas exchange has occurred in the alveoli, oxygen and carbon dioxide are transported from and back to the lungs by the bloodstream. This process is ***respiratory gas transport***.

The fourth phase of respiration is **internal respiration**. This occurs within the cells of the body when oxygen and carbon dioxide are exchanged within the capillaries.

## Mechanics of Breathing

Breathing is a mechanical process because it depends on the change in the volume of air within the lungs with the contraction or relaxation of the chest muscles. This movement either increases or decreases pressure on the air, and as pressure increases, the volume of air decreases, and as the pressure decreases, the volume of air increases.

Pulmonary ventilation occurs by movements of the muscles of the thoracic cavity and the diaphragm, which is a thick muscle that separates the thoracic cavity from the abdominal cavity. The process of pulmonary ventilation has two phases: inspiration and expiration (see Fig. 9–7).

During inspiration, or inhalation, the diaphragm pulls downward causing the intercostal muscles of the thoracic cavity to pull the chest upward and outward. The lungs are attached to the pleura of the thoracic cavity so the lungs stretch as the chest enlarges. This stretching creates space for the gases within the lungs to spread out and decrease the lung pressure. The decrease in pressure makes a partial vacuum, which sucks air into the lungs because gases move from a place of high concentration to a place of lower concentration. The lungs fill until the pressure inside and outside of the lungs is equal.

Expiration, or exhalation, expels the air from the lungs. When the diaphragm relaxes, it pushes upward, and the intercostal muscles relax and allow the chest to move downward. This movement creates a smaller space as the lungs are pushed closer together. The gases in the smaller space are pushed closer together causing the internal pressure to increase, and air is forced out. This cycle repeats with every breath.

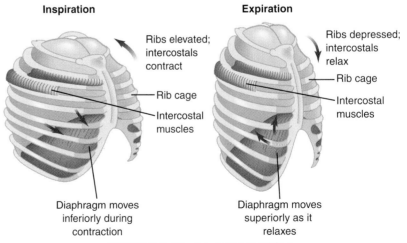

**Inspiration**

Ribs elevated; intercostals contract

Rib cage

Intercostal muscles

Diaphragm moves inferiorly during contraction

**Expiration**

Ribs depressed; intercostals relax

Rib cage

Intercostal muscles

Diaphragm moves superiorly as it relaxes

**FIGURE 9–7 Mechanical breathing.**

## Respiratory Capacities and Volumes

The normal amount or volume of air within the lungs is called the **vital capacity** and equals about 4000 to 6000 mL (see Fig. 9–8). The actual amount present depends on age, gender, weight, and activity level. How much air the lungs can hold is the capacity. The normal amount of air that goes into and out of the lungs with one breath is called the **tidal volume**. This amount is about 500 mL of air. More air can be taken into the lungs past the normal tidal volume. This is the **inspiratory reserve volume**, and it can range from 2000 to 3200 mL.

**Expiratory reserve volume** is the amount of air that is expired with one maximum breath. This is a breath that forces air out of the lungs longer than a normal expiration. On average, 1200 mL of air can be forced out of the lungs.

Because gas exchange must occur constantly regardless of how much air is expelled, some air must remain in the lungs. The amount of air always present is called the **residual volume**. This amount is about 1200 mL.

All air present in the lungs—meaning the residual volume and the vital capacity combined—is the **total capacity** of the lungs. Respiratory capacity is often measured for patients with asthma or other obstructive disorders of the lungs to determine the amount of gas exchange in the lungs.

Infectious diseases of the respiratory system can also cause a change in respiratory capacity (see Box 9–1).

Table 9–1 describes the different volumes of air found in the lungs.

*Flashpoint*

Pulmonary function tests (PFTs) measure how well lungs take in and release air. Spirometry is a PFT that measures how much and how quickly air moves out of the lungs using an instrument called a spirometer.

## Variations of Respiration

The rate and depth of breathing change as a result of such factors as age, exercise, weather, stress, emotion, and medications (see Table 9–2). Normal breathing is called eupnea (normal breathing), the general term **dyspnea** (bad breathing) refers to any abnormal change or difficulty in breathing.

Hyperpnea refers to an increased rate and increased depth during breathing. This type of breathing occurs during exertion, such as exercise, when the body needs more oxygen to make ATP to sustain the muscles. A decrease in rate and depth is **hypopnea**. Hypopnea is slow, shallow breathing that results in a lack of oxygen. Hypopnea commonly occurs because of an obstruction in the airway

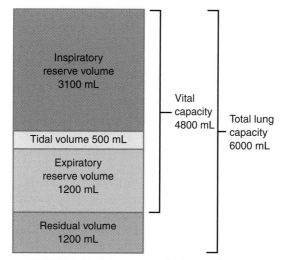

FIGURE 9–8  Average respiratory volumes.

## Box 9-1 Infectious Respiratory Disorders

Communicable, or infectious, respiratory diseases are spread by inhalation of droplets from an infected person by a cough or sneeze. These diseases are most often spread in close environments such as the home, workplace, or school.

Tuberculosis is caused by bacteria that most often attacks the lungs, but can affect any body part. Many people who have come in contact with the bacteria do not develop symptoms, but can be carriers capable of spreading the disease. Symptoms include chest pain, coughing blood, fever, swollen lymph nodes, and weight loss. If the bacteria is in the lungs, it destroys the lung tissue, and eventually death occurs from respiratory failure. Treatment is long-term (6 to 12 months) use of antibiotics to kill the bacteria.

Influenza (the flu) is caused by the influenza virus. Symptoms are fever, sore throat, muscle aches, headache, coughing, and weakness. The flu can affect any age group, but elderly adults and young children are at greatest risk. Most people recover, but death can occur, especially in people in the high-risk groups. Treatment is supportive with fluids, rest, and oral medication to relieve pain. A vaccine does exist, but because the influenza virus changes quickly, a new vaccine is needed every year.

Pertussis (whooping cough) is a bacterial infection that occurs most often in children younger than 6 months of age, but it can occur in older children and adults. The main symptom is severe coughing bouts in which the cough makes a whooping sound on inhalation. Pneumonia may develop after infection, and death can occur from respiratory failure. Treatment is with antibiotics to kill the bacteria. A vaccine is available and given routinely as part of childhood vaccination series.

### TABLE 9-1
### AIR VOLUMES OF THE LUNGS

| Term | Definition |
| --- | --- |
| Tidal volume | Amount of air taken in a normal single breath |
| Expiratory reserve volume | Amount of air expelled in one maximum breath past normal exhalation |
| Residual volume | Amount of air left in the lungs after maximum expiration |
| Total capacity | Total amount of residual volume and vital capacity |
| Vital capacity | Amount of air exchanged during normal breathing |
| Inspiratory reserve volume | Amount of air taken in past the normal inhalation |

that decreases the flow of air. A lack of oxygen to the tissues for any reason is called **hypoxia.**

**Hyperventilation** is different from hyperpnea because it is an increased rate, but not an increased depth. This breathing is fast and shallow. The short breaths cause an increase in oxygen, and carbon dioxide levels in the blood decrease. Someone who is hyperventilating may feel faint. To increase the carbon dioxide, breathing into a bag causes the exhaled carbon dioxide to be breathed back in, increasing the blood levels. Crying, especially in children, can cause a quick intake of air and cause hyperventilation (see Box 9-2). **Hypoventilation** is also a decrease in rate and depth, but in contrast to hypopnea, the amount of air to the lungs is decreased enough to cause a decrease of gas exchange by the alveoli. The result is an increased amount of carbon dioxide in the blood,

*Flashpoint*
More than 35 million Americans have a chronic lung disease.

## TABLE 9–2
### TYPES OF RESPIRATION

| Term | Definition |
| --- | --- |
| Apnea | Lack of breathing |
| Dyspnea | Painful or difficult breathing |
| Eupnea | Normal breathing |
| Hyperpnea | Increased depth and rate of breathing, usually a result of exercise |
| Hyperventilation | Increased rate and depth of breathing that causes a decrease of carbon dioxide in the blood; tingling in the limbs or fainting may occur |
| Hypopnea | Slow, shallow breathing, usually caused by an obstructed airway |
| Hypoventilation | Slow and shallow breathing that decreases gas exchange by the alveoli, resulting in an increase of carbon dioxide in the blood |

## Box 9–2 Common Disruptions of Respiration

Respiratory rate and depth can change as a result of disorders or diseases of the respiratory system or increased activity. Breathing can also change by other movements of the respiratory tract that are not related to disease.

Yawning is the involuntary opening of the mouth and drawing in of air into the lungs to capacity and then exhaling immediately. Little is known about why we yawn, but one of the common theories is that it is done to bring in more oxygen and expel a buildup of carbon dioxide. Yawning can also be done to relieve fatigue or boredom. The other unusual property about yawns is that they are contagious. Seeing someone yawn or even talking about yawns causes others to do the same. (Bet you are yawning right now.)

Coughing, or tussis, is a sudden repetitive spasm of the thoracic cavity forcing the air out of the lungs. It is usually done to clear the breathing passages of irritants or to clear mucus from the trachea.

Sneezing is a convulsive explosion of air from the lungs. A sneeze occurs because irritants entering the nasal passage trigger the brain to create the sneeze to clear the nasal cavity. Air from a sneeze can move at 150 mph. A sneeze is so powerful because it not only involves the nasal cavity, but also the muscles of the mouth, throat, and chest.

Hiccoughs (or hiccups) are the result of spasms of the diaphragm. The sound of a hiccough is caused by the sudden rush of air into the lungs, which snaps the epiglottis closed. Hiccoughs can be caused by crying, laughing, eating quickly, or inhaling an irritant. Hiccoughs usually stop on their own.

Crying is an inspiration followed by release of air in a series of short breaths. This change in respiration is emotionally induced.

Laughing actually has the same change in respiration as crying with an inspiration followed by bursts of short breaths. Laughing is also an emotionally induced change in respiration.

decreasing the amount of oxygen. Hypoxia occurs. Hypoventilation is a symptom of many obstructive pulmonary disorders.

A lack of breathing is **apnea**. It can be voluntary, such as holding your breath, or involuntary. Extended apnea causes insufficient oxygen to reach the tissues, and **cyanosis,** or blueness, of the skin may occur.

For a summary of diseases and disorders of the respiratory system, see Table 9–3.

### TABLE 9–3
### PATHOLOGY TERMS FOR THE RESPIRATORY SYSTEM

| | |
|---|---|
| Asthma | Chronic attacks of dyspnea caused by spasms of the bronchi; symptoms include wheezing, tightness of the chest, and shortness of breath; usually starts in childhood, but can begin at any age; the exact cause is unknown, although it has been linked to genetics, respiratory infections, and airborne irritants such as dust and cigarette smoke |
| Bronchitis | Inflammation of the bronchi; can be caused by bacterial or viral infection; chronic bronchitis is due to inhaled irritants, such as cigarette smoke |
| Chronic obstructive pulmonary disease (COPD) | General term for obstruction of the lung tissue resulting in loss of airflow |
| Cystic fibrosis | Genetic disorder inherited from both parents; causes an overproduction of mucus that clogs the lungs and digestive system; death occurs from infection or respiratory failure; life expectancy previously was early childhood, but with antibiotics and other treatments patients with cystic fibrosis can live well into adulthood |
| Emphysema | Irreversible expansion of the alveoli most often caused by cigarette smoke; oxygen and carbon dioxide cannot be exchanged because of limited exhalation; symptoms include COPD, chronic cough, fatigue, and shortness of breath |
| Pneumonia | Alveoli become filled with fluid because of infection; can be caused by bacteria, viruses, trauma, or mold; symptoms include fever, chills, productive cough, chest pain when coughing, and shortness of breath |

# Practice Exercises

## Multiple Choice

1. The amount of air inspired and expired during normal breathing is _____.

   a. residual volume

   b. vital capacity

   c. total volume

   d. tidal volume

2. The piece of tissue that stops food and liquids from entering the nasal cavity is the _____.

   a. epiglottis

   b. adenoids

   c. uvula

   d. tonsils

3. The voice box is the common name for the _____.

   a.  larynx

   b.  pharynx

   c.  trachea

   d.  bronchus

4. _____ respiration occurs when oxygen and carbon dioxide are exchanged in the lungs.

   a.  internal

   b.  external

   c.  inspiratory

   d.  expiratory

5. The serous membrane that lines that thoracic cavity is the _____ pleura.

   a.  pulmonary

   b.  parietal

   c.  visceral

   d.  thoracic

## Fill in the Blank

1. The respiratory system is responsible for the intake of
   _____ and the outtake of _____.

2. _____ is the medical term for normal breathing.

3. One inspiration and one expiration are known as the
   _____.

4. Sound is created when air moves over flaps of tissue called the
   _____.

5. The _____ and _____ are parts of
   both the digestive system and the respiratory system.

6. Gas exchange in the lungs is done by tiny structures called
   _____.

7. Oxygen is used by cells to make an energy source called
   _____.

8. The waste product produced by cells is called _____.

9. _____ is the air that remains in the lungs after an exhalation.

10. The right lung has _____ lobes, and the left lung has _____ lobes.

## Matching

1. _____ Medical name for nostrils

2. _____ Difficult respiration

3. _____ Another term for exhalation

4. _____ Increased shallow breathing resulting in too much carbon dioxide

5. _____ Substance found in the lungs that prevents alveoli from collapsing

6. _____ Slow, shallow breathing

7. _____ Medical term for the throat

8. _____ Increased rate and depth of respiration

9. _____ Another term for inhalation

10. _____ Absence of respiration

a. hyperventilation

b. dyspnea

c. hypopnea

d. surfactant

e. expiration

f. apnea

g. pharynx

h. nares

i. inspiration

j. hyperpnea

## Short Answer

1. **Describe the different respiratory volumes and lung capacities.**

# Labeling

*Fill in the blanks with the appropriate anatomical terms.*

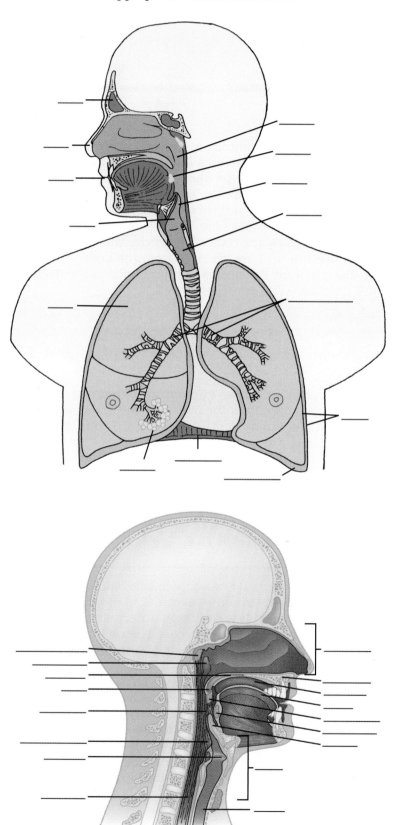

# 10 THE DIGESTIVE SYSTEM

One of the things needed to sustain life is food. Food gives us the nutrients our cells need to grow, repair, and reproduce the tissues that make up our body. The digestive system is responsible for the functions of ingestion, digestion, absorption, and excretion. These are the processes through which this system takes food in through the mouth and then breaks that food down in the stomach, changing it into its basic molecules. These molecules are drawn into the small intestines to be used by the cells of the body. Waste products move through the large intestine and are removed from the body.

This chapter discusses the structures and functions of the digestive system. Metabolism and nutrients also are summarized.

## Structure of the Digestive System

The digestive system is also called the **alimentary canal** or gastrointestinal (GI) tract. It is one continuous tube from the mouth to the anus (see Fig. 10–1). It begins with the mouth and extends to the pharynx, which is continuous with the esophagus to the stomach. From the stomach, the GI tract continues to the small intestine, then to the large intestine, and ends with the anus. In addition to the organs that make up the alimentary canal, there are several accessory, or helper, organs that aid the digestive system. The accessory organs of the digestive system are the teeth, tongue, salivary glands, appendix, pancreas, gallbladder, and liver.

## Mouth

The process of turning food into its basic molecules starts with **ingestion**, which is taking food and fluids into the mouth. The **mouth**, or oral cavity, is lined with mucous membranes. It is protected anteriorly by the lips, or labia, and laterally by skin referred to as the cheeks. The roof of the mouth consists of the hard palate, which is the anterior portion, and the soft palate, which is the posterior portion.

The mouth is the first place of **digestion**, which is the process of breaking down food. Breaking down, or chewing, of food is known as **mastication**. The tongue and teeth aid in digestion, and the **salivary glands** provide a fluid containing digestive enzymes called saliva. The **tongue** is a skeletal muscle that contains sensory receptors for taste and aids in mastication of food. As food is masticated by the teeth, the tongue pushes the food together, and the saliva helps bind it. The result is a mass of chewed food and saliva called a **bolus**.

*Flashpoint*

The digestive system maintains homeostasis by providing the body with nutrients.

*Flashpoint*

The salivary glands make 1 to 3 pints of saliva a day.

Key Terms—cont'd

mineral

nutrient

peristalsis

protein

vitamin

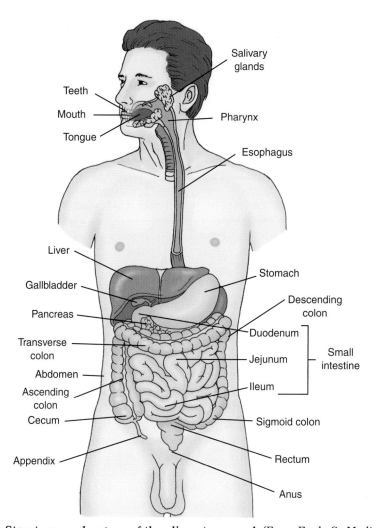

**FIGURE 10–1 Structures and organs of the alimentary canal.** (From Eagle S. *Medical Terminology in a Flash!* Philadelphia: FA Davis; 2006:121.)

## Teeth

**Teeth** are used to tear and chew food. The **crown** of the tooth is visible above the gums and is made of a substance called **enamel**, which is the hardest substance in the body. Inside the tooth is a **pulp cavity** that contains the blood vessels. The base of the tooth is the **root**, and it is located in a socket found within the upper and lower jaw bones. The root is held in place by a substance called **cementum**.

The first teeth are called **deciduous** (falling off) or baby teeth. Deciduous teeth start erupting at about 3 months of age and finish by age 2. Children have 20 teeth when all have surfaced. Deciduous teeth are pushed out of the sockets by the growing permanent teeth. They eventually fall out of the sockets and are lost. The permanent, or adult, teeth start to come in around age 6, and all 32 teeth usually erupt by age 18. The 32 adult teeth consist of 12 molars, 8 premolars, 4 canines, and 4 incisors (see Fig. 10–2). The last molars to surface are commonly called "wisdom teeth" and often do not fully surface but crowd the other teeth pushing them out of alignment. These molars are often surgically removed.

Flashpoint
Dental decay or caries is caused by bacteria that damage the enamel and the inner structures of the tooth. These bacteria can also cause gum disease and abscesses and increase the incidence of heart disease and blood clots.

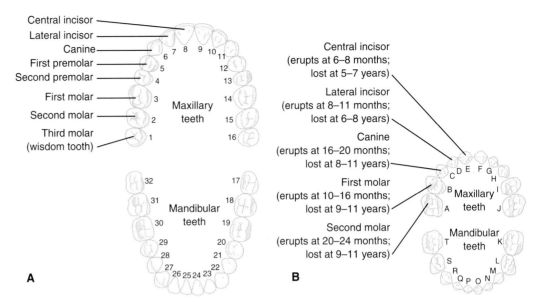

FIGURE 10-2  *(A)* **Adult teeth.** *(B)* **Deciduous teeth.**

## Pharynx

The masticated bolus is pushed by the tongue into the throat, or *pharynx*. The pharynx, also part of the respiratory system, is divided into three sections. The upper section is the *nasopharynx*, located behind the nasal cavity; the middle section is the *oropharynx*, located behind the oral cavity; and the lower section is the *laryngopharynx*, located within the neck.

The bolus moves from the oral cavity into the oropharynx and down into the laryngopharynx. At the back of the mouth is a punching bag–shaped flap of tissue called the *uvula*. The uvula covers the entrance to the nasopharynx when swallowing to prevent food or liquid from entering the nasal cavity. The pharynx is continuous with another tube of cartilage called the esophagus that allows the bolus to travel to the stomach. Figure 10–3 shows the structures of the oral cavity and pharynx.

## Esophagus

The *esophagus* is a tube about 10 inches long, and it is continuous with the laryngopharynx. This tube, also called the gullet, is made of cartilage and connects the oral cavity to the stomach. It moves the bolus along by wavelike movements called *peristalsis*. The movement of food should be one-way. There are times when food or liquid comes back up the esophagus. This is done by reverse peristalsis and is called *regurgitation,* or vomiting.

## Stomach

From the esophagus, the bolus is pushed through the entrance to the stomach (see Fig. 10–4). This entrance is a ring of muscle called a sphincter. This sphincter is known as the *cardiac sphincter* or cardioesophageal sphincter. Sphincters in the stomach prevent stomach juices from entering

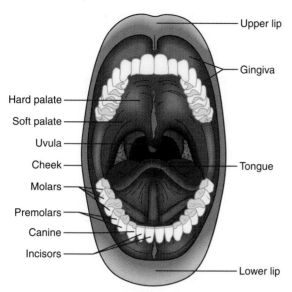

FIGURE 10-3  **Oral cavity and pharynx.**

Upper lip

Gingiva

Hard palate

Soft palate

Uvula

Cheek

Molars

Premolars

Canine

Incisors

Tongue

Lower lip

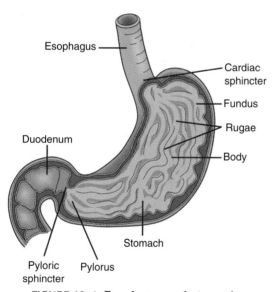

FIGURE 10-4  **Esophagus and stomach.**

Esophagus

Cardiac sphincter

Fundus

Rugae

Body

Duodenum

Stomach

Pyloric sphincter

Pylorus

the esophagus or intestines and prevent food from entering or leaving the stomach too quickly.

After pushing through the sphincter, the bolus is now in the ***stomach***. This is the major site of digestion. The stomach is a muscular sac about 12 inches long and 6 inches across at its widest point. It is divided into three sections. The section connected to the esophagus is the ***fundus***, the middle section is the ***body***, and the lower section is the pylorus.

An empty stomach resembles a deflated balloon with the tissue folding into itself. These folds are called ***rugae***. The rugae stretch to accommodate the chewed food, but can only stretch so far. The stomach can hold about a quart of food. If the stomach is filled past its normal size, the result is pain and discomfort in the abdominal region.

*Flashpoint*

The procedure for surgically decreasing the size of the stomach is a gastric bypass. The stomach is reduced and the small intestine is reattached so that the first portion of the intestine is bypassed. Weight is lost because only small amounts of food can be consumed, and fewer calories can be reabsorbed.

In the stomach, the bolus is churned with gastric juices that break it down further into a semiliquid called **chyme**. Gastric juices are a combination of acids and enzymes. Some of the digestive fluids are pancreatic juices provided by the pancreas. The stomach is a highly acidic environment with a pH of 2.0 to 3.0. The secretions of the stomach are the following:

- Hydrochloric acid is produced by parietal cells of the gastric mucosa. This acid breaks down proteins.
- Pepsin is an enzyme that begins as pepsinogen, but is changed by the stomach acids to pepsin. This enzyme breaks down the amino acids, which are a result of protein digestion.
- Renin is an enzyme that breaks down milk protein. Renin is produced in large amounts in infants, but decreases with age.
- Pancreatic juices are a combination of enzymes that break down fat and sugar.

The juices enter the stomach by a duct connected to the pancreas. Production of gastric juices is stimulated by the sight, smell, or even thought of food. This is a parasympathetic response, or an unconscious response, that stimulates cells within the stomach lining to produce gastrin. This is a hormone that stimulates the secretion of gastric juices so that the stomach has gastric juice present when food is ingested.

The stomach is lined with mucous cells. These cells secrete mucus that coats the stomach lining and protects it from erosion by the gastric juices. Sometimes an oversecretion of hydrochloric acid or an underproduction of mucus causes the stomach lining to come in contact with the gastric juices. Erosion of the lining results. This condition is called a **gastric ulcer** (see Fig. 10–5). Gastric ulcer can occur because of an increased amount of stomach acids being produced, by the use of nonsteroidal anti-inflammatory drugs (NSAIDs), such as aspirin, or by bacteria called *Helicobacter pylori*. All of these conditions or a combination of them weakens the lining of the GI tract. The ulcer usually heals with a few weeks of antibiotic treatment. If untreated, the erosion can break through the lower lining and rupture the blood vessels, which causes bleeding. If the ulcer erodes through the stomach lining, the gastric contents leak into the abdominal cavity creating a condition called **peritonitis**.

See Box 10–1 for a description of some digestive disorders caused by diet.

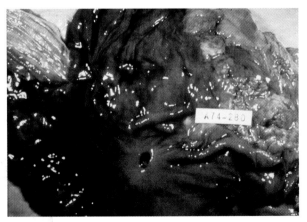

**FIGURE 10–5  Gastric ulcer.** (From Masters RA, Gylys BA. *Medical Terminology Specialties.* Philadelphia: FA Davis; 2003:195.)

## Box 10-1 Digestive Disorders Caused by Diet

Many disorders and diseases of the digestive system are due to diet and lifestyle. Most can be easily treated without permanent damage to the digestive system.

Gastroenteritis is also called "stomach flu," although it is not related to influenza. It is caused by toxins or microorganisms in food or fluids that have been ingested. These microorganisms can come from improperly cooked or prepared food or contaminated water. Symptoms are nausea, diarrhea, abdominal pain, and cramps. Anyone can get gastroenteritis, but elderly adults and small children are most susceptible, and death can occur because of dehydration or shock. Treatment is fluid and electrolyte replacement. If needed, antidiarrheal and antinausea drugs can be prescribed.

Indigestion, also called dyspepsia or "upset stomach," occurs from eating too much or too fast. Symptoms include nausea, bloating, gas, and heartburn. Treatments are antacids and digestive enzyme capsules. Persistent indigestion may be a symptom of another digestive disorder and requires further medical treatment.

Acid reflux, also called "heartburn," refers to stomach acid in the esophagus resulting from the cardiac sphincter not closing properly. Acid can splash upward into the esophagus. Symptoms are burning pain below the sternum and difficulty swallowing. Coffee, acidic foods, milk, and large meals can cause heartburn. Short-term treatment is antacids taken before meals or when symptoms occur. Long-term treatments are prescription medications that lessen the amount of stomach acid produced and dietary changes.

Constipation is a lack of bowel movements because of the stool becoming hard and dry. Symptoms include pain when passing stool, bloating, and a sensation of fullness in the bowel. The most common reason for constipation is lack of fiber in the diet. Treatment includes eating more vegetables, fruits, and whole grains and drinking more water. Fiber supplements can be added to the diet, and for short-term relief laxatives can be prescribed.

## Small Intestine

Chyme leaves the stomach by moving through another opening called the **pyloric sphincter** and enters into the small intestine (see Fig. 10-6). The small intestine is about 23 feet long and has three sections: the duodenum, the jejunum, and the ileum. The small intestine is the site of **absorption**. Here the nutrients in the chyme are absorbed for use in the body by **microvilli**, which are finger-like projections lining the small intestine. After the nutrients are absorbed, the leftover material is waste, and it leaves the small intestines and enters into the large intestine.

At the entrance to the intestines is another accessory organ called the **gallbladder**. The gallbladder is a storage container for **bile**, which is a substance made by the liver, another accessory organ. Bile is secreted into the **duodenum** and is responsible for **emulsification**, or the breaking down of fat contained in the chyme.

See Box 10-2 for a description of hernias.

*Flashpoint*
It can take 4 hours for chyme to pass through the small intestine.

## Gallbladder

The **gallbladder** is a small green sac inferior to the liver and is an accessory organ to the liver and the stomach. It is the storage area for bile produced by the liver. When fatty foods enter the duodenum from the stomach, the gallbladder

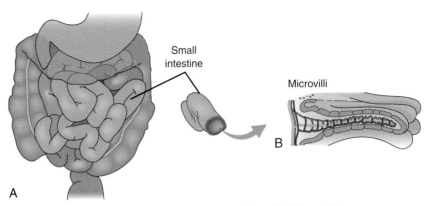

**FIGURE 10-6** *(A)* **Small intestine.** *(B)* **Microvilli.**

## Box 10-2 Disorders Affecting the Liver

Many disorders or diseases may cause the liver to function improperly or to cease all functions. As with any malfunctioning organ, infection, trauma, and genetic abnormalities can be the cause, but because the liver is the detoxifying organ, medications, alcohol, and drug use must also be considered as causes.

Cirrhosis is a chronic liver disease that results in degeneration and scarring of the liver tissue. As the scar tissue replaces healthy tissue, blood flow is impeded, and loss of liver function eventually results. The most common causes of cirrhosis are alcoholism and hepatitis C. Obesity is also becoming a cause of cirrhosis. Symptoms are loss of appetite, nausea, fatigue, weakness, and weight loss. Damage to the liver cannot be reversed. As cirrhosis progresses, it leads to other complications, such as jaundice, splenomegaly (enlarged spleen), insulin resistance, Type 2 diabetes, and ascites or fluid in the abdomen. Treatment is to abstain from drinking alcohol and maintain a healthy diet. Medications may help with complications of cirrhosis. A liver transplant may be needed if complications cannot be controlled.

Hepatitis is an inflammation of the liver resulting from a bacterial infection, toxin, or, more commonly, viral infection. The viruses that cause hepatitis are named hepatitis A, hepatitis B, and hepatitis C.

Hepatitis A is spread through fecal contamination of water and food. Symptoms are jaundice, nausea, diarrhea, fatigue, and dark urine. This is the milder form of hepatitis and does not become chronic. There is no true treatment for hepatitis A. Bed rest, a healthy diet, and treatment of symptoms is recommended. The virus usually clears the body in 3 to 6 months.

Hepatitis B is the most common type of hepatitis in the United States. The virus is spread through blood, body secretions, sexual intercourse, tattooing, and body piercing. It may also be spread from a mother to an unborn child. Symptoms of hepatitis B vary. Some infected individuals show no symptoms, and others may just have mild flulike symptoms that last about 2 to 3 weeks. The liver is cleared of the virus in about 4 to 6 months. Many infected individuals recover without any medical intervention. Other individuals may become carriers of the virus and infect others. Of these carriers, 1% to 3% progress to chronic liver damage. For patients with acute illness, recommended treatment is bed rest and a low-protein diet. Patients who develop chronic liver damage may be treated with antiviral medications; eventually, a liver transplant is needed.

## Box 10-2 Disorders Affecting the Liver—cont'd

Hepatitis C is spread by exposure to contaminated blood. This exposure can occur through sharing needles, tattooing, body piercing, and sexual activity, and from a mother to an unborn child. Hepatitis C is less common than hepatitis B, but most individuals who are infected develop chronic liver damage. Infected individuals may show no symptoms for many years, becoming symptomatic only when cirrhosis has developed. Hepatitis C is treated by injection of the medications ribavirin and interferon-alfa.

There are vaccines against hepatitis A and hepatitis B. The hepatitis A vaccine is recommended for children younger than 2 years and any adult traveling to China, South America, or Africa. Hepatitis B vaccine is recommended for all health-care workers and is given in a series of three injections. It is now routinely given to infants with the first injection given at birth.

Some medications can cause liver damage or failure. Medications account for 10% of all hepatitis cases in adults, known as drug hepatotoxicity or drug-induced hepatitis. Medications can cause acute or chronic symptoms, including jaundice, liver tumors, and liver failure.

More than 1000 medications are known to be hepatotoxic, and mixing any of these with alcohol increases the risk. Most drugs show toxicity within 5 to 90 days after beginning the medication. Some more commonly prescribed drugs that may cause liver malfunction are acetaminophen, naproxen, penicillin, tricyclic antidepressants, anabolic steroids, and oral contraceptives.

The most effective treatment is to stop taking the medication causing the problem. The liver resolves the damage itself in most cases. Liver transplant is needed in other cases if the damage is too severe or cannot be reversed.

contracts and releases bile through the bile ducts into the small intestine. Bile emulsifies, or breaks down, the fat that cannot be digested in the stomach. Bile is made of water, bile salts, cholesterol, and bilirubin. It has a yellowish green color because of bilirubin, a pigment released from the breakdown of red blood cells that is excreted from the liver.

**Cholelithiasis** is the accumulation of bile salts and cholesterol into stones that block the bile ducts. If bile cannot be released, fat cannot be digested. The bile obstruction can cause pain and discomfort in the upper right quadrant that could spread to the back and right shoulder. The lack of fat digestion can lead to nausea, indigestion, **jaundice** (yellowing of the eyes and skin), and clay-colored stool. Stones usually require removal of the gallbladder to alleviate symptoms.

## Large Intestine

The opening between the small intestine and the large intestine is the ileocecal valve. The **large intestine** (see Fig. 10–7) is about 5 feet long and is responsible for absorption of water back into the body and excretion of solid waste. Bacteria in the intestine aid the body by producing vitamin K.

The first section of the large intestine, which is attached to the ileum, is the **cecum**, a pouch that collects the solid waste that cannot be digested or absorbed. Attached to this section of the intestine is the **appendix**.

Flashpoint
Vitamin K helps to clear calcium deposits from the arteries, and it is needed by the liver to make blood clotting proteins.

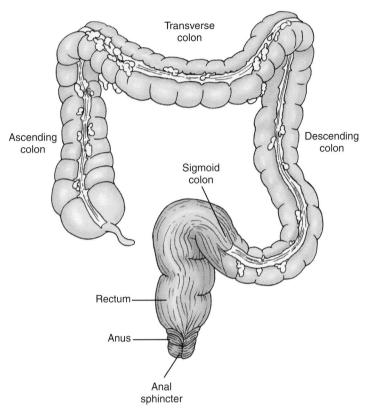

Ascending colon

Transverse colon

Descending colon

Sigmoid colon

Rectum

Anus

Anal sphincter

**FIGURE 10–7  Large intestine.** (Adapted from Eagle S. *Medical Terminology in a Flash!* Philadelphia: FA Davis; 2006:129.)

The waste leaves the cecum and moves into the ***ascending colon***, then into the ***transverse colon***, and then down into the ***descending colon***. This portion is continuous with the sigmoid colon and ***rectum***. In the rectum, the waste pauses until the body is ready to remove it. When the waste is released, it moves into the last area of the large intestine called the ***anus***. From the anus, the solid waste is released from the body in a process called ***defecation***. The ***anal sphincter*** is the last structure of the alimentary canal, and it voluntarily controls the removal of waste from the body.

## Appendix

The ***appendix*** is a small wormlike tube attached to the entrance of the cecum. This organ is considered an accessory organ to the digestive system, although it is a vestigial organ or an organ that has little or no function. It is theorized that the appendix was at one time a functioning organ that aided in digestion when uncooked or undercooked meat was part of the human diet.

The appendix has no known aid to us now, but it can de deadly. Bacteria can clog the appendix and cause it to become inflamed and enlarged in a disorder called appendicitis. If ***appendicitis*** occurs, the appendix is removed in a procedure called an appendectomy. If the appendix is not removed, it can burst and spread bacteria throughout the body.

## Pancreas

The **pancreas** is about 6 inches in length and located in the upper right abdominal cavity between the duodenum and the spleen. The pancreas performs several distinctly different functions and is part of two different systems: the endocrine system and the digestive system. As part of the endocrine system, the pancreas is similar to an endocrine gland secreting insulin into the bloodstream. In the digestive system, the pancreas is responsible for **excretion**, or eliminating substances. The pancreas excretes pancreatic enzymes through the pancreatic duct to the stomach to aid in digestion. Pancreatic enzymes are as follows:

- Amylase breaks down starch into the sugar maltose.
- Lipase emulsifies fats. The bile salts from the gallbladder aid the lipase so that it works faster.
- Trypsin begins as trypsinogen, but when it leaves the stomach it is changed to trypsin in the duodenum. Trypsin digests polypeptides into amino acids.
- Bicarbonate neutralizes the acid in the gastric juice as it enters the duodenum so that it does not damage the lining of the small intestine.

## Liver

The **liver** is an organ of many varied functions. It is the largest of the internal organs and consists of two lobes. The liver is reddish brown in color and is triangular in shape. It is found in the upper right abdominal cavity just below the diaphragm. The liver is the only organ able to regenerate itself. Because the liver has so many functions, it is an accessory to many systems (see Table 10–1). In the digestive system, it produces bile that is stored in the gallbladder to emulsify fat. Other functions of the liver include:

- Amino acid metabolism: The liver is responsible for regulation of blood amino acid levels. There are 20 amino acids, and 12 of them are synthesized or produced by the liver. The other eight amino acids come from diet. Amino acids are used to build new proteins.

**TABLE 10–1**

**FUNCTIONS OF THE LIVER**

| | |
|---|---|
| Amino acid metabolism | Regulates amino acid levels in the blood—creates 12 of the 20 amino acids |
| Carbohydrate metabolism | Regulates blood glucose metabolism—converts glucose to glycogen and glycogen back to glucose |
| Lipid metabolism | Synthesizes cholesterol and forms lipoproteins that act as carriers for other substances |
| Plasma protein synthesis | Produces blood proteins to maintain blood volume, form clots, and act as transport |
| Formation of bilirubin | Removes bilirubin for red blood cells and secretes it into the bile |
| Storage | Stores vitamins A, D, E, K, and $B_{12}$; minerals; and water |
| Detoxification | Detoxifies harmful substances such as alcohol and drugs |

- Carbohydrate metabolism: The liver is responsible for blood glucose regulation. It converts excess glucose to glycogen when blood glucose is high. When blood glucose levels are low, it converts the glycogen back to glucose.
- Lipid metabolism: The liver synthesizes cholesterol and forms lipoproteins that transport fats from the blood to the tissues.
- Plasma protein synthesis: The liver produces many of the proteins in the blood. Albumin is the most common blood protein, and it maintains blood volume by removing tissue fluid from the capillaries. Prothrombin and fibrinogen are clotting proteins made by the liver that stop bleeding. The liver also creates globulins that act as carriers for other molecules.
- Formation of bilirubin: The liver removes the pigment bilirubin, which is formed from the breakdown of old red blood cells. It is excreted into the bile giving it a yellowish green color. Bilirubin is eventually excreted by the body through the feces.
- Storage: The liver stores the fat-soluble vitamins A, D, E, and K and the water-soluble vitamin $B_{12}$. It also stores the minerals iron and copper for the production of hemoglobin.
- Detoxification: The liver synthesizes enzymes that detoxify harmful substances. Alcohol is changed to acetate that can be used in the body. Medications are broken down in the liver and changed to create therapeutic effects. Ammonia is a toxic substance produced by bacteria in the colon. Ammonia is converted to urea and excreted by the kidneys.

See Figure 10–8 for an illustration of the pancreas, gallbladder, and liver. A flowchart of the structures of the alimentary canal is shown in Figure 10–9. See Box 10–3 for information about disorders of the liver.

*Flashpoint*

The liver filters 1 liter of blood per minute.

## Metabolism

**Metabolism** is a general term for all the chemical reactions that occur in the body. This process includes **catabolism**, which is breaking down substances into smaller ones, and **anabolism**, which is forming or binding together smaller molecules to make larger ones. An example of catabolism is breaking down

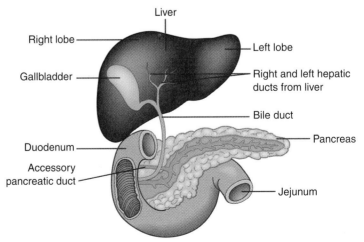

**FIGURE 10–8  Liver gallbladder and pancreas.**

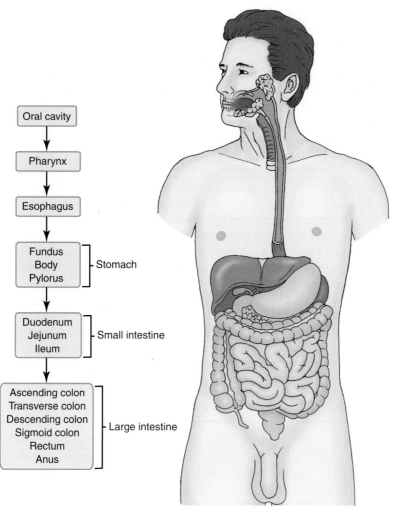

FIGURE 10–9  **Pathway through the digestive system.**

## Box 10–3 Hernias

A hernia is a protrusion of part of an organ into tissue where it is not normally contained. The term hernia is usually used to describe bulges through the abdominal wall. There are several different abdominal hernias—inguinal, umbilical, and femoral. Other common nonabdominal hernias are hiatal and incisional.

Of the abdominal hernias, inguinal hernia is the most common. This type of hernia is a protrusion of the intestine or bladder into the groin area. Umbilical hernia is most common in newborns and occurs when the intestine protrudes into the abdomen near the navel. A femoral hernia is a protrusion of the intestine into the area of the femoral artery. It is most common in women who are pregnant or obese.

A hiatal hernia occurs when the stomach protrudes into the hiatus, which is an opening in the diaphragm through which the esophagus passes. An incisional hernia is a result of the intestine passing through the site of an abdominal surgery. This type of hernia occurs more often in elderly adults and patients who are sedentary after surgery.

The only way to repair a hernia is through surgery. Most repairs can be done laparoscopically on an outpatient basis. If hernias are not repaired, they can cause pain, limit activity, cause a blockage of the bowel, and lead to necrosis, or death, of the intestine.

protein into individual amino acids. The individual amino acids are used in anabolism to make new proteins.

Metabolism also frees energy that can be converted to ATP by the cells. Different foods have different amounts of energy in them. The energy value of food is called a *calorie*. Calories come from food groups called carbohydrates, protein, and fats. The digested forms of these food groups are generally called nutrients.

## Nutrients

*Nutrients* are the essential substances the body needs to grow, repair, and sustain life functions. Most of these essential nutrients come from food or supplements. Nutrients can be classified according to size and molecular structure. By size, there are two types of nutrients: macronutrients and micronutrients. *Macronutrients* are needed in large quantities by the body; they include protein and glucose. *Micronutrients* are needed in small quantities by the body and include most minerals.

Nutrients can also be thought of structurally as organic or inorganic. *Organic nutrients* are complex molecules that contain carbon and hydrogen. Examples are carbohydrates, proteins, and fats. *Inorganic molecules* are simpler structures usually composed of only one or two molecules. Water and oxygen are the best examples of inorganic nutrients needed by the body.

## Carbohydrates

*Flashpoint*

The U.S. Department of Agriculture recommends 45% to 65% of total caloric intake come from carbohydrates.

*Carbohydrates* are the preferred source of fuel for cells to make ATP. From every gram of carbohydrate, the body can make 4 calories. Carbohydrates are digested into their simplest form, which is glucose. The hormone insulin carries glucose to the cells. The cells break down glucose in an action called glycolysis. The energy created from glycolysis is added to oxygen in the process of cellular respiration. When glucose and oxygen are mixed, they produce ATP, and they create the waste products water and carbon dioxide. The water is recycled by the body, and the carbon dioxide is released into the bloodstream to be expelled by the lungs.

## Proteins

*Flashpoint*

Each person needs 1 gram of protein for each kilogram (2.2 lb) of body weight.

*Proteins* are found throughout the body. They form skin, muscles, and ligaments; maintain blood volume; allow blood to clot; are a component of hemoglobin, antibodies, and hormones; aid in digestion; and make up the enzymes that control all reactions within the body. The simplest form of a protein is an amino acid. Of the 20 amino acids, 12 are made by liver and are considered nonessential because they do not need to be ingested in food. The other eight are essential amino acids because they need to be ingested. Amino acids are mainly used to make new proteins. If new proteins are not needed, amino acids can be metabolized and used for energy. For every gram of protein, 4 calories are produced. Excess amino acids are broken down and changed into carbohydrates that are converted into glycogen for storage. Carbohydrates not used for energy are changed to fat and stored in the adipose tissue.

## Fats

**Fats** are used for energy production, are a component of cell membranes, and are stored for insulation and cushioning. Fat stores can also be used in place of glucose if none is available. From every gram of fat consumed, 9 calories are produced. Fats are a type of lipid and are broken down into triglycerides that are used by the liver as an energy source for the cells. They are also used to form cell membranes. Excess triglycerides are stored as adipose for thermal insulation and to protect the bones and organs from shock.

Fats can either be saturated or unsaturated. Saturated fats are found in butter, lard, meat, and dairy foods. Too much saturated fat raises the level of cholesterol in the blood. Unsaturated fats are found in vegetable oils, olive oil, nuts, and seeds. These fats do not raise the levels of cholesterol.

**Cholesterol** is another type of lipid that is made by the liver and ingested through diet. Cholesterol made by the liver is called endogenous (made within) cholesterol, and cholesterol obtained from the diet is exogenous (made outside) cholesterol. Cholesterol is also used by the liver. It is soluble in the blood and comes in two forms. One form is high-density lipoproteins (HDL), which are the "good" lipids. They transport excess cholesterol to the liver to be excreted. HDL can also remove some cholesterol from the arteries. The other form of cholesterol is low-density lipoproteins (LDL), which are the "bad" lipids. These lipids get stored in the body and build up in the arteries increasing the risk of coronary artery disease and myocardial infarction, or heart attack.

## Vitamins

**Vitamins** are organic molecules needed only in small amounts by the body. Vitamins are either water-soluble or fat-soluble. Water-soluble vitamins can dissolve in water. They include vitamin $B_1$ (thiamine), vitamin $B_2$ (riboflavin), vitamin C, and folic acid. These vitamins cannot be stored in the body, and whatever is not used is excreted in the urine. Fat-soluble vitamins include vitamins A, D, E, and K. They are dissolved in the adipose tissue, and some can be stored in the body (see Table 10–2).

In the body, vitamins function as coenzymes or antioxidants. Coenzymes assist other enzymes to function. Antioxidants prevent damage from free radicals, which are molecules that can degrade DNA, cell membranes, and organelles.

Each vitamin has a specific level that the body needs to maintain. Deficiency in a vitamin often results in disease. A deficiency of vitamin C results in **scurvy**, a disease that causes deterioration of the skin and mucous membranes. Vitamin D deficiency causes abnormal bone growth called **rickets**. A lack of vitamin $B_{12}$ results in a blood disease called **pernicious anemia**.

Amounts of vitamins over the normally needed amount can also result in damage or disease. Increased vitamin A can cause liver damage and hair loss. High levels of vitamin D can cause stones to form in the organs because of increased calcium absorption. Nerve damage can be a result of excessive amounts of vitamin $B_6$.

**TABLE 10–2**

**VITAMINS**

| Vitamin Water-soluble | Function | Source |
|---|---|---|
| B$_1$ (thiamine) | Synthesis of sugars and acetylcholine | Meat, legumes, eggs, green leafy vegetables |
| B$_2$ (riboflavin) | Aids in cell respiration | Milk, cheese, meat, whole grains |
| B$_3$ (niacin) | Aids in cell respiration and fat metabolism | Meat, fish, whole grains, legumes |
| B$_5$ (pantothenic acid) | Aids in energy production from fat and amino acids | Meat, fish, whole grains, legumes |
| B$_6$ (pyridoxine) | Metabolism of amino acids; synthesis of protein | Meat, fish, whole grains, yogurt, yeast |
| B$_7$ (biotin) | Synthesis of nucleic acids | Liver, eggs, yeast |
| B$_9$ (folic acid) | Aids in blood cell development; aids in development of fetal nervous system | Liver, whole grains, legumes, green leafy vegetables |
| B$_{12}$ (cobalamin) | Synthesis of DNA; metabolism of amino acids | Liver, fish, meat, cheese, milk |
| C (ascorbic acid) | Synthesis of collagen for wound healing; aids in iron absorption; antioxidant | Citrus fruit, tomatoes, potatoes |
| Fat-soluble | | |
| A | Maintenance of epithelial tissues; aids in bone calcification | Yellow and green vegetables, liver, milk, eggs |
| D | Aids in absorption of calcium and phosphorus; aids in immune response | Fortified milk, egg yolks, fish oil |
| E | Aids with wound healing; aids in detoxification in liver; antioxidant | Nuts, wheat germ, seeds |
| K | Synthesis of clotting factors | Liver, spinach, cabbage |

## Minerals

**Minerals** are inorganic substances needed in small or trace amounts by the body. They are needed for bone and tooth formation, synthesis of DNA, metabolism, and nerve conduction. Some minerals needed by the body are calcium, phosphorus, potassium, sulfur, sodium, chloride, and magnesium (see Table 10–3).

See Table 10–4 for a summary of pathological conditions of the digestive system.

### TABLE 10–3
### MINERALS

| Mineral | Function | Source |
| --- | --- | --- |
| Calcium | Formation of bones and teeth; blood clotting | Milk, cheese, shellfish, leafy green vegetables |
| Chlorine | Part of hydrochloric acid | Table salt |
| Cobalt | Part of vitamin $B_{12}$ | Liver, meat, eggs |
| Copper | Synthesis of hemoglobin and melanin | Liver, whole grains, nuts, legumes |
| Iodine | Needed for synthesis of triiodothyronine and thyroxine | Table salt, seafood |
| Iron | Component of hemoglobin | Meat, shellfish, legumes, eggs |
| Magnesium | Formation of bone | Green leafy vegetables, legumes, seafood, milk |
| Manganese | Synthesis of fatty acids and cholesterol; aids in bone formation | Green leafy vegetables, legumes, nuts |
| Phosphorus | Formation of bones and teeth | Milk, cheese, meat, fish |
| Potassium | Aids in nerve impulse transmission and muscle contraction | Most foods |
| Sodium | Aids in nerve impulse transmission and muscle contraction | Table salt |
| Sulfur | Part of $B_1$ and $B_7$ | Meat eggs |
| Zinc | Part of enzymes for protein digestion; aids in wound healing | Meat, whole grains legumes, seafood |

### TABLE 10–4
### PATHOLOGY TERMS FOR THE DIGESTIVE SYSTEM

| | |
| --- | --- |
| Cholecystitis | Inflammation of the gallbladder most often caused by gallstones; symptoms include nausea, upper right quadrant pain, jaundice, and fever |
| Cholelithiasis | Gallstones; caused by cholesterol and bile pigments that accumulate in the bile; stones can be the size of a grain of sand or as large as a golf ball; they can block bile production and clog the bile and hepatic ducts causing inflammation and pain |
| Crohn disease | Swelling of the ileum that causes diarrhea, abdominal pain, rectal bleeding, and weight loss; can occur at any age, but most often diagnosed in adults 20–30 yr old |
| Diarrhea | Loose, watery stools caused by bacteria, viruses, medications, or intestinal disorders |
| Diverticulitis | Inflammation of one or more diverticula or pouches that have formed in the wall of the colon; symptoms include severe abdominal pain, nausea, fever, constipation, or diarrhea; if a pouch ruptures, peritonitis can occur |

*Continued*

## TABLE 10–4

## PATHOLOGY TERMS FOR THE DIGESTIVE SYSTEM—cont'd

| | |
|---|---|
| Diverticulosis | Condition in which diverticula or pouches form in the wall of the colon; caused by low-fiber diet that causes more pressure to move stool through the large intestine, which causes weak spots in the wall. Usually discovered only if symptoms of abdominal pain and cramping on the left side develop; occurs most often in adults older than 40 |

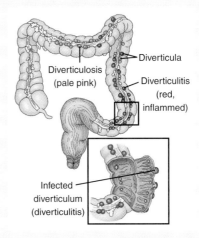

Diverticulosis (From Eagle S. *Medical Terminology in a Flash!* Philadelphia, PA: FA Davis; 2006:129.)

| | |
|---|---|
| Gastroenteritis | Symptoms are watery diarrhea, abdominal cramps, nausea, vomiting, and low-grade fever; most often occurs from microorganisms in food or water |
| Gastrointestinal reflux disease (GERD) | Improper closure of cardiac sphincter that causes stomach acid to back up into the esophagus; symptoms in adults include heartburn, cough, hoarseness, and nausea; symptoms in children include vomiting, weight loss or poor weight gain, and refusal to eat |
| Hemorrhoids | Swollen veins either in the anal canal or near the anal sphincter; pressure secondary to constipation, pregnancy, or obesity can cause the veins to swell, become painful, itch, or bleed |
| Irritable bowel syndrome (IBS) | Symptoms are lower abdomen pain and bouts of diarrhea and constipation; also called spastic colon; occurs more commonly in women younger than 35 |
| Pyloric stenosis | Affects infants; narrowing of the pylorus so that digested food cannot enter the duodenum; causes projectile vomiting, weight loss, and dehydration; can be corrected by surgery |
| Ulcers | Erosion of the stomach lining, esophagus, or small intestine because of increased stomach acid and possibly by the bacteria *H. pylori* |

# Practice Exercises

## Multiple Choice

1. The act of bringing food into the body is _____.

   a. digestion

   b. mastication

   c. ingestion

   d. defecation

2. The simplest form of a carbohydrate is _____ .

   a.  glucose

   b.  maltose

   c.  lactose

   d.  glycogen

3. The gallbladder stores bile made by the _____ .

   a.  liver

   b.  pancreas

   c.  appendix

   d.  stomach

4. _____ are the folds of the stomach.

   a.  microvilli

   b.  rugae

   c.  uvula

   d.  sphincters

5. Baby teeth are also called _____ teeth.

   a.  adult

   b.  small

   c.  deciduous

   d.  semipermanent

6. Finger-like projections in the small intestine are called _____ .

   a.  microvilli

   b.  rugae

   c.  appendages

   d.  uvula

7. _____ are nutrients that can be either water-soluble or fat-soluble.

   a.  minerals

   b.  vitamins

   c.  proteins

   d.  carbohydrates

8. The flap of tissue that stops food and fluid from entering the nasal cavity is the _____ .

   a.  uvula

   b.  epiglottis

   c.  microvilli

   d.  pharynx

9. Detoxification of alcohol and medication is done by the _____.

   a. gallbladder

   b. stomach

   c. liver

   d. appendix

10. Amino acids form _____.

   a. fats

   b. sugars

   c. carbohydrates

   d. proteins

## True or False

1. True   False     Another name for bile is gall.

2. True   False     Organic nutrients are large molecules.

3. True   False     Permanent teeth are also called deciduous teeth.

4. True   False     Mastication is the process of chewing food.

5. True   False     Fats are stored in the body as lipids.

6. True   False     HDL is the healthy cholesterol.

7. True   False     Cilia are the finger-like projections lining the small intestine.

8. True   False     Nutrients are essential substances needed by the body.

9. True   False     The liver is the smallest organ of the body.

10. True   False     The pancreas aids in digestion.

## Fill in the Blank

1. The stomach has _____ that allow the stomach to expand.

2. The small intestine has microvilli to absorb _____.

3. Chewed food and saliva form a mass called a _____.

4. _____ is the breakdown of fat.

5. The _____ is no longer a functional organ.

6. Bile is produced by the _____ and stored in the

   _____ .

7. The esophagus moves food by a process called _____ .

8. Digested food that moves into the small intestine is called

   _____ .

9. The _____ sphincter is the doorway between the

   stomach and small intestine.

10. The act of bringing food into the body is _____ .

## Matching

1. _____ The middle section of the small intestine

2. _____ The first section of the stomach

3. _____ The last section of the large intestine

4. _____ The first section of the small intestine

5. _____ The middle section of the large intestine

6. _____ The last section of the stomach

7. _____ The middle section of the stomach

8. _____ The last section of the small intestine

a. fundus

b. transverse colon

c. ileum

d. ascending colon

e. body

f. descending colon

g. jejunum

h. cecum

i. pylorus

j. duodenum

9. _____ The first
section of the
large intestine

10. _____ The pouch at
the entrance to
the large intestine

## Short Answer

1. **Name the accessory organs of the digestive system.**

2. **Name the four functions of the digestive system.**

## Labeling

*Fill in the blanks with the appropriate anatomical terms.*

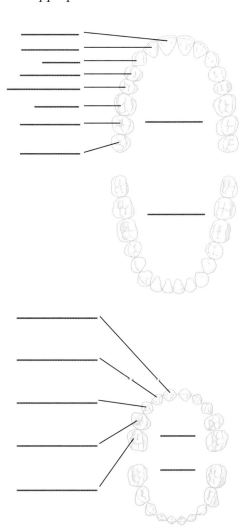

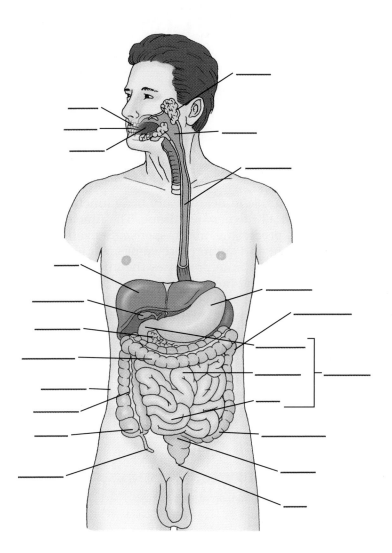

# 11

# THE NERVOUS SYSTEM

## Key Terms

autonomic nervous system

brain

central nervous system

cerebrospinal fluid

cranial nerves

gyri

lobe

meninges

neuroglia

neuron

neurotransmitters

parasympathetic nervous system

peripheral nervous system

*Continued*

The nervous system plays a role in nearly every body function. It consists of the brain, spinal cord, and all the nervous tissue. The functions of the nervous system are interpretation, processing, and response. Sensations, or sensory input, are taken to the brain and are interpreted or identified to determine the cause of the sensation. The brain processes the information to understand the meaning of the sensation and how the body should react. Then the brain creates the appropriate response or reaction to the sensation. For example, a tickling sensation on the skin may be interpreted by the brain as the crawling of an insect, the brain processes this information and determines an act to remove the insect, and the body responds by moving the arm to shake it off. In addition to interpretation, processing, and response, the nervous system also coordinates muscle activity and organ function.

This chapter examines the different cells of the nervous system and their functions. The different structures and functions of the nervous system are also explored.

## Cells of the Nervous System

The nervous system consists of two types of cells: neurons and glial cells. Neurons conduct stimuli from one part of the body to another. The strength of the stimuli varies by the effect of the stimuli on individual neurons. This effect is regulated by a process called the action potential. Glial cells provide support to the brain and spinal cord. These support cells are the most abundant type of nervous system cell.

### Neurons

Nerve cells are also called **neurons**. All neurons direct an impulse in one direction starting at the point where the stimulus occurred. Depending on the type of stimulus, it ends at the brain or spinal cord.

Neurons differ in structure, size, and function. There are three types of neurons: sensory, motor, and mixed.

#### Types of Neurons

**Sensory neurons**, or afferent neurons, are a one-way relay for stimuli to the central nervous system (CNS). **Motor neurons**, also called efferent neurons,

*Flashpoint*

The nervous system maintains homeostasis in the body by acting as the communication system that detects, interprets, and responds to internal and external changes.

*Flashpoint*

Neurons are so small that 30,000 can fit on the head of a pin.

carry impulses on a one-way path away from the CNS. ***Mixed neurons***, or interneurons, can carry impulses to and from the CNS on the same nerve tract.

Sensory neurons and motor neurons have similar structures (see Fig. 11–1). Each has a ***cell body*** that houses the nucleus and other organelles. Motor neurons have additional antenna-like structures called ***dendrites*** (branches) attached to the cell body to collect the incoming stimuli. Both types of neurons have a long tail-like structure made of conductive tissue called an ***axon***. The axon is wrapped

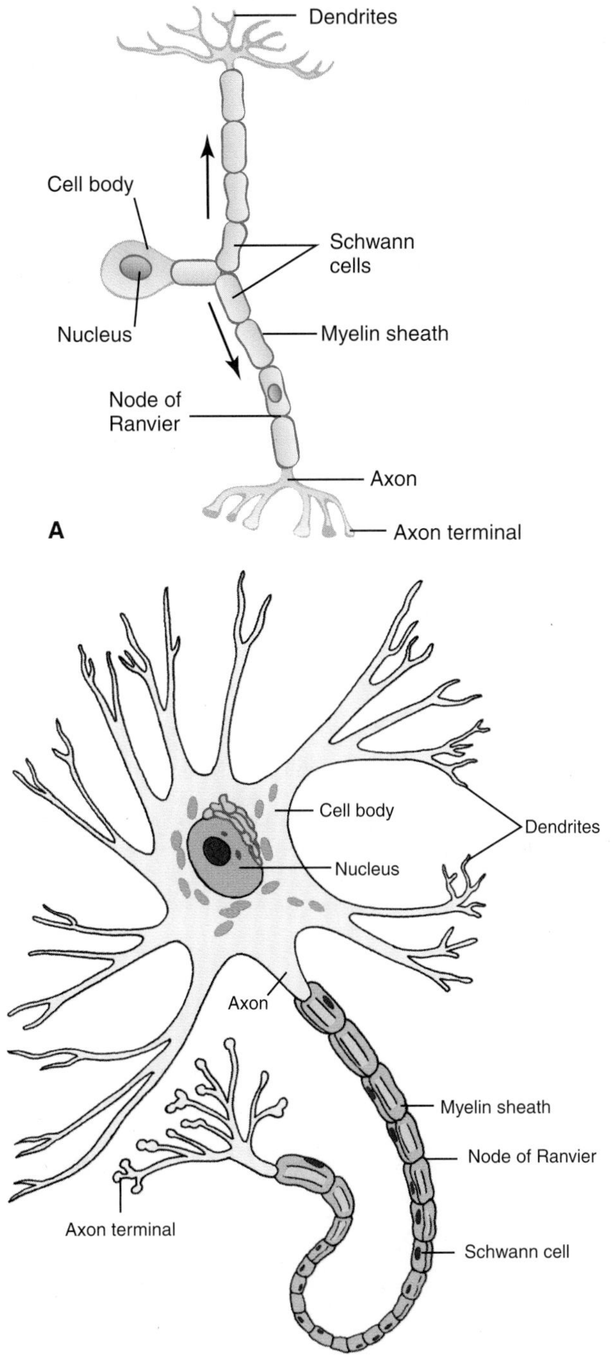


FIGURE 11–1 **Structure of a neuron. *(A)* Sensory neuron. *(B)* Motor neuron.** (*B* adapted from Eagle S. *Medical Terminology in a Flash!* Philadelphia: FA Davis; 2006:49.)

## Key Terms—cont'd

reflex

somatic nervous system

spinal cord

spinal nerves

sulci

sympathetic nervous system

ventricles

### Flashpoint

The time it takes nerve impulses to travel along the nerves can vary. Transmission of an impulse ranges from 0.5 to 120 m per second. Traveling at 120 m per second is equivalent to moving 268 miles an hour.

in a protective coating called **myelin**. The myelin is not one continuous sheath, but forms in a beadlike pattern along the axon. These beads are called **Schwann cells**, and the exposed axon between each Schwann cell is referred to as a **node of Ranvier**. Myelinated axons have a grayish color, and unmyelinated axons appear white. Clusters of myelinated neurons are referred to as gray matter, and clusters of unmyelinated neurons are white matter.

Neurons are not connected to one another. They are separated by a space called a **synapse**. At the end of the axon are **axon terminals**, which are bulb-shaped structures that contain chemicals. These chemicals are called **neurotransmitters** (see Table 11–1). These axon terminals are stimulated by the nerve impulse and release the neurotransmitters. They cross the synapse to the dendrites of the next neuron to continue the impulse along the nerve tract (see Fig. 11–2).

Each neurotransmitter can produce a different response in the body. Lack of a neurotransmitter or a change in the release or absorption of a

## TABLE 11–1
### NEUROTRANSMITTERS

| Transmitter | Function |
|---|---|
| Acetylcholine | Activates muscles; part of the autonomic nervous system |
| Epinephrine (adrenaline) | Increases heart rate, respiration, and blood pressure; allows more glucose to be given to the skeletal muscles; part of the sympathetic nervous system |
| Norepinephrine | Causes alertness and arousal; aids epinephrine in the sympathetic response |
| Gamma-aminobutyric acid (GABA) | Regulates nerve excitability |
| Dopamine | Controls motor function, memory, mood, attention, and learning |
| Serotonin | Regulates metabolism, mood, anger, aggression, and sleep |
| Endorphin (endogenous morphine) | Regulates pleasure and pain |

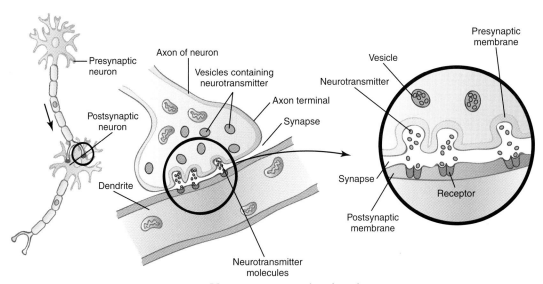

FIGURE 11-2  Motors neurons showing the synapse.

neurotransmitter in the brain can result in conditions such as depression, mania, and obesity (see Box 11–1).

## Neuroglia

The nervous system has several cells collectively called **neuroglia** (nerve glue) that aid the neurons in some way (see Fig. 11–3). These neuroglias are the astrocytes, microglia, oligodendrocytes, and ependymal cells (see Table 11–2).

- **Astrocytes** (star cells) have branched shapes that resemble stars. These cells act as support for the neurons. They also create the blood-brain

### Box 11-1 Disorders Caused by Neurotransmitter Levels

Neurotransmitters are the chemicals secreted by neurons to relay messages, cause a reaction, or slow down a reaction. In the brain, an increase or a decrease of a neurotransmitter can result in a change in mood, addiction, or a disease. Many of these conditions can be reversed with medications to control the release of a neurotransmitter or slow the absorption or reuptake of a neurotransmitter.

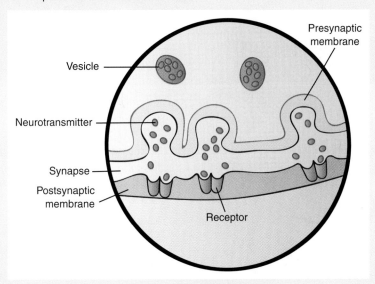

Gamma-aminobutyric acid (GABA) regulates the excitability of nerves. Low levels of GABA in the brain can result in anxiety disorders, and if specific areas of the brain lack GABA, epilepsy results. Diazepam (Valium) is used to treat anxiety because it enhances the effects of GABA. Alcohol and barbiturates also increase the effects of GABA.

Acetylcholine controls muscle movement. Lack of acetylcholine results in paralysis. Type A botulinum toxin (Botox) can be used cosmetically to relax muscles that cause wrinkles and to relax the muscles of the head and neck to relieve migraines. Botox blocks the acetylcholine, paralyzing the muscles into which it is injected. Patients with Alzheimer disease have also shown a loss of acetylcholine levels in the brain.

Dopamine controls mood and memory and stimulates the reward centers of the brain. An increase in dopamine has been linked to schizophrenia, and drugs that block release of dopamine are used to treat this condition. Patients with Parkinson disease show low levels of dopamine. A synthetic form of dopamine called levodopa (L-Dopa) is used to treat Parkinson disease and other conditions caused by low levels of dopamine. The drugs cocaine, heroin, opium, and alcohol increase dopamine release and stimulate the reward centers. Addiction occurs because these drugs can overstimulate the receptors until they lose sensitivity or cause more receptors to be

*Continued*

## Box 11-1 Disorders Caused by Neurotransmitter Levels—cont'd

made, needing more dopamine to fill them. More of the drug is needed to force more dopamine to be made to get the same stimulation.

Serotonin regulates mood and controls anger and aggression. Low levels of serotonin have been linked to depression, lack of anger control, obsessive-compulsive disorder, and suicide attempts. There are many treatments for depression and other mood disorders. Monoamine oxidase (MAO) inhibitors such as tranylcypromine (Parnate) block the breakdown of serotonin and norepinephrine, which is another neurotransmitter that regulates mood. Another drug class is the selective serotonin reuptake inhibitors (SSRIs), which stop absorption of serotonin. Examples are fluoxetine (Prozac) and paroxetine (Paxil). These drugs are also used to treat panic disorder and anxiety. Tricyclics are a drug class used to prevent reuptake of serotonin and norepinephrine. The most common tricyclic drug is amitriptyline (Elavil). A new class of drug called bupropion (Wellbutrin) blocks reuptake of norepinephrine, epinephrine, and serotonin. It is also used to stop smoking addiction.

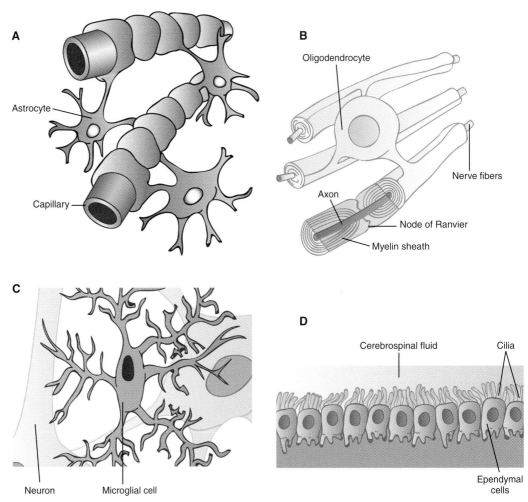

**FIGURE 11-3** Neuroglia. *(A)* Astrocytes. *(B)* Oligodendrocytes. *(C)* Microglia. *(D)* Ependymal cells.

**TABLE 11–2**

**NEUROGLIA**

| | Function |
|---|---|
| Astrocytes | Support neurons and contribute to blood-brain barrier |
| Microglia | Phagocytes that clear damaged cells and debris |
| Oligodendrocytes | Produce the myelin that protects and insulates the axon |
| Ependymal cells | Line the ventricles of the brain and have cilia that circulate the cerebrospinal fluid |

barrier, which is a network of capillaries that keep harmful substances, such as microorganisms and toxins, from entering the brain.

- *Microglia* (little glue) is able to move in and out of the nerve tissues. These cells are phagocytes (cell eaters) that collect and destroy bacteria and cell debris found within the cerebrospinal fluid.
- *Oligodendrocytes* (few branches) are found along the outside of the neurons. They resemble the astrocytes but have fewer branches. These cells produce the myelin that insulates and protects the axons.
- *Ependymocytes* (covering) also called ependymal cells form the lining inside the cavities of the brain and spinal cord. These cells have cilia that circulate the cerebrospinal fluid to keep it fresh.

# Action Potential

All neurons have two main functions: excitability and conductivity. The ability to respond to a stimulus is *excitability*, and the ability to transmit the stimulus to other neurons is *conductivity*. These abilities are part of the *action potential*, or nerve impulse (see Fig. 11–4). For a nerve cell to respond, it needs to go from a state of rest to a state of activity. Changes need to occur inside and outside of the cell for the action potential to occur.

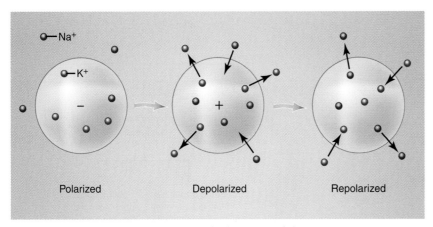

FIGURE 11–4  Action potential.

The exterior of a cell is positively charged and contains more sodium ions (Na⁺). The inside of a cell is negatively charged and contains more potassium ions (K⁺). In this state, the cell is *polarized*, or at rest. When an electrical current stimulates the cell, the state of the cell changes, allowing K⁺ to flow out of and Na⁺ to flow into the cell. As the change in Na⁺ and K⁺ occurs, the inside of the cell becomes positively charged, and the outside becomes negatively charged. The cell is now *depolarized*, or stimulated, and is capable of producing an action. When a cell is stimulated, it cannot be stimulated again until it goes back to a resting state. Na⁺ inside the cell must flow out and K⁺ must flow back in changing the inside again to a negative charge and the outside to a positive charge. The act of the cell changing back to resting is called *repolarization*.

## Divisions of the Nervous System

The nervous system has two divisions: the *central nervous system* (CNS) and the *peripheral nervous system* (PNS) (see Fig. 11–5). The CNS comprises the brain and spinal cord. The PNS comprises the nerves attached to the brain and spinal cord.

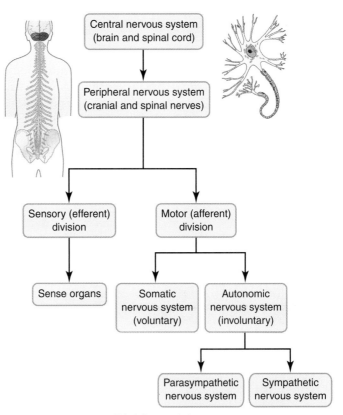

FIGURE 11–5 Divisions of the nervous system.

## Central Nervous System

The CNS oversees the entire nervous system. It consists of the brain and spinal cord. In a developing fetus, the CNS begins to develop at about the third week of gestation and is referred to as a neural tube. By 12 weeks of gestation, the fetus has a functional brain, nerves, and spinal cord. The brain and spinal cord are responsible for interpretation, processing, and response to all information detected inside and outside of the body. This information is also called *stimuli*.

### Brain

The **brain** is the control center of the body (see Fig. 11–6). It directs all other systems and is the site of consciousness, memory, reason, and emotion. The highly complex brain is divided into four sections: brainstem, cerebellum, diencephalon, and cerebrum.

The **brainstem** is the site where the spine attaches to the brain. It is about 3 inches in length. Here all the functions that maintain life, such as breathing, heartbeat, and digestion, are regulated. There are thee parts of the brainstem: medulla oblongata, pons, and midbrain.

- **Medulla oblongata** joins the brain to the spinal cord. This part of the brain is responsible for vital functions such as regulating heart rate, blood pressure, and breathing. The medulla oblongata also controls the reflexes of the head, such as swallowing, sneezing, coughing, and vomiting.
- **Pons** (bridge) is a rounded knoblike area above the medulla. This structure acts as a relay station between the cerebrum and the cerebellum. The pons also aids the medulla oblongata in regulating breathing. The pons has been

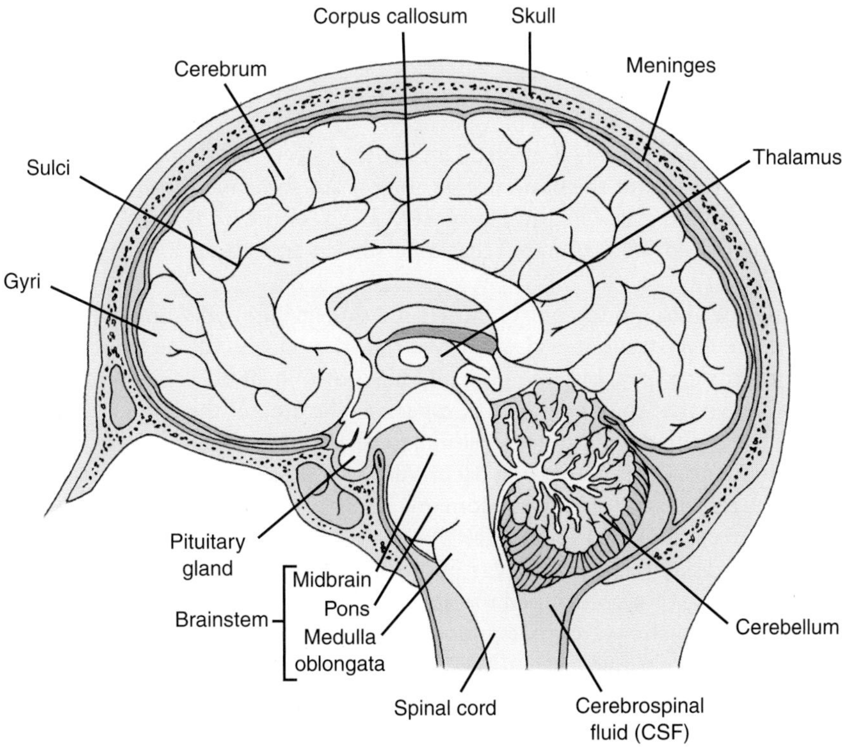

*Flashpoint*
The brain contains more than 100 billion neurons.

**FIGURE 11-6 Sections of the brain.** (Adapted from Eagle S. *Medical Terminology in a Flash!* Philadelphia: FA Davis; 2006:47.)

shown to play a role in dreaming, although the full function is not yet understood (see Box 11–2).

- *Midbrain* consists of two nerve tracts that convey sensory and motor impulses. Within the midbrain is a tunnel that connects the third and fourth ventricles. Visual and auditory reflexes are controlled here. An example of a visual reflex is blinking if something comes toward the eye. Turning toward a loud sound is an auditory reflex.

The *cerebellum* is located at the base of the skull. This cauliflower-shaped structure maintains balance and posture and coordinates movement. The cerebellum along with the midbrain uses the receptors in the ear to regulate equilibrium or balance.

The *diencephalon* or interbrain is directly above the brainstem in the interior of the brain. This structure is saddle-shaped and acts as the relay station for all incoming stimuli. It also controls body temperature, sleep patterns, and whether a person feels hungry or full. The diencephalon is made of three structures: thalamus, hypothalamus, and epithalamus.

- *Thalamus* is found in the third ventricle of the brain and is a relay station for sensory impulses to the cerebrum. As sensations pass through the thalamus, they are recognized as individual sensations, but they can also be interpreted

## Box 11–2 Dreams

Dreams are the thoughts, images, feelings, and sounds one experiences when asleep. Why we dream is not fully understood, and there are many theories. Some theories for the purpose of dreams are that they allow us to gain control of waking emotions, compensate for waking attitudes, uncover memories, find solutions to problems, or act like a delete mechanism that erases extra stimuli from the mind.

Where dreams form in the brain is also poorly understood. It is known that when we dream we are in a state of rapid eye movement (REM) sleep. In this state, the brain is highly active, although the body is at rest. During REM sleep, breathing, heart rate, and blood pressure increase, but the brain decreases levels of some neurotransmitters to keep the body still. The brain cycles in and out of REM sleep, so the body changes between deeper and lighter sleep. It is estimated that a person dreams about 2 hours over the course of the night.

The pons has been found to control muscle movement during dreaming and allow rapid eye movement to occur. It is also believed that the pons sends out random signals that the brain turns into dreams. The parietal lobe is also involved in creating dreams. Research has shown that the parietal lobe, especially the area of the limbic system, which is responsible for emotions and urges, is stimulated. Also stimulated is the occipital lobe, where perception and abstract thinking occur. All of these stimuli being processed together may be responsible for the random images and seemingly senseless activities in dreams.

Damage to the dream-producing areas of the brain has changed the types of dreams experienced by people or even stopped the ability to dream. Lack of REM sleep and lack of dreaming have been shown to affect mood and coordination. They have been linked to depression, obesity, chronic fatigue, and poor memory.

Whatever the purpose of dreams, humans are not the only ones that dream. Other mammals such as dogs, cats, elephants, and horses have been found to produce dreams during REM sleep. Even fish have shown signs that they are in a dream state.

as being together. For example, a fluffy towel just taken from the dryer feels both warm and soft. The thalamus recognizes both sensations and allows both to be felt at the same time. The thalamus is also responsible for blocking some sensations, such as the movements of others in a room or the sound of the air-conditioning, allowing a person to concentrate on one thing at a time.

- *Hypothalamus* is located below the thalamus and above the pituitary gland. This structure is the center for regulation of body temperature, hydration, and metabolism. The hypothalamus is also part of the limbic system, which comprises several structures within the brain and controls emotion. Drives and emotions controlled by the hypothalamus include thirst, hunger, pleasure, and pain.

- *Epithalamus* creates the roof of the third ventricle. This structure forms the pineal gland and the choroid plexus. The choroid plexus comprises a mesh of capillaries that produce cerebrospinal fluid.

- The largest section of the brain is the **cerebrum**. It has two halves or hemispheres held together by a tough yet flexible tissue called the **corpus callosum**. The cerebrum resembles a walnut, and the place where a walnut would be broken into halves is the corpus callosum.

To provide more surface area, the tissue of the cerebrum is folded. The folds are called **gyri**, and the grooves in between are **sulci**. The cerebrum is the structure that makes us human. It holds all learned information and stores memories, creates thoughts, provides the ability to reason, and provides the ability to form language. These functions along with all bodily functions are controlled from different **lobes**, or areas of the brain. Each lobe is named for the cranial bone under which it is located. The lobes are parietal, occipital, temporal, and frontal (see Fig. 11–7).

- *Parietal lobe* is located behind the frontal lobes and is the mid-section of the brain. The functions of this lobe are the least understood, but it is known that it interprets stimuli from the receptors of the skin and allows us to recognize sensations such as pain, temperature, and textures. Areas of the parietal lobe also allow us to read and do arithmetic. Because damage to this lobe may result in **optic ataxia**, which is difficulty in reaching for and grasping an object, this lobe is believed to aid in hand-eye coordination and depth perception.

> Flashpoint
>
> There are 1 million brain injuries a year. The Glasgow Coma Scale rates injury severity and determines how responsive the person is to behavioral measures. The Glasgow Outcome Scale is used at various points after an injury to determine the prognosis or likelihood of the person regaining his or her independence.

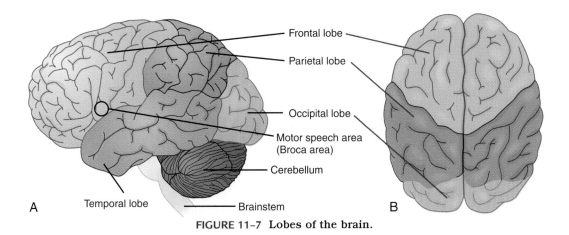

A

B

Frontal lobe
Parietal lobe
Occipital lobe
Motor speech area (Broca area)
Cerebellum
Temporal lobe
Brainstem

**FIGURE 11–7 Lobes of the brain.**

- *Occipital lobe* is located in the back of the brain and is the smallest of the lobes. Visual stimuli are interpreted here. This lobe is also believed to aid in hearing. Injury to this lobe can result in visual hallucinations, color blindness, and **agraphia**, which is the inability to write.
- *Temporal lobes* are found on each side of the cerebrum. These lobes are responsible for hearing, perception, and recognition. Stimuli from the olfactory receptors in the nose are also interpreted in this area. Damage to a temporal lobe can result in loss of the ability to remember words, recognize visual images, and recognize human faces, which is a condition called **prosopagnosia.** Impairment of long-term memory may also occur.
- *Frontal lobe* is located behind the frontal bone or forehead. This part of the cerebrum has many diverse functions. The frontal lobe is responsible for language, problem solving, and the ability to reason. It allows us to plan and make judgments. This lobe is responsible for impulse control and causes us to worry. This area controls motor function and allows us to move the skeletal muscles voluntarily. The ability to speak comes from a specialized area of the cerebrum called Broca's area. This section of the brain is usually found in the left hemisphere only. Damage to this area may result in aphasia, which is the inability to form words into sentences. Frontal lobe injury can result in varied symptoms, such as impaired movement, loss of intellect, altered personality, an increase in high-risk activities, and mood changes.

*Flashpoint*

The brain and spinal cord are surrounded by about 125 to 150 mL of cerebrospinal fluid.

Deep inside the middle of the brain are four chambers called **ventricles**. They are filled with a clear fluid produced by the ependymocytes called **cerebrospinal fluid**. This fluid also circulates around the brain and spinal cord and protects them from shock. Nutrients that are filtered from the blood are also found in the cerebrospinal fluid.

The outer brain is protected by three layers of tissue called **meninges** (see Fig. 11–8). The innermost layer is the **pia mater** (thin mother), which is a thin wrapping that lies directly against the brain. The next layer is a fibrous, weblike tissue called the **arachnoid mater** (spider mother), and the outermost layer is composed of thick, fibrous connective tissue called the **dura mater** (tough mother). Together, these layers form a fluid-filled barrier to protect the CNS.

Attached to the brain are 12 pairs of **cranial nerves** (see Table 11–3). These nerves create the movement of the head, neck, and abdomen. Cranial nerves are also responsible for detection of sensory information that is interpreted as sight, sound, smell, and taste, and reflexes such as swallowing, blinking, and saliva production.

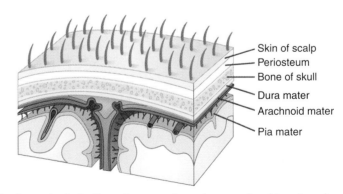

Skin of scalp
Periosteum
Bone of skull
Dura mater
Arachnoid mater
Pia mater

**FIGURE 11–8** Meninges include three layers: pia mater, arachnoid mater, dura mater (from innermost to outermost).

## TABLE 11–3

## CRANIAL NERVES

| Number | Name | Function |
|---|---|---|
| I | Olfactory | Sense of smell |
| II | Optic | Sense of vision |
| III | Oculomotor | Movement of the eyelid; constriction of pupil |
| IV | Trochlear | Movement of the eyeball |
| V | Trigeminal | Chewing, sensation of face, scalp, and teeth |
| VI | Abducens | Movement of the eyeball |
| VII | Facial | Contraction of facial muscles; production of saliva; sense of taste |
| VIII | Vestibulocochlear (acoustic) | Sense of hearing; sense of equilibrium |
| IX | Glossopharyngeal | Sense of taste; reflexes for heart, lungs, and blood pressure; contraction of pharynx |
| X | Vagus | Speaking; decreases heart rate; peristalsis; increases digestive juices |
| XI | Accessory | Contraction of neck and shoulder muscles; speaking |
| XII | Hypoglossal | Movement of the tongue |

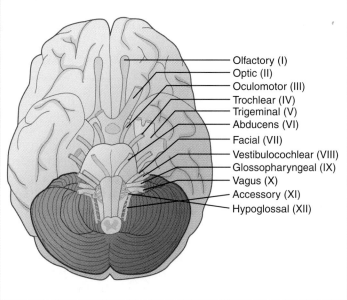

All the spinal nerves originate in the ventral portion of the brain. The first four pairs of nerves are the olfactory, optic, oculomotor, and trochlear, and they begin in the frontal lobe. The next four pairs are the trigeminal, abducens, facial, and vestibulocochlear. All four pairs are connected to the pons. The last four pairs of nerves are the glossopharyngeal, vagus, accessory, and hypoglossal, and they attach to the medulla oblongata.

### Spinal Cord

The **spinal cord** is composed of two bundles, or tracts, of nerves that transmit impulses to and from the brain. These tracts are the ascending tract, which takes sensory information to the brain, and the descending tract, which takes impulses away from the brain and sends them throughout the body. An example of this transmission occurs when you touch a hot object. The impulses travel from the sensory receptors in the fingertip to the ascending tract of the spinal cord and then to the brain, which interprets the impulse as heat. An impulse from the brain travels to the descending tract to cause you to move your finger away from the hot object.

The spinal cord resides inside the spine, which is a column of 24 separate bones called vertebrae. Attached to the spinal cord are 31 pairs of **spinal nerve**s. These nerves are located in different regions of the spinal column and in the bones inferior to the vertebrae called the sacrum and coccyx. The first 8 pairs of nerves are found in cervical vertebrae, the thoracic vertebrae have 12 pairs of nerves, and the lumbar vertebrae have five pairs of nerves. The next five pairs of nerves are found at the sacrum, and there is one pair of nerves at the coccyx (see Fig. 11–9). Each pair of nerves has two branches or roots that leave the spine on either side of the bone to which they are attached. These roots create the nerves of the PNS.

## Peripheral Nervous System

The PNS is found outside the CNS and consists of the spinal nerves that carry impulses to and from the spinal cord and the cranial nerves that carry impulses to and from the brain.

The PNS has several divisions. First, the PNS is divided into the somatic (body) nervous system and the autonomic (self-controlled) nervous system. The **somatic nervous system** controls the voluntary functions of the body, which includes muscle movement. The **autonomic nervous system** controls involuntary bodily functions, such as heart rate, breathing, and digestion. The autonomic nervous system is divided further into the sympathetic and parasympathetic nervous systems.

The **sympathetic nervous system** increases heart rate, respiration, and blood pressure so that more oxygen can be given to the tissues; it dilates the pupils; and it slows digestion. This response is called the *"fight or flight"* response, and it prepares the body to act quickly in a stressful situation. You can feel this response if you are sitting in the classroom and the fire alarm sounds. The sudden loud sound startles you, and your heartbeat and respiration immediately increase. When you realize what the sound is, your heart rate slows, and you begin to breathe normally. Sometimes you may feel a little nauseous or tired after this response because of the sudden increase and decrease of neurotransmitters.

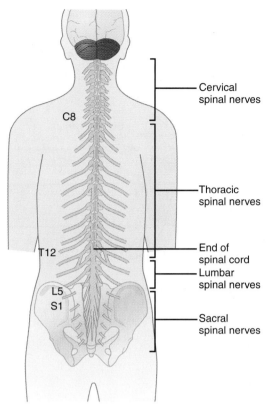

Cervical
spinal nerves

Thoracic
spinal nerves

End of
spinal cord

Lumbar
spinal nerves

Sacral
spinal nerves

C8

T12

L5
S1

FIGURE 11–9  Spinal nerves.

*Epinephrine*, or adrenaline, is a chemical that acts as a hormone and a neurotransmitter, and it controls the functions of the body during the sympathetic
response. Epinephrine is aided by another stress hormone called norepinephrine, which also can act as a neurotransmitter. *Norepinephrine* directly
increases heart rate and speeds the release of glucose to be used for energy to
fuel the skeletal muscles.

The **parasympathetic nervous system** slows down the sympathetic response
and returns the body to its normal state. It uses the hormone *acetylcholine*
to counter the effects of epinephrine from the sympathetic response. It also regulates the body during its normal functioning.

# Reflexes

Because many responses of the body must be done repeatedly, some nerve
pathways are programmed so that certain stimuli get the same response every
time. These types of responses are called **reflexes,** and they are rapid, involuntary, and predictable (see Fig. 11–10). There are two types of reflexes: somatic
reflexes that control body responses and autonomic reflexes that control involuntary responses. Reflexes can use brain and spinal neurons or just spinal
neurons for an even faster response.

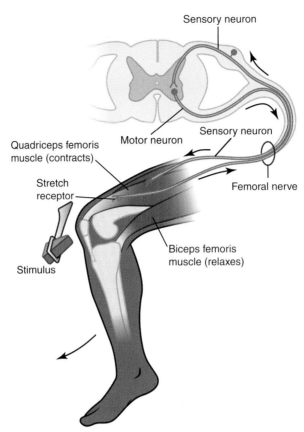

FIGURE 11-10  Patellar reflex.

*Somatic reflexes* are ones that stimulate the skeletal muscles. An example of a somatic reflex is the withdrawal reflex, such as pulling away from a hot object. Another is the patellar reflex, which occurs when the knee tendon is struck and the lower leg jerks upward. *Autonomic reflexes* regulate activities of the smooth muscles and are responsible for body functions such as sweating, urination, and digestion.

See Table 11–4 for a summary of pathological conditions of the nervous system.

### TABLE 11-4

#### PATHOLOGY TERMS OF THE NERVOUS SYSTEM

| | |
|---|---|
| Amyotrophic lateral sclerosis (ALS) | Progressive weakness and wasting of the muscles caused by degeneration of the motor neurons; eventually the muscles become paralyzed; usually begins as weakness in the muscles of the arms and muscles involved in swallowing and speech; also called Lou Gehrig disease |
| Aphasia | Defective or absent language functions because of disease or injury of Broca area in the frontal lobe of the brain |
| Ataxia | Motor dysfunction because of disease or injury to the brain causing loss of coordination and unsteady gait |
| Dementia | Progressive loss of cognitive and intellectual function of the brain; causes include brain injury, depression |

**TABLE 11–4**

**PATHOLOGY TERMS OF THE NERVOUS SYSTEM—cont'd**

| | |
|---|---|
| Epilepsy | Group of disorders characterized by recurrent seizures |
| Huntington chorea | Inherited disease that causes speech disturbances, muscle tics, and degeneration of the cerebral cortex. Effects at 30-50 years old |
| Meningitis | Inflammation of the covering of the brain and spinal cord caused by virus or bacteria |
| Parkinson disease | Progressive degeneration of the neurons of the brain that causes tremors, stiff joints, and unblinking eyes; usually occurs in adults older than 60 |
| Spina bifida | Congenital malformation in which the spine fails to close; it can occur in the occult form, where the spine appears closed from the outside, or in the most severe form, where the spinal cord within the meninges is outside the body |
| Tourette syndrome | Neurological disorder characterized by spasms, tics, uncontrolled vocal sounds, and inappropriate verbal responses |

# Practice Exercises

## Multiple Choice

1. The neuroglia that act as phagocytes are the _____.

    a. astrocytes

    b. microglia

    c. oligodendrocytes

    d. ependymal cells

2. A _____ is the space between one neuron and another.

    a. gap

    b. neural space

    c. synapse

    d. synaptic space

3. The tough outer layer of tissue surrounding the brain is called the _____.

    a. pia mater

    b. arachnoid mater

    c. soma mater

    d. dura mater

4. Visual stimuli are processes in the _____ lobe.

    a. occipital

    b. parietal

    c. frontal

    d. temporal

5. The _____ regulates body temperature and hydration.

    a. epithalamus

    b. hypothalamus

    c. pons

    d. cerebrum

6. The _____ aids the medulla oblongata in regulating breathing.

    a. epithalamus

    b. pons

    c. cerebellum

    d. hypothalamus

7. _____ form the support for neurons and create the blood-brain barrier.

   a.   astrocytes

   b.   microglia

   c.   oligodendrocytes

   d.   ependymal cells

8. _____ are responses that are rapid, involuntary, and predictable.

   a.   senses

   b.   reflexes

   c.   nerves

   d.   neuroglia

9. The chemicals that cross the synaptic space are _____.

   a.   hormones

   b.   neural enzymes

   c.   neurotransmitters

   d.   impulses

10. The _____ controls balance, posture, and muscle coordination.

   a.   cerebellum

   b.   cerebrum

   c.   hypothalamus

   d.   pons

## True or False

1. True   False      The cerebellum regulates body temperature.

2. True   False      The meninges cover the brain and spinal cord.

3. True   False      Myelin is produced by the astrocytes.

4. True   False      The somatic nervous system controls involuntary movement.

5. True   False      The PNS is made up of the brain and spinal cord.

6. True   False      There are 31 pairs of cranial nerves.

7. True   False      The sympathetic nervous system is responsible for the "fight or flight" response.

8. True   False      The corpus callosum joins the two hemispheres of the brain.

9. True   False     Nerve cells are also called neurons.

10. True   False     The brainstem is the area of the brain that controls thought, memory, and language.

## Fill in the Blank

1. The _____ neurons take impulses to the CNS, and _____ neurons take impulses away from the CNS.

2. A _____ is the space between one neuron and another.

3. The nucleus of a nerve cell is in the _____.

4. The folds of the brain are _____ and the folds are _____.

5. The _____ nervous system speeds up the body, and the _____ nervous system slows it down.

6. Electrical impulses are carried from one neuron to the next by the _____.

7. The _____ have cilia that circulate the cerebrospinal fluid.

8. The fluid within the ventricles of the brain is the _____.

9. Afferent neurons are also called _____ neurons.

10. Oligodendrocytes produce _____, which is the protective covering around the neurons.

## Short Answer

1. **Compare and contrast the sympathetic and parasympathetic nervous systems.**

2. **Compare and contrast the autonomic and somatic nervous systems.**

## Labeling

*Fill in the blanks with the appropriate anatomical terms.*

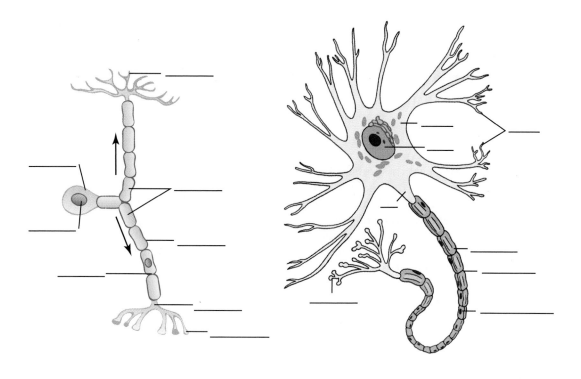

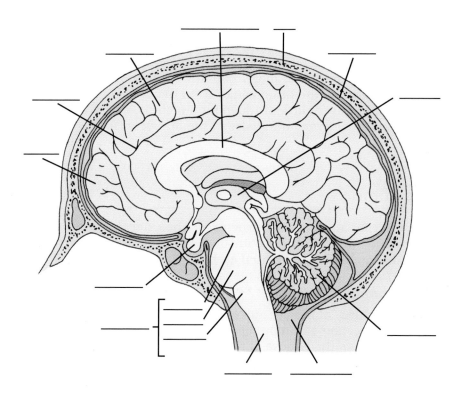

# 12 THE SENSES

The senses provide the stimuli the nervous system interprets to give the body information about the internal and external environment. Sight, hearing, smell, taste, and touch are the senses that provide a way for the body to detect these changes. All senses have sensory receptors that are triggered and start the stimulus along the peripheral nervous system to the brain. There are two types of sensory receptors: special and general. The receptors for sight, hearing, smell, and taste are referred to as "special senses" and are found in specific areas of the body. Touch is a general sense because the sensations felt are scattered throughout the body.

This chapter discusses the physical structures of the eye, ear, nose, tongue, and skin and the different receptors responsible for each sense. In addition, the differences in vision and the different of types of deafness are described.

## Sight

The organ of sight is the *eye*. The eye provides ***vision***, which is a means of interpreting light waves and changing them into images the brain can recognize. Of all the sensory receptors in the body, the eye contains the largest amount. Humans rely on vision more than any other sense because most information processed by the brain comes from the eye.

The eyeball changes very little throughout a lifetime. At birth, eyeballs are about 18 mm, and they grow to full size in the first year. A full-sized eyeball is 24 mm.

### Structures of the Eye

The eye has external and internal structures. The external structures do not contribute to vision, but aid the eye in some way. The internal structures are the layers and chambers of the actual eyeball.

#### External Structures

The external structures of the eye surround the eye; they do not provide vision, but they aid in protection and movement of the eye. These external structures are often referred to as the adnexa of the eye. They include the tissue surrounding the eye, the glands, and muscles (see Fig. 12–1).

*Flashpoint*

The senses maintain homeostasis by detecting and interpreting stimuli so that the other body systems can respond accordingly.

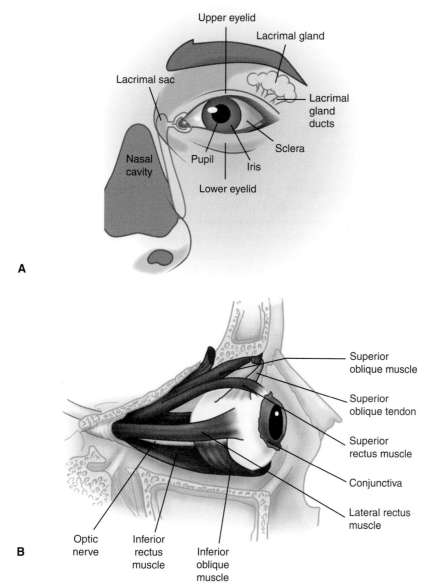

FIGURE 12–1  **External structures of the eye.** *(A)* Anterior view. *(B)* Sagittal view

The eye is located in an orbit of bone that is set back in the skull, so it is protected by the facial bones. The eye is further protected by tissue covering it called the eyelid. The hairs attached to the eyelid are the eyelashes; they help keep debris from the eye.

Located between the nose and the eyeball are the **lacrimal glands**, which produce tears to lubricate the eye and flush out debris. Tears also keep the eye moistened and provide lubrication for the eyelids. Within tears is an enzyme called lysozyme that destroys bacteria and immunoglobulins that protect against microorganisms that may try to enter the body through the eye. The lacrimal glands drain into the nasal cavity to prevent the eyes from overflowing with tears. This overflow into the nasal cavity is what causes the nose to "run" when crying.

Attached to the eyeball by tendons are six extrinsic (external) muscles. These muscles control the movement of the eye. Each muscle is responsible for one primary movement, but several may act together if needed. The extrinsic muscles are:

- Lateral rectus: Moves the eye to the sides
- Medial rectus: Moves the eye to the middle
- Superior rectus: Raises the eye
- Inferior rectus: Lowers the eye
- Inferior oblique: Raises the eye and turns it to the side
- Superior oblique: Lowers the eye and turns it to the side

### Internal Structures

The internal structures of the eye are the parts of the eyeball itself. All these structures contribute to vision. These structures include the sclera, the cornea, the lens, the retina, and the chambers (see Fig. 12–2).

The eyeball is composed of three separate layers of tissue. The outermost layer is the *sclera*, a tough, fibrous membrane that creates what is called the "white of the eye." The anterior portion of the sclera is transparent to allow light to enter the eye, and this portion is called the *cornea*. The sclera is covered in a clear membrane called the *conjunctiva*. This tissue provides protection to the eye. The conjunctiva can become inflamed and red because of an allergy or from a bacterial infection. This condition is called *conjunctivitis*, or "pink eye."

Under the sclera is the middle layer of the eye called the *choroid layer*. This layer is where the bloods vessels are located. Anteriorly, the choroid layer forms *ciliary bodies*, which are armlike structures that hold another structure called the *lens* in place. The lens, also called the crystalline lens, can stretch or thicken to focus on near or far objects. The lens is located posterior to the

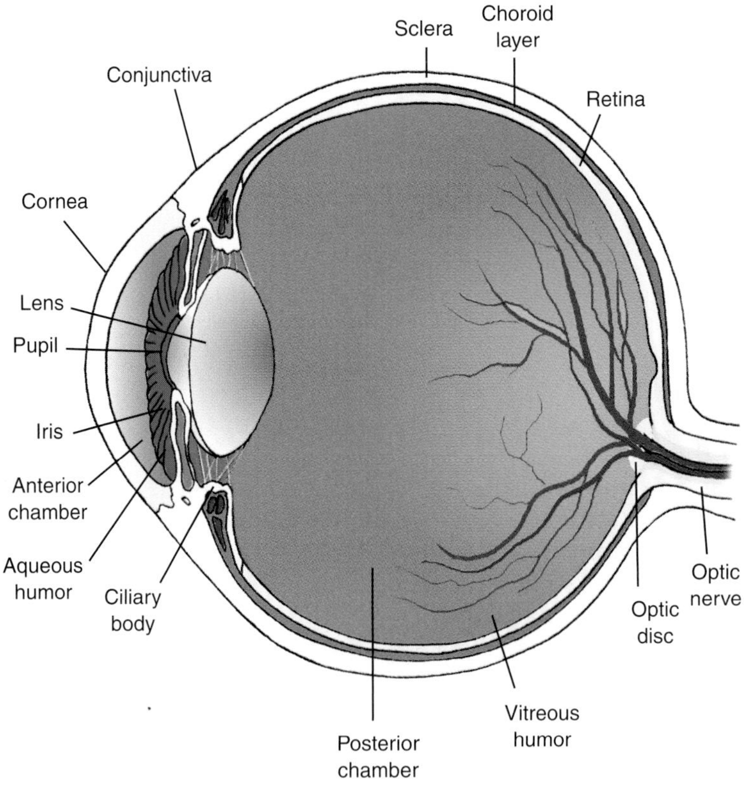

*Flashpoint*

The cornea is the same thickness as a dime.

FIGURE 12–2 **Internal structures of the eye.** (Adapted from Eagle S. *Medical Terminology in a Flash!* Philadelphia, PA: FA Davis; 2006:249.)

*iris* (rainbow), which is the colored portion of the eye. The iris surrounds the *pupil*, which opens and closes, depending on the availability of the light and the closeness of an object.

The innermost layer of the eye is the **retina**. The retina contains the photoreceptors responsible for vision. There are two types of photoreceptors: cones and rods.

**Cones** provide color perception. There are three types of cones, and each is sensitive to a different wavelength of light that would be interpreted as a color. There are red, green, and blue cones. When light hits the retina, it stimulates one of these cones. To see a color other than these three, two different cones are stimulated, such as blue and red to make purple. If all three cones are activated at once, the color seen is white. The cones themselves do not actually interpret the colors. The brain takes the stimuli from the cones, and it recognizes the color of an object.

**Rods** distinguish between shadows. These receptors also allow us to see different shades of gray. They are also responsible for peripheral vision, or the ability to see objects from the side of the eye.

The eye also contains two chambers. The first is the anterior chamber located behind the cornea. Inside this chamber is the **aqueous humor** (watery fluid), a clear, watery fluid that contains nutrients derived from the blood. This fluid is constantly replenished to supply nutrients to the eye tissues. Within the eyeball is the posterior chamber. It contains a thicker fluid called **vitreous humor** (glassy fluid). This fluid gives the eyeball its shape and its firm, yet springy texture. Because this fluid provides no nutrients, it is not replenished.

Posterior to the eyeball is the **optic nerve** that sends visual stimuli to the brain. There are no rods or cones where the optic nerve attaches to the retina. This area is the optic disc, commonly called the "blind spot" because when an image hits this spot, there are no visual receptors to conduct the stimuli to the brain. The medulla oblongata in the midbrain is responsible for interpreting visual stimuli from the optic nerve.

*Flashpoint*
There are 1.2 million nerve fibers in the optic nerve.

## Process of Vision

For sight to occur, light must first enter the eye. Light enters through the cornea and passes through the pupil and into the lens. The cornea bends, or refracts, the light from an object, and the image is reversed and turned upside down. Light travels through the lens, then through the vitreous humor, and stops at the retina. As the light moves through the lens, it forms into a point. This single point of light lands somewhere on the retina. The photoreceptors take the stimulus created by the light to the optic nerve, which takes the stimulus to the brain. The eye "sees" the image of light right side up even though it enters the eye upside down. This occurs because the brain not only interprets what the light image is, but also compensates for the **refraction** so that the image is correctly perceived (see Fig. 12–3).

See Fig. 12–4 for a flowchart of the pathway of light through the eye.

### Variations of Vision

Any change in the shape of the lens affects how light enters the eye. From a distance, light enters the eye as parallel rays, so the lens does not need to change to get the image into the eye. Light entering the eye from a close object causes the light to scatter, so the lens must shorten and bulge slightly to get the light into a tighter form to correct the image. This change in the eye is called **accommodation**. When the lens changes normally in response to the distance of objects, this vision is called **emmetropia** (harmonious vision).

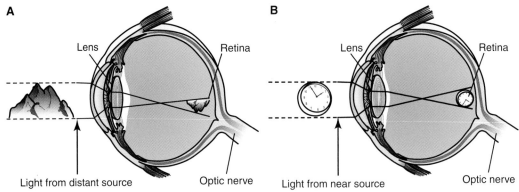

**FIGURE 12–3 Refraction of light in the eye.** *(A)* **Distant vision.** *(B)* **Near vision.**

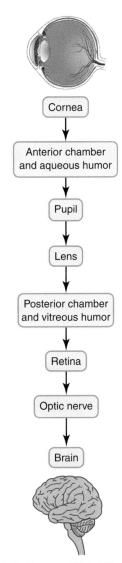

**FIGURE 12–4 Pathway of light through the eye.**

If the lens cannot accommodate properly because the lens is not shortening or stretching enough, the eye cannot focus correctly. These are refractive defects and cause changes in visual acuity or the ability to see (see Box 12–1). One type of refractive defect causes myopia (short vision), or nearsightedness, where the eye cannot focus on far objects and they appear blurry. With myopia, the cornea is too curved, or the eyeball is elongated and cannot change to accommodate far-away objects. Correction is with a lens that has a concave shape that spreads the light that enters the eye. Another refractive defect causes *hyperopia* (far vision) or farsightedness, where the eye cannot focus on objects that are close. In this case, the cornea is too flat and cannot thicken to focus on near objects, so they appear blurry. Correction is a convex lens that brings the light closer together as it enters the eye. As eyes age, they lose the ability to accommodate. *Presbyopia* (old vision) is the natural-occurring inability to focus on near objects. Many people need glasses to read as they age to correct this change.

Some corneas have an unequal curvature. This is called *astigmatism* (not pointed). With astigmatism, light entering the eye does not form a point, but enters as a straight line, so the image cannot be focused. Because the defect is uneven, it is more difficult to correct, but a lens shaped more like a cylinder can be used. See Figure 12–5 for illustrations of refractive defects.

Vision can also be impaired by changes in the photoreceptors. *Nyctolopia*, or night blindness, occurs because the rods no longer respond to light, so the difference between shadows is impaired in the darkness.

*Color blindness* is an impairment of the cones so that differences in some colors cannot be perceived. The most common type is red-green color blindness, in which the colors red, yellow, and green cannot be distinguished. A rare type of color blindness is called *monochromacy*, where all color vision is gone, and sight is only in shades of gray. Color blindness is more common in males than females because a defect on the X chromosome is responsible for this condition. A female has two X chromosomes, and a male only has one. If a female inherits a faulty X chromosome, the other normal one compensates. In a male, there is nothing to compensate for the defective chromosome, so color blindness occurs. It is possible for a female to be color blind if her father is color blind and her mother is a carrier and she receives two defective X chromosomes.

See Table 12–1 for the different types of vision.

Flashpoint

Laser assisted in situ keratomileusis, or LASIK, is a procedure that uses a laser to cut and reshape the cornea to correct refractive vision defects.

## Box 12–1 Visual Acuity Testing

Visual acuity, or the ability to see, is measured in several ways. The most common method is by using a Snellen chart. This wall chart uses 11 lines of letters of decreasing sizes. The largest line is the single letter E. Each line also designates a certain acuity.

Normal visual acuity is considered 20/20. This means that the average person standing at 20 feet from the chart sees the same line clearly. The upper number is the 20-foot distance from the chart and stays the same for each line. The bottom number shows acuity. The vision becomes more difficult below 20/20 and easier above 20/20. Someone with 20/15 vision sees better than normal, and someone with 20/200 vision sees poorer than normal. A person with 20/15 vision can see a line of letters at 20 feet that someone else would be able to see only at 15 feet. A person with 20/200 vision sees a line of letters at 20 feet that someone else could see at 200 feet away from the chart. People with 20/200 vision are considered to be legally blind and are able to see only the top line of the Snellen chart, which is the single E.

*Continued*

## Box 12–1 Visual Acuity Testing—cont'd

For children who cannot read, there is a Snellen chart with pictures of stars, cups, crosses, hearts, hands, and boats that a child could easily recognize. The largest image is a single boat. As with the adult chart, the lines of images change in order and decrease in size.

A measurement of the ability to see written print is called a Jaeger test. Eleven paragraphs of decreasing size are written on a single card. The patient holds the card 14 to 16 inches away from his or her eyes and reads as far as the print remains clear.

Color acuity is tested using the Ishihara chart. This chart is actually a book containing a series of 14 different plates. Each plate is a circle created by colored dots. A number or shape in the middle of the plate is created by another series of dots in a different color. If the number or shape cannot be seen, the person is deficient in that color and considered to be color blind.

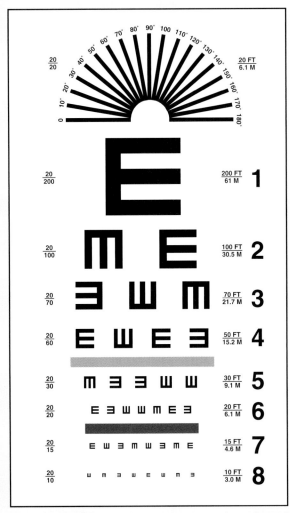

Snellen chart. (From Eagle S, Brassington C, Dailey C, Goretti C. *The Professional Medical Assistant.* Philadelphia, PA: FA Davis; 2009:763.)

## Box 12-1 Visual Acuity Testing—cont'd

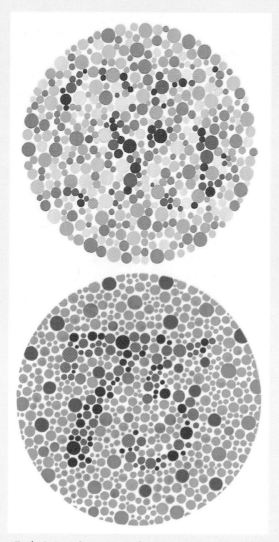

Ishihara plate. (From Eagle S, BrassingtonC, Dailey C, Goretti C. *The Professional Medical Assistant.* Philadelphia, PA: FA Davis; 2009:766.)

## Reflexes of the Eye

A reflex is a rapid, involuntary, and expected response to a stimulus. The pupil of the eye has two types of reflexes: photopupillary response and accommodation pupillary response. The ***photopupillary response*** causes the pupil to constrict when the eyes are suddenly exposed to bright light. This constriction protects the photoreceptors from being damaged by the sudden flood of light into the eye. Light suddenly entering the eye can be painful and causes momentary blindness. You notice this reflex when you step out of a dark building into the bright sun and you are blinded for a few seconds. This occurs because the pupil did not have a chance to accommodate the sudden change in light.

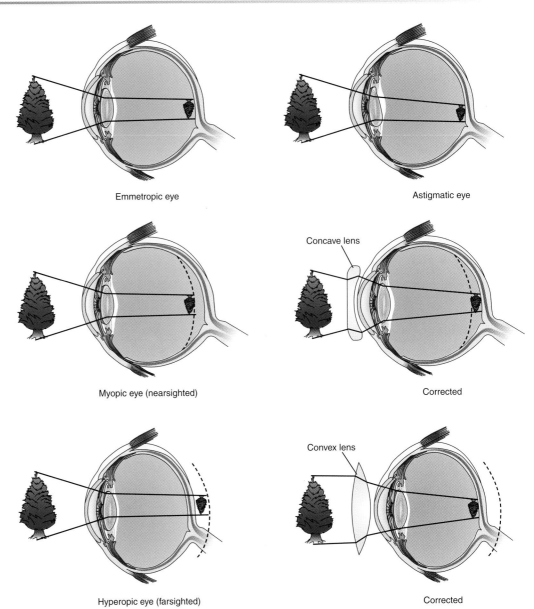

Emmetropic eye

Astigmatic eye

Myopic eye (nearsighted)

Concave lens

Corrected

Hyperopic eye (farsighted)

Convex lens

Corrected

**FIGURE 12–5  Refraction defects**

| TABLE 12–1 | |
|---|---|
| **TYPES OF VISION** | |
| Hyperopia | Refractive defect where the eye is too short or the cornea is too flat; objects in the distance are clear, but close objects are blurred; also called farsightedness |
| Myopia | Refractive defect where the eye is too long or the cornea is too thick; near objects are seen clearly, but objects in the distance are blurred; also called nearsightedness |
| Nyctolopia | The rods of the eye have lost the ability to respond to light, so vision at night is impaired; also called night blindness |
| Presbyopia | Progressive loss of ability to focus on near objects because of aging |
| Astigmatism | Unequal curvature of the cornea so that light entering the eye does not form a point, but enters as straight lines |
| Color blindness | Genetic defect that causes the loss of color differentiation; usually affects the ability to see the difference between red, yellow, and green |

The pupils also constrict when focusing on very near objects. Closing of the pupil causes sharper focus of the lens and is called the *accommodation pupillary reflex*. The muscles of the ciliary body and the muscles of the iris also constrict to produce this reflex. Eventually, these muscles fatigue as the constriction is maintained and cause the eyes to ache. This is called eyestrain.

# Hearing

The *ear* is the structure that provides the sense of hearing by bringing sound stimuli to the brain for interpretation. In contrast to the other "special senses" that use chemical reactions to change stimuli into a form the brain can understand, the ear uses a mechanical process to transmit sound to the nervous system. In addition to hearing, the ear is responsible for maintaining equilibrium or balance.

## Structures of the Ear

Before a sound can be interpreted, vibrations in the air must be brought into the ear and pass through several structures before it reaches the brain (see Fig. 12–6). The ear is divided into three sections: the outer ear, the middle ear, and the inner ear.

### Outer Ear

The outer ear consists of the *auricle*, or pinna, which is the structure on the outside of the skull. This structure is commonly referred to as the ear even though it is only the external portion. The auricle is constructed of cartilage, and every individual has a uniquely shaped ear. Attached to the auricle and located within the skull is a tube called the *auditory canal*. Within the canal are ceruminous glands, which are specialized sweat glands that make *cerumen* or earwax, which acts a lubricant.

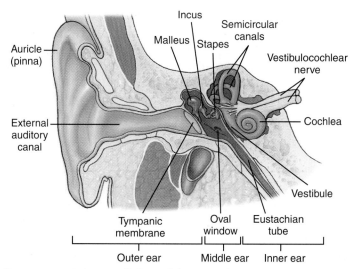

**FIGURE 12–6 Structures of the ear.** (Adapted from Eagle S. *Medical Terminology in a Flash!* Philadelphia, PA: FA Davis; 2006:250.)

Sound is funneled into the canal by the auricle, and it bounces against the *tympanic membrane*, or eardrum. The tympanic membrane is the division between the outer and middle ear.

### Middle Ear

The middle ear consists of three small bones collectively called **ossicles**. These bones are the smallest in the human body, and all three bones together take up less space than a dime. When the tympanic membrane vibrates, it sends the sound to the first ossicle called the **malleus** (hammer), which strikes against the second ossicle called **incus** (anvil). The incus sends vibrations to the third ossicle called the **stapes** (stirrups). The stapes connects to the inner ear by going through an opening called the **oval window**. Also in the middle ear is the **eustachian tube**, or auditory tube, which connects the ear to the throat. This tube plays no role in hearing, but maintains air pressure on the eardrum. It is this tube in which you feel a popping sensation when changing altitudes as the tube changes shape to accommodate the difference in air pressure.

### Inner Ear

The inner ear comprises a series of connecting tubes and chambers collectively called a **labyrinth** (maze). Inside the labyrinth are the **semicircular canals** and the **cochlea** (shell). Sound goes from the stapes into the semicircular canals and then to the cochlea.

Inside the cochlea is the **organ of Corti**, a small chamber that contains **hair cells**. These hairs vibrate and send the stimulus to the **vestibulocochlear nerve**, or auditory nerve, which takes the stimulus to the temporal lobe of the brain for interpretation of the sound.

See Figure 12–7 for a flowchart tracing the pathway of sound through the ear.

## Sound

Sound is created by vibrations called waves. The number of vibrations in a sound wave is called **frequency**, and it is measured in Hertz (Hz), where 1 Hz is equal to one sound wave per second. When sound enters the ear, the sensation caused by that sound is its **pitch**. Frequency and pitch are related to one another, so the higher the frequency of a sound, the higher the pitch, and the lower the frequency of a sound, the lower the pitch. The range of human hearing is 20 to 20,000 Hz. Often we can feel the vibration of a sound that is too low for us to hear, and sounds that are too high can be painful. The ability to hear higher-frequency sounds decreases as we age. To determine the ability to hear, auditory acuity testing is done. This type of testing uses different methods of introducing sound waves to the ear to measure the ability of the ear to conduct sound or to transmit nerve impulses (see Box 12–2).

## Types of Hearing

Hearing occurs by two different processes: conduction and sensorineural. **Conduction** is the process of sound waves being funneled into the auricle and traveling through the outer, middle, and inner ear and arriving in the cochlea. The sound stimulates the tympanic membrane and ossicles, so the vibrations continue until they reach the hair cells within the cochlea. The

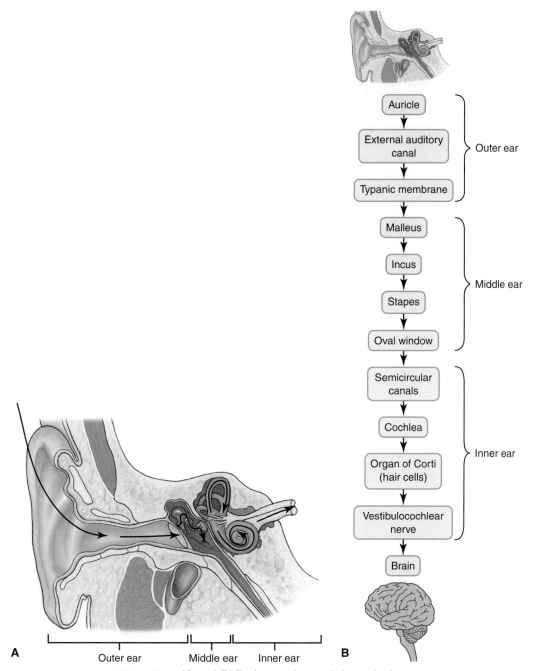

**FIGURE 12-7** *(A and B)* Pathway of sound through the ear.

hair cells vibrate and transmit that vibration to the nervous system. Conduction deafness occurs when sound is inhibited anywhere along the path from the auricle to the cochlea (see Fig. 12–8). This type of deafness may be caused by impacted earwax, frequent ear infections, and inherited diseases that change the ability of the ossicles to transmit sound.

***Sensorineural*** hearing begins in the hair cells located inside the cochlea. These cells take the stimulus of the sound wave and convert it to an electrical

## Box 12–2 Auditory Acuity Testing

Auditory ability can be measured by several different methods. The testing can be simple or complex.

Simple methods to test hearing ability include whispering by the ear, listening to a ticking watch, or using a tuning fork. When using a tuning fork, hearing is determined by placing a vibrating tuning fork behind the ear and on top of the head. The vibration should be heard and felt by the patient. This is done to identify nerve and conduction deafness.

Complex procedures include the use of an audiometer or a tympanometer. Audiometry is a procedure for overall hearing. During testing, the patient wears earphones and the sits facing away from the audiometer. This instrument can produce sounds of varying intensity and length. The patient raises his or her hand to indicate in which ear the sound is heard. Sounds start from the lowest pitch and get increasingly higher.

Tympanometry is a procedure to measure the ability of the middle ear to transmit sound. A probe is inserted into the ear canal, and the pressure within the ear is compared with the pressure within the room. This test is commonly done to diagnose middle ear infections and conduction deafness.

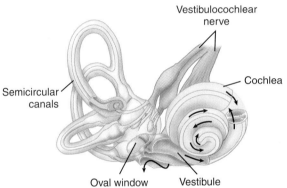

FIGURE 12–8 **Structure of the cochlea.**

impulse. That impulse travels the vestibulocochlear nerve to the brain. Hair cells can be damaged by excessive vibrations from loud sounds. When the hairs are damaged, they cannot conduct the sound impulse to the brain. Damage to hair cells can result in temporary hearing loss, such as after a concert, or permanent hearing loss resulting from constant exposure to loud sound. Injured hair cells produce a ringing sound called tinnitus. The ringing subsides with temporary hearing loss, but may be constant with permanent damage.

See Box 12–3 for a summary of childhood illnesses that cause blindness and deafness.

*Flashpoint*

Hearing loss is found in 1 out of 10 Americans. It occurs in 29% of people older than age 65.

## Equilibrium

The ear not only interprets sound, but also interprets the motion of the body and its position. **Equilibrium** is the process of maintaining balance or stability. The ear maintains two types of equilibrium: static and dynamic.

The vestibule, a small chamber located between the semicircular canals, and the cochlea are responsible for maintaining balance by monitoring the movement

## Box 12-3 Childhood Causes of Blindness and Deafness

Many cases of blindness and deafness are due to childhood illnesses. Each year, 500,000 new cases of childhood blindness occur worldwide. Blindness occurs more often in developing countries.

In poorer nations, the main causes of blindness are vitamin A deficiency and disease. Lack of vitamin A causes the cornea to dry out and scar. Measles, a common illness in children, can also cause scarring of the cornea.

Eye infections can also lead to blindness. Trachoma is a common bacterial infection. Repeated trachoma infections cause scarring underneath the upper eyelid making it turn inward. The eyelashes scratch the cornea and cause blindness.

Blindness resulting from structural defects is common in developed and poorer countries. Amblyopia, or "lazy eye," is a misalignment of the eyes that causes loss of vision in the weaker eye. Amblyopia can be corrected with glasses or surgery to correct the weak extrinsic muscles. After surgery, an eye patch over the strong eye forces the weaker one to focus and increase the strength of the muscles.

All of these causes of blindness can be treated and corrected if medication and health care are available.

Deafness in childhood is not linked to poverty the way blindness is. Deafness can be either conductive, where sound does not move through the ear, or sensorineural, where the hair cells or auditory nerve are affected.

In the United States, deafness in children commonly results from repeated ear infections. Conduction deafness can be a result of otitis externa, also called "swimmer's ear." This is an infection of the auricle and auditory canal. Wetness in the ear leads to bacterial growth, which causes redness and swelling of the tissue. Frequent occurrence of otitis externa can lead to scarring and thickening of the ear, preventing sound from entering the middle ear. Otitis media, also called "glue ear," can also cause conduction deafness. Otitis media is caused by a bacterial infection of the middle ear, and fluid buildup can cause temporary deafness. Continuous middle ear infections can lead to scarring and fluid retention in the ear. Both of these symptoms can prevent sound from conducting through the middle ear.

The best treatment is prevention. By keeping the ears dry and clean, cases of otitis externa can be reduced. Antibiotics can be prescribed to treat both types of infections.

Sensorineural deafness is a defect in the hair cells of the cochlea. Some children may be born with defective or absent hair cells. Maternal illness with syphilis or rubella can damage the ears of the developing fetus and lead to sensorineural deafness. This type of deafness may be treated with hearing aids or cochlear implants.

Although rare, deafness and blindness can be the result of maternal illness or can be genetically inherited. The combination of blindness and deafness can be a result of maternal rubella infection during pregnancy. Usher disease is genetically inherited from the mother and father and results in blindness and deafness.

of the head. Inside the vestibule are receptors that react to changes in gravity. The type of balance monitored by the vestibule is *static equilibrium*. This equilibrium tells the body its position in space and detects changes in acceleration. Static equilibrium tells you which way is up or down. This equilibrium is especially important when diving into water where other senses may not be useful in finding the surface. The body still knows which way is up because of static equilibrium.

The semicircular canals have receptors that respond to circular or sideways motions of the head. Within the canals is a fluid called endolymph that signals the receptors that the head is engaged in angular or circular movement. Keeping the body upright when in this type of motion is called *dynamic equilibrium*. This type of balance tries to keep us upright after spinning in a circle.

# Smell

The *nose* is the structure that forms the sense of smell by bringing odors to the brain to interpret (see Fig. 12–9). In contrast to light and sound waves, odors must be converted to a chemical form before they can become a stimulus. Although humans can recognize approximately 10,000 different odors, smell is the weakest sense. Our ability to smell is easily distorted by an overproduction of mucus caused by a cold or an allergy.

## Structure of the Nose

Odors enter the nose through the nares, or nostrils, and flow into the sinus cavities. Here the odors reach the mucous membranes on the roof of the nasal cavity. Within the mucous membranes are *olfactory receptors*. Humans have about 5 million of these receptors, which may seem like a lot, but in comparison, a dog has about 250 million. Olfactory receptors are a type of chemoreceptor because these receptors transform odors into chemicals that are absorbed through the mucous membrane. The chemicals of an odor are absorbed by olfactory hairs within the mucous membrane that are attached to the olfactory receptors. From the receptors, they travel along the tracts of the *olfactory nerve* to the brain. The area of the brain called the temporal lobe identifies the odor.

Olfactory receptors are extremely sensitive, and only a few molecules of an odor can trigger them. Air helps to intensify an odor. By sniffing, more air enters the nasal cavity with the odor, increasing the chances that the odor will be detected.

The sense of smell is also very closely tied to memory and emotion. The briefest whiff of a scent can cause the recall of a memory related to that scent.

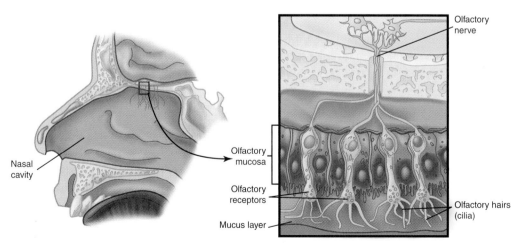

FIGURE 12–9 Structures of the nose.

For example, the smell of roses may remind you of a garden from childhood, or sugar cookies may remind you of a grandmother who often baked them. We tend to prefer smells that remind us of good things and dislike odors that cause unpleasant reactions.

Olfactory receptors are so sensitive they can adapt to a constant stimulus. An unchanging odor eventually causes the olfactory receptors to become less sensitive to that scent and can make it unnoticeable. This is why the scent of perfume can be unbearable to someone who just stepped into a room, but is not noticed by the wearer.

# Taste

The **mouth** is the location for the sense of taste. The tongue is the major taste organ (see Fig. 12–10). Similar to odor, tastes must be changed to chemical form before they can be perceived by the brain.

## Structure of the Tongue

The tongue is covered with bumps called papillae. Along the surface of the papillae are **taste buds**. Most taste buds are scattered along the tongue, but they can also be found on the walls of the throat and on the roof of the mouth. Humans have approximately 10,000 taste buds, and each contains about 50 to 150 **gustatory receptors**, which are another type of chemoreceptor. There are different gustatory receptors to recognize the tastes: salt, sweet, sour, and bitter. These taste receptors are localized in different areas of the tongue. The tip of the tongue is most sensitive to sweet, the back of the tongue is most sensitive to bitter, and the sides of the tongue are most sensitive to sour; salt receptors are more scattered throughout the tongue.

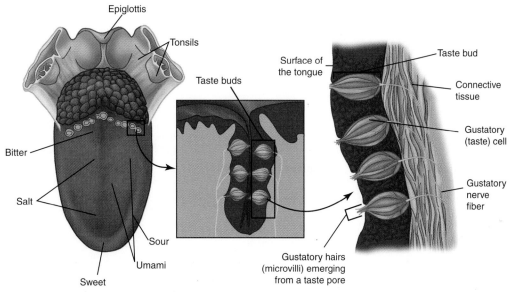

**FIGURE 12–10  Structures of the tongue.**

Flashpoint

Taste buds decrease as we age. By middle age, the number decreases to about 8000, and by age 65 people only have about 5000 taste buds.

A fifth taste bud has been identified. It is called umami and provides identification for the flavors of meat and cheese. These taste buds are also more scattered throughout the tongue. See Table 12–2 for a summary of the taste buds.

For the taste buds to detect a "flavor," the food must be broken down into chemical molecules and dissolved in saliva. The dissolved molecules bind with the taste buds and stimulate the gustatory receptors. The stimulus is then sent along the *facial* and *glossopharyngeal nerves* to the brain. Taste is interpreted in the parietal region of the brain.

The nose also plays a large part in the ability to taste. The odor of food enhances taste, and food tastes bland without the ability to smell. As we age, we begin to lose the sensitivity to smell and taste. This is why foods we enjoyed as children may not taste the same as we remember. Elderly people often have a loss of appetite because they may be unable to smell or taste the food. Older individuals often overly season or salt their food or lose their appetites for certain foods.

Taste can also be affected by temperature or texture. Overly heated or spicy foods can cause pain receptors to react and override the taste. Cold can make food taste bland or change the texture. Texture is sometimes more important than the actual taste, and foods can be objectionable because of a rubbery, gritty, or pasty texture.

# Touch

The greatest number sensory receptors found outside the "special senses" are found in the skin. These receptors are called *somatosensory receptors*, and they detect the sensations of heat, cold, pain, pressure, and vibration (see Fig. 12–11).

## Sensations

*Sensations* are feelings that the brain interprets, depending on the receptor that receives the stimulus. The somatosensory receptors are located in the dermis or middle layer of the skin. There are five different sensory receptors that provide sensations:

- *Pain receptors* are stimulated by tissue damage.
- *Chemoreceptors* are stimulated when there is a change in chemical concentrations of the body.

**TABLE 12–2**

**LOCATION OF TASTE BUDS**

| Type of Taste Bud | Location |
| --- | --- |
| Sweet | Tip of tongue |
| Sour | Sides of tongue |
| Bitter | Back of tongue |
| Salt | Scattered over tongue |
| Umami | Scattered over tongue |

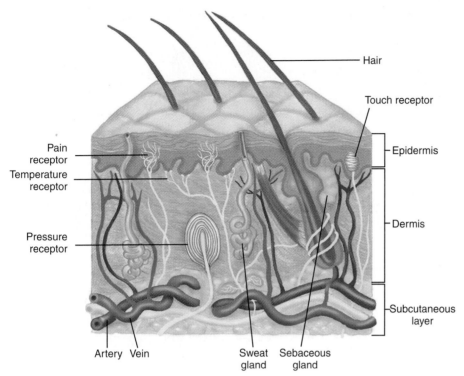

**FIGURE 12–11** **Sensory receptors.** (Adapted from Eagle S. *Medical Terminology in a Flash!* Philadelphia, PA: FA Davis; 2006:25.)

- ***Thermoreceptors*** detect changes in temperature.
- ***Photoreceptors*** respond to changes in light.
- ***Mechanoreceptors*** detect changes in movement or pressure.

The receptors for hot, cold, and pain are free nerve endings, meaning the endings are exposed. These nerves respond to any intense stimulus; this is why extreme cold can be felt as pain, as can intense pressure. The receptors for touch, pressure, and vibration have a covering over the nerve endings and are called encapsulated.

All somatoreceptors provide information about the skin and the external environment. Most of the sensations that these receptors detect are not consciously processed because somatoreceptors, similar to chemoreceptors in the nose, become desensitized or used to the sensation. Desensitized sensations can become conscious sensations if a change occurs in the stimulus. For example, you become unaware of how your shoes feel on your feet after putting them on. If your sock falls down or a pebble gets inside the shoe, the change in stimulus makes you aware of not only the sock or pebble, but also the feel of the shoe.

How intensely we are aware of a sensation depends on the type of somatoreceptors triggered and how concentrated those receptors are in a particular area of the skin. The hands and face have the most receptors per area of skin, so they are the most sensitive parts of the body and detect the most stimuli.

See Table 12–3 for a summary of pathology terms associated with the senses.

*Flashpoint*

Wetness or humidity is a feeling that comes from a combination of touch, pressure, and temperature receptors being triggered simultaneously.

## TABLE 12–3

## PATHOLOGY TERMS RELATED TO THE SENSES

| | |
|---|---|
| Ageusia | Loss of sense of taste |
| Agnosia | Loss of ability to recognize objects, shapes, sounds, persons, or smells; usually due to brain trauma |
| Amaurosis | Blindness usually occurring from a lesion in the optic nerve, brain, or spinal cord |
| Anacusis | Total deafness |
| Anosmia | Loss of sense of smell |
| Color blindness | Inability to perceive some or all colors; most often due to genetic defect of the X chromosome, so boys are more likely to be affected |
| Exophthalmos | Bulging of the eyes; can be due to trauma or from a disease process such as Graves disease |

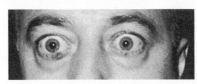

Exophthalmos (From Tamparo CD, Lewis MA. *Diseases of the Human Body*, 4th ed. Philadelphia, PA: FA Davis; 2005:339.)

| | |
|---|---|
| Hordeolum | Infection of the sebaceous glands of the eyelid; a yellowish, painful bump develops at the site; also called a sty |
| Motion sickness | Nausea or dizziness that occurs when the sense of movement and the sense of sight are not in agreement |
| Strabismus | Inability of the eyes to align so that one or both eyes turn in, out, up, or down. Commonly called "cross-eyes" |

Esotropia

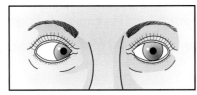

Exotropia

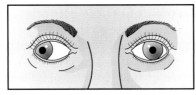

Strabismus

| | |
|---|---|
| Tinnitus | Ringing in the ears caused by damage to the hair receptors in the inner ear; may be temporary or permanent |
| Vertigo | Sensation of moving or spinning usually a result of disturbance in the inner ear causing a loss of balance |

# Practice Exercises

## Multiple Choice

1. The colored portion of the eye is the _____.

   a. cornea

   b. iris

   c. lens

   d. sclera

2. Taste buds are a type of _____.

   a. photoreceptor

   b. sensory receptor

   c. chemoreceptor

   d. olfactory receptor

3. Hair cells are found in the _____.

   a. cochlea

   b. retina

   c. ossicles

   d. skin

4. _____ equilibrium is maintained by the vestibule of the ear.

   a. dynamic

   b. rotational

   c. static

   d. transitional

5. The _____ adjusts to allow the eye to focus or near or far objects.

   a. retina

   b. cornea

   c. iris

   d. lens

## True or False

1. True  False    The bones of the middle ear are the auricles.

2. True  False    The optic disc is the "blind spot."

3. True  False    Vitreous humor is constantly replenished.

4. True  False    The colored portion of the eye is the iris.

5. True  False    Olfactory bulbs detect taste.

6. True  False    The external and middle section of the ear is separated by the tympanic membrane.

7. True  False    Light is reflected when it enters the eye.

8. True  False    The ear has three sections.

9. True  False    Static equilibrium maintains balance and detects motion.

10. True  False   The retina is the outermost layer of the eye.

## Fill in the Blank

1. The _____ provide color vision, and the _____ provide shadow vision.

2. The _____ is located under the cornea.

3. The tongue is covered with _____ that detect salt, sweet, sour, and bitter.

4. _____ receptors give clues about the external environment.

5. The _____ or _____ is the external portion of the ear.

6. _____ is the sense of taste for meat and cheese.

7. The _____ is the structure of the ear that provides hearing and balance.

8. Tears are produced by _____ glands.

9. The white of the eye is the _____.

10. Sensations are felt by _____ receptors.

## Short Answer

1. **Describe the different types of taste buds.**

2. **List the five different sensory receptors.**

## Labeling

*Fill in the blanks with the appropriate anatomical terms.*

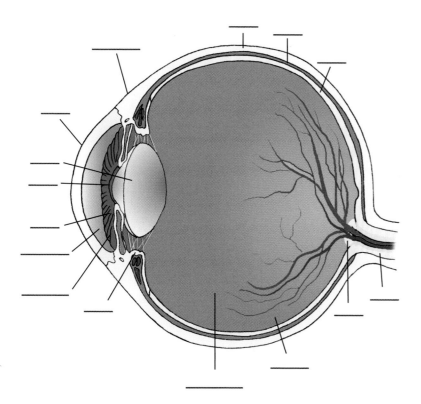

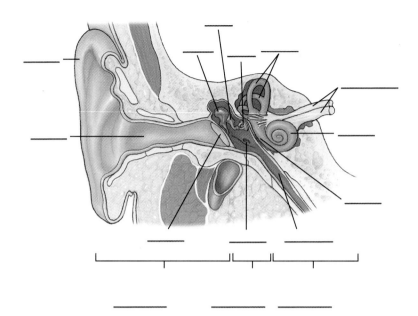

# THE URINARY SYSTEM

The urinary system consists of the kidneys, ureters, urinary bladder, and urethra. Its functions include removal of soluble wastes and secretion of various hormones to maintain blood volume, hydration, and blood pressure and to stimulate the production of red blood cells.

The kidneys process the fluid waste from the blood and remove it from the body in the form of urine. They also monitor the level of total blood in the body and can retain more fluid or release extra fluid to maintain proper blood volume. Secretion of several hormones by the kidneys maintains blood pressure, red blood cell production, and constriction of blood vessels.

This chapter discusses the structures of the urinary system and the production of urine. The other functions of the kidneys and the hormones that are responsible for fluid balance and renal failure also are described.

## Key Terms

extracellular fluid

filtration

intracellular fluid

micturition

nephron

nitrogenous wastes

reabsorption

renal filtrate

secretion

urine

urochrome

## Structures of the Urinary System

The human urinary system consists of four separate structures. There are two kidneys that remove wastes from the blood and form urine. Attached to each kidney is a ureter, which is a tube through which urine is transported. Both ureters attach to the urinary bladder. The last structure is the urethra, a small tube through which urine leaves the body. Figure 13–1 shows the structures of the urinary system.

### Kidney

Each body contains a pair of **kidneys**, which are located one on each side of the vertebral column usually between the 12th thoracic and 3rd lumbar vertebrae. They are located beneath the diaphragm and posterior to the liver and are partially protected by the ribs. Each kidney is about 3 to 4 inches in length. The right kidney sits lower in the abdominal cavity because of the shape of the liver, which is wider on the right side than the left. Both kidneys are surrounded by adipose tissue that acts as a cushion and provides protection.

A kidney has a convex outer side and a concave inner side (see Fig. 13–2). The outer, darker layer of tissue is the **renal cortex**, and the inner portion of tissue is the **renal medulla**. The tissue of the medulla is arranged in triangular patterns referred to as **renal pyramids**. The tissue of the innermost curve of the kidney is the **renal pelvis**. The curve itself is the **hilus**. At the hilus, the

*Flashpoint*

The urinary system maintains homeostasis in the body by controlling blood pressure and fluid output.

*Flashpoint*

Of the world population, 0.07% is born with more than two kidneys, and 0.02% is born with only one kidney.

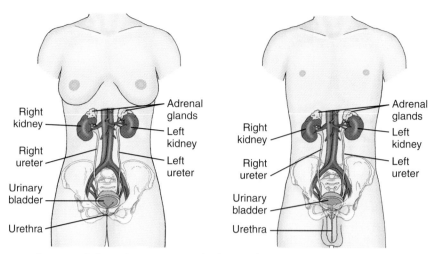

**FIGURE 13–1  Organs of the urinary system.** (Adapted from Eagle S. *Medical Terminology in a Flash!* Philadelphia, PA: FA Davis; 2006:147.)

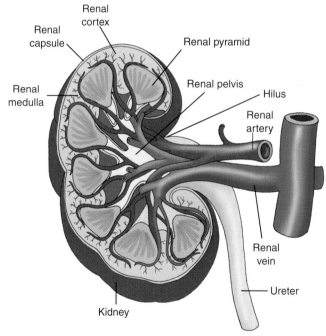

**FIGURE 13–2  Sagittal view of the kidney.** (Adapted from Eagle S. *Medical Terminology in a Flash!* Philadelphia, PA: FA Davis; 2006:148.)

renal artery and renal vein enter and exit the kidney. It is also the place of attachment for the ureter.

## Nephron

The kidney is filled with approximately 1 million small structures called **nephrons**. The nephrons filter waste from the blood and process it to leave the body in a form called urine. A nephron resembles the plumbing system found under a kitchen sink. All the pipes are connected, but each section has an individual name and plays a different role in the production of urine.

The first step of creating urine begins at the portion of the nephron called the *glomerulus* (ball) (see Fig. 13–3). These structures work like filters and are located in the renal cortex. The blood supply for the kidney flows through the cortex, and the glomerulus filters the blood as it passes and brings it into the nephron. From the glomerulus, the blood flows to the *glomerular capsule*, or Bowman capsule, a cup-shaped structure in which the glomerulus sits. The capsule is joined to a coiled tubule called the *proximal convoluted tubule*.

The tubules of the nephron are located in the renal pelvis. The proximal convoluted tubule extends downward and forms a bend called the *loop of Henle*. It then extends upward and forms another coiled tubule called the *distal convoluted tubule*. The distal convoluted tubule joins with several other distal convoluted tubules from neighboring nephrons. These tubules merge into one larger *collecting duct*. All collecting ducts flow to the renal pelvis where they join together. The urine carried in the ducts enters the ureters, which carry the urine to the urinary bladder.

## Ureters

Each kidney has a *ureter*, which starts as a funnel-shaped attachment at the renal pelvis. The ureters are muscular tubes about 12 inches long that bring urine from the collecting ducts of the nephron to the urinary bladder. Urine is moved through the ureter by *peristalsis*, a wavelike movement that is also used by the esophagus. Where the ureter attaches to the urinary bladder, a flap of membrane covers the opening. This cover prevents backflow of the urine and limits the speed at which the bladder fills. Peristalsis not only moves the urine, but the wavelike motion also forces it through the flap in spurts instead of a continuous flow.

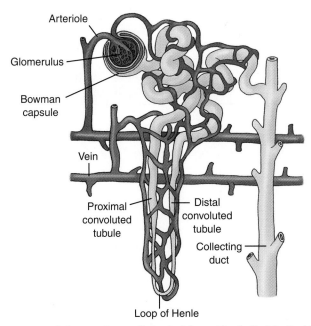

**FIGURE 13–3  Structures of the nephron.** (Adapted from Eagle S. *Medical Terminology in a Flash!* Philadelphia, PA: FA Davis; 2006:148.)

## Urinary Bladder

The **urinary bladder** is a storage area for the urine. The bladder is a muscle that can stretch to accommodate the urine. It is a slightly triangular pouch that, similar to the stomach, collapses into folds when empty. These folds stretch as the bladder fills. Also similar to the stomach, the bladder can stretch only so far before it becomes painful.

An empty bladder is about 2 to 3 inches long, and when full it extends to about 5 inches. A full bladder holds about 500 mL of urine. It is capable of stretching to a maximum of about 10 inches and holding 1000 mL of urine. When the bladder is this full, it feels firm if pushed and painful.

The bottom triangular portion of the bladder is called the **trigone**. Urine flows downward through the trigone and leaves by a small funnel called the neck, which is the place of connection to the urethra (see Fig. 13–4).

*Flashpoint*

Cigarette smoking doubles the risk of developing bladder cancer.

## Urethra

The urethra is the tube through which urine leaves the body. Within the urethra are two valves that control urine flow. The **internal sphincter** is a band of muscle that acts as an opening into the urethra, and the **external**

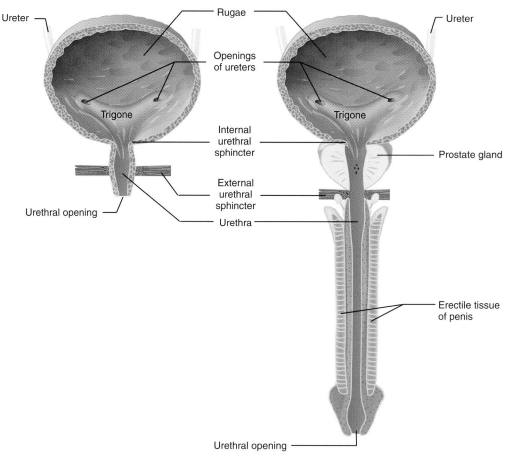

**FIGURE 13–4  Urinary bladder and urethra.**

*sphincter*, located about 1 inch into the urethra, is the second opening. Both sphincters are voluntarily controlled. When the bladder is full, the sphincters release, and urine leaves the body in a process called micturition.

The urethra of the male and female differ in size. The female urethra is about 1.5 inches long, and the male urethra averages about 8 inches. The male urethra is also part of the reproductive system acting as the passageway for sperm to leave the body. Because of the short length of the female urethra, it is prone to collect bacteria resulting in a common ailment called a urinary tract infection (UTI) (see Box 13–1).

### Micturition

Voiding urine from the body, or **micturition**, is a reflexive and a voluntary action. As the urinary bladder fills with urine, the walls of the bladder begin to stretch. When the bladder fills to about 200 mL of fluid, it is stretched far enough to activate sensory receptors in the bladder. These receptors carry impulses to the nerves of the sacral region of the spinal cord. The spinal cord

> *Flashpoint*
> Urethral stricture is a narrowing of the urethra caused by infection or trauma. It is treated by inserting an instrument into the urethra to stretch it.

## Box 13-1 Common Disorders of the Urinary System

Urinary system disorders and diseases are quite common, and most are easily treatable. Women tend to have urinary ailments more often than men.

One of the most common ailments is urinary tract infection (UTI). Symptoms include pain, burning during urination, redness, and swelling of the vulva. UTI is most often caused by bacteria that enter the urethra. More women than men have UTIs; because of the short length of the urethra, microorganisms can gain access to a woman's body more easily. Treatment includes oral prescription medications and topical medications to relieve the external irritation.

Incontinence is the inability to hold urine in the bladder usually when laughing, sitting, coughing, or lifting. It can be a result of pregnancy, abnormal nerve signals to the bladder, weakening of the pelvic muscles, UTI, or a disease of the urinary system. Treatment includes exercise or surgery to strengthen the surrounding bladder muscles, prescription medications, and restricting fluids such as coffee and tea.

A kidney stone, or renal stone, is a hard mass of urine crystals that forms because of excess amounts of crystals in the urine that are not flushed from the bladder. Excess crystals can be due to diet, UTI, or urinary blockage. Stones occur more often in white men in their 40s, but they can occur in anyone. Symptoms include sharp and extreme abdominal pain, blood in the urine, and painful urination. Usually the stone is allowed to pass by itself, but if it becomes obstructed or is too large to pass, surgery is required to remove it.

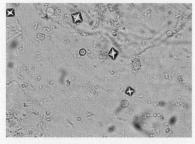

Calcium oxalate crystals in urine. (From *Taber's Cyclopedic Medical Dictionary*. 21st ed. Philadelphia, PA: FA Davis; 2009:339.)

transmits a stimulus back to the bladder that causes the bladder to go into reflexive contraction. These contractions force urine past the internal urethral sphincter into the upper urethra.

At this point, the person is aware that the bladder is full and feels the urge to urinate. The skeletal muscles of the pelvis surround the external urethral sphincter and keep the sphincter closed until it is voluntarily opened. When the muscles relax, urine is released down into the urethra. If the urge to void is ignored, the contractions stop after several minutes, but the bladder continues to fill. The bladder contracts again after another 200 to 300 mL of urine enters. The bladder is now full, and if the urge to void is still ignored, the bladder continues filling past the 500- to 600-mL full point. When this occurs, the bladder becomes overstretched and uncomfortable. It becomes painful, and eventually the skeletal muscles are no longer able to control the force of urine in the sphincter, and urine is involuntarily released.

If the external sphincter cannot be voluntarily controlled, it is called **incontinence**. In children younger than 2 years, incontinence is normal because they have not learned voluntary control of the urethral sphincter. Some older children sleep so soundly that even though they are able to control micturition when awake, they are unaware of bladder contractions when asleep, and the skeletal muscles involuntarily release. This is **nocturnal enuresis**, commonly called bedwetting. In adults, incontinence can be caused by occurrences such as pregnancy, stroke, weakening of the pelvic muscles after childbirth, and spinal cord injuries.

## Urine Production

Urine production depends on three processes: filtration, reabsorption, and secretion. Each of the three processes occurs in a different section of the nephron.

The production of urine begins with the act of the glomerulus bringing blood into the nephron. Blood first enters the kidney through the renal artery, which branches into arterioles within the renal cortex. From the arterioles, blood pressure pushes plasma and substances dissolved in the plasma into the glomeruli. This is called **filtration**, or glomerular filtration. Glomerular filtration rate (GFR) is the amount of fluid filtered from the kidneys and into the Bowman capsules in 1 minute. Normal GFR is 60 to 70 mL/min. This test is commonly done to check renal function.

From the glomerulus, the plasma, now called **renal filtrate**, is passed into the proximal convoluted tubule. Here substances the body needs, such as glucose, hormones, salts, and amino acids, flow back into the blood. Waste products are dissolved in the filtrate, so they remain in the tubule. The process of the proximal convoluted tubules returning some substances to the blood and keeping others is **reabsorption**, or tubular reabsorption. Approximately 99% of the filtrate is reabsorbed from the distal convoluted tubule back into the blood. The nephrons produce about 180 liters of filtrate a day. The cleansed blood leaves the nephrons by venules that flow to the renal vein.

The remaining renal filtrate takes a turn at the loop of Henle and travels to the distal convoluted tubule. In the distal convoluted tubules, hydrogen ions ($H^-$) and sodium ions ($Na^+$) are released back into the blood supply as needed to maintain blood pH. Water is also taken from or added to the renal filtrate. This process is called **secretion**, or tubular secretion. After secretion, the fluid in the distal convoluted tubule is called urine.

## Urine

**Urine** is the final product of the processes of filtration, reabsorption, and secretion of the nephron. Urinalysis is the evaluation of a urine sample, which has physical, chemical, and microscopic characteristics. These characteristics include amount, color, pH, specific gravity, components of urine, and nitrogenous wastes.

- Amount: The body makes about 1 to 2 liters of urine a day. Output changes because of age, gender, medications, exercise, and diet. The amount of fluid taken in should equal the amount of fluid excreted from the body.
- Color: Urine gets its color from **urochrome**, a pigment obtained from the breakdown of bile. This pigment originally comes from the breakdown of red blood cells in the liver, which then excretes it into the bile. Other pigments from red blood cells leave the body in the solid waste. The color of urine depends on the concentration of the wastes and varies from pale yellow to straw to amber.
- pH: The pH range of normal urine is 4.0 to 8.0 with an average of 6.0. Diet plays a role in urine pH. Vegetarians tend to have more alkaline urine (>7.0), and people who eat more meat and protein have more acidic urine (<7.0).
- Specific gravity: Specific gravity is a measurement of the concentration of urine compared with distilled water, which has no substances dissolved in it. The specific gravity of distilled water is 1.000. Urine has an average concentration of 1.010 to 1.030. Normally, the first urine of the day is more concentrated than urine produced later in the day. Urine becomes more dilute as more fluid is ingested.
- Components of urine: Urine is composed of water and nitrogenous wastes. Water is about 95% of the total volume of urine. The rest of the composition is the solutes, which are waste products that can be dissolved in fluid. These wastes are called **nitrogenous wastes** and salts.
- Wastes: These wastes are called nitrogenous wastes and are water-soluble; they include urea, creatinine, and uric acid. Urea is excreted by the liver from the breakdown of amino acids. Creatinine is the result of the breakdown of creatine phosphate during muscle metabolism. Uric acid is a result of the breakdown of nucleic acids. Other substances that are soluble in the urine and excreted as waste are ammonia, phosphates, carbohydrates, sodium, potassium, and other minerals.

Table 13–1 describes the normal characteristics of urine.

Flashpoint

Urine has historically been used as an antiseptic to clean wounds.

# Water Volumes

The human body seems solid, but it is mostly water. About 55% to 75% of a person's total body weight is water. This water comes from two sources: intracellular fluid and extracellular fluid. About two-thirds of the total water content

## TABLE 13–1
### NORMAL CHARACTERISTICS OF URINE

| Characteristic | Normal Range |
| --- | --- |
| Amount | 1–2 liters per day |
| Color | Pale yellow, straw, or amber |
| pH | 4.0–8.0 |
| Specific gravity | 1.010–1.030 |
| Components | 95% water and 5% solutes (salts and waste) |
| Wastes | Urea from amino acid breakdown<br>Creatinine from muscle metabolism<br>Uric acid from nucleic acid breakdown |

of the body is ***intracellular fluid***, meaning it is the fluid found within the cells. The other one-third is ***extracellular fluid*** found outside the cells. The extracellular fluid includes the fluids found in plasma, lymph, and tissues; surrounding the brain and spinal cord; and within the joints.

Because so much water is used by the body, it needs to be ingested daily. The average water requirement for an adult is about 2500 mL, or 2.5 liters per day. Most water, about 1600 mL, comes from the ingestion of liquids, and another 700 mL can come from food. Water is also a waste product of cellular metabolism. The cells make about 200 mL a day that the body reabsorbs.

In a healthy body, input of fluids is equal to the output of fluids. Water leaves the body in several ways. The greatest amount, about 1500 mL a day, is excreted as urine. Another 500 mL leaves as sweat, and about 300 mL is exhaled as water vapor. Excretion of feces also removes another 200 mL of fluid a day. Total output of fluid should be about 2500 mL (see Fig. 13–5). If the output increases, such as during exercise when more water is lost through sweat and respiration, more fluids need to be ingested. If more fluids are ingested than needed, more fluid is removed in the form of urine.

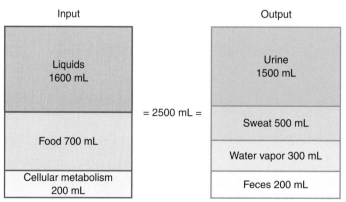

FIGURE 13–5 **Fluid balance.**

## Other Kidney Functions

The kidneys perform many important functions besides urine formation, including maintaining the pH of blood, secretion of renin, production of erythropoietin, and activation of vitamin D.

- pH: Normal blood pH is 7.4. If the pH decreases or becomes too acidic, the body is in a state of acidosis. To increase the pH of the blood, the kidneys secrete more $H^-$ into the filtrate and return more bicarbonate ions ($HCO_3^-$) to the blood until the pH becomes normal. If the pH increases or becomes alkaline, the body enters alkalosis. To decrease the blood pH, the kidneys secrete more $HCO_3^-$ into the urine and return $H^-$ ions to the blood until the pH decreases to normal.
- Renin secretion: If blood pressure decreases, the arterioles of the kidneys produce renin, which is an enzyme that changes the blood protein angiotensinogen into angiotensin. Angiotensin causes vasoconstriction, or constriction of the veins, and stimulates the adrenal glands to produce aldosterone, which increases the blood pressure.
- Erythropoietin secretion: The hormone erythropoietin influences the production of red blood cells by the bone marrow. If the body becomes hypoxic or loses oxygen, erythropoietin stimulates the increase in red blood cell output until the oxygen level in the blood is increased to normal.
- Vitamin D activation: The kidneys convert vitamin D to calcitriol, a highly active form of the vitamin. Calcitriol increases the absorption of calcium and phosphate in the small intestine.

## Hormones That Maintain Fluid Balance

Hormones are chemicals secreted by glands that influence the actions of another gland or organ. The hormones that influence the maintenance of blood pressure and blood volume are aldosterone, atrial natriuretic peptide (ANP), and antidiuretic hormone (ADH) (see Table 13–2).

- Aldosterone: Aldosterone is secreted by the adrenal glands and stimulates the reabsorption of $Na^+$ in response to high potassium ($K^+$) levels in the

**TABLE 13–2**

**HORMONES THAT AFFECT KIDNEY FUNCTION**

| Hormone | Function |
|---|---|
| Aldosterone | Increases reabsorption of $Na^+$ ions from the filtrate to the blood, causing more water reabsorption to maintain blood pressure and volume |
| Atrial natriuretic peptide (ANP) | Decreases reabsorption of $Na^+$ ions, bringing more water into the filtrate to be excreted |
| Antidiuretic hormone (ADH) | Increases reabsorption of water from the filtrate if more water is needed in the body or decreases reabsorption, so excess water is excreted |

blood, low sodium levels, or a decrease in blood pressure. The reabsorption of Na⁺ from the nephron causes water also to leave the filtrate and return to the blood, which maintains the blood volume and pressure.

- Atrial natriuretic peptide: ANP is secreted by the atria of the heart when excess blood volume or increased blood pressure causes the atria to stretch under the pressure. ANP stimulates the kidneys to decrease the reabsorption of Na⁺ so that the sodium and water remain in the filtrate. By eliminating more water and sodium, the blood pressure and blood volume are decreased.
- Antidiuretic hormone: ADH is a hormone released by the pituitary gland when the body becomes dehydrated or loses water. ADH causes the distal convoluted tubules and collecting ducts to pull water out of the urine and return it to the blood. This increases blood pressure and blood volume and causes urine to concentrate. If the body has an increased amount of water, such as with a large quantity of fluid intake, ADH decreases and allows the kidneys to dilute the urine and eliminate more water until the volume returns to normal.

## Renal Failure

*Renal failure* occurs when the kidneys are no longer functioning. Failure of the kidneys can be due to another medical condition that affects the renal output or to a malfunction of the kidneys themselves. Renal failure can be acute or chronic.

### Acute Renal Failure

Acute renal failure is a rapid decline in the function of the kidney. This can occur for many reasons, including trauma; infection; hypovolemia; or shock from blood loss, toxins, and medications. It is diagnosed by high levels of creatinine and urea in the blood and *oliguria*, which is a decrease in urine output. With treatment, the condition can be reversed. Treatment includes catheterization to remove the urine, diuretics to increase fluid output, and control of blood pressure. If the kidney cannot be revived, it is in renal failure, and the patient needs dialysis to cleanse the blood or a kidney transplant.

### Chronic Renal Failure

Chronic renal failure is a progressive loss of renal function over months or years. The progression is measured in five stages, each stage measuring the level of the inability of the glomeruli to function. It is also monitored by the increase of creatinine in the blood. Symptoms of chronic renal failure are *hypertension* (an increase in blood pressure); accumulation of urea, potassium, and creatinine in the blood; fluid buildup in the body; anemia; and possible cardiac arrhythmias. Chronic renal failure is usually due to another disease process, such as hypertension, diabetes, and polycystic kidney disease. Symptoms are treated with iron supplements, blood pressure–lowering medications, and drugs to increase manufacture of red blood cells. Because the damage cannot be reversed for full recovery, dialysis or kidney transplantation is needed (see Box 13–2).

# Box 13–2 Dialysis

Dialysis is the mechanical means of performing the function of a healthy kidney. It is used when a patient has reached end-stage renal failure, and the patient's own kidneys are no longer able to function. Dialysis removes nitrogenous wastes, salts, and excess fluid from the body. It also helps to maintain normal fluid levels and blood pressure. There are two types of dialysis: hemodialysis and peritoneal dialysis.

In hemodialysis, a machine is used as an artificial kidney. A catheter is placed in the vessels of a patient, and the blood is pulled from the body and through the hemodialyzer and then back into the body. The artificial kidney cleanses the blood and removes excess fluid. The whole process takes 3 to 4 hours and must be done at least three times a week.

With peritoneal dialysis, a catheter is placed in the abdomen into the peritoneal cavity. A fluid called dialysate is slowly drained into the cavity. Wastes and extra fluid are drawn from the veins and arteries that surround the peritoneum into the dialysate. The dialysate is drained from the body by the catheter.

There are two kinds of peritoneal dialysis. One type is continuous ambulatory peritoneal dialysis (CAPD). In CAPD, the patient drains about 2 quarts of dialysate from a bag into the cavity and leaves it for 3 to 4 hours. The patient then drains the fluid back into the bag. This must be done about four times a day.

The other type of peritoneal dialysis is continuous cycling peritoneal dialysis (CCPD). CCPD is done by the patient placing dialysate into the peritoneal cavity and then attaching tubing from a machine called a cycler to the catheter. The machine removes the fluid and cleanses it and then replaces it back into the cavity about every 90 minutes. This is usually done at night while sleeping.

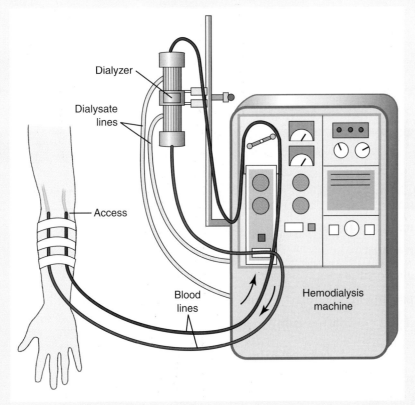

Hemodialysis. (From Eagle S. *Medical Terminology in a Flash!* Philadelphia, PA: FA Davis; 2006:149.)

See Table 13–3 for a summary of other pathological conditions of the urine.

**TABLE 13–3**

**PATHOLOGY TERMS OF THE URINARY SYSTEM**

| | |
|---|---|
| Anuria | Lack of urine production or inability to void urine |
| Hematuria | Blood in the urine |
| Maple syrup urine disease | Inherited disorder in which the body is unable to process certain proteins, resulting in urine that smells like maple syrup. Without treatment, the child has seizures, slow growth, and mental delays |
| Nocturia | Frequent urination at night |
| Nocturnal enuresis | Involuntary urination while sleeping usually occurs in children younger than 6 who have not learned voluntary control of urination; also called bedwetting |
| Oliguria | Decreased amount of urine production; decrease in voiding urine; causes include dehydration, kidney damage, or blockage |
| Polycystic kidney disease | Genetic disorder in which numerous cysts form in the kidneys, resulting in enlarged kidneys and reduction of renal function |
| Polyuria | Increase in urine production; increase in voiding urination; causes include increased fluid intake, diabetes, or diuretic drugs |
| Pyuria | Pus in the urine; sign of inflammation in urinary tract |
| Renal calculi | Hardened mineral deposits that form in kidneys; also called kidney stones |
| Renal failure | Loss of ability of kidneys to function; can be due to trauma or a disease process; may be acute or chronic |
| Uremia | Urine in the blood caused by urine backing up into the bloodstream because it is unable to leave the body through the urethra |

# Practice Exercises

## Multiple Choice

1. Bowman capsule is another name for the _____.
   a. renal capsule
   b. glomerulus
   c. proximal convoluted tubule
   d. distal convoluted tubule

2. The _____ connects the kidney to the urinary bladder.
   a. ureter
   b. urethra
   c. uterus
   d. uremia

3. The bottom portion of the bladder is the _____.

   a.   digone

   b.   sphincter

   c.   trigone

   d.   urethra

4. The enzyme that influences vasoconstriction and increase in blood pressure is _____.

   a.   aldosterone

   b.   renin

   c.   antidiuretic hormone

   d.   erythropoietin

5. The pigment _____ gives color to urine.

   a.   bilirubin

   b.   angiotensin

   c.   urochrome

   d.   bile

6. Tubular reabsorption occurs in the _____ of the nephron.

   a.   glomerulus

   b.   distal convoluted tubule

   c.   proximal convoluted tubule

   d.   collecting duct

7. Specific gravity of urine is compared with that of _____.

   a.   distilled water

   b.   bile

   c.   whole blood

   d.   serum

8. The _____ is the structure through which urine leaves the body.

   a.   urethra

   b.   ureter

   c.   collecting duct

   d.   renal capsule

9. The blood supply of the kidney runs through the _____.

    a.  hilus

    b.  renal cortex

    c.  renal medulla

    d.  renal pyramids

10. Tubular secretion occurs in the _____ of the nephron.

    a.  glomerulus

    b.  distal convoluted tubule

    c.  proximal convoluted tubule

    d.  collecting duct

## True or False

1.  True    False    The normal range of urine pH is 4.0 to 8.0.

2.  True    False    The male urethra is part of the urinary and reproductive systems.

3.  True    False    Renal filtrate is produced in the proximal convoluted tubule.

4.  True    False    Nephrons are the functional units of the bladder.

5.  True    False    The loop of Henle carries urine from the nephrons to the ureter.

## Fill in the Blank

1.  The hormone _____ is released when the body becomes dehydrated.

2.  Another term for urination is _____.

3.  The filter of the nephron is the _____.

4.  The portion of the bladder connected to the urethra is the _____.

5.  The act of bringing blood into the glomerulus is called _____.

6.  Collecting ducts transfer urine to the _____.

7. Renal pyramids are found in the _____.

8. _____ is the act of keeping wastes and returning substances back to the body.

9. The inner curve of the kidney is the _____.

10. Uric acid, ammonia, and urea are examples of _____.

## Short answer

1. **Describe the structures and functions of the nephron.**

## Labeling

*Fill in the blanks with the appropriate anatomical terms.*

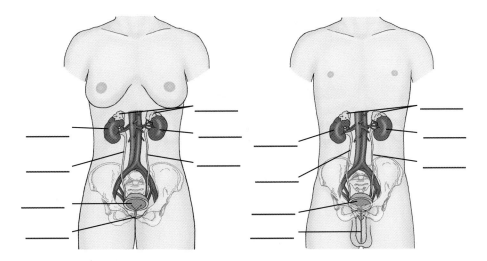

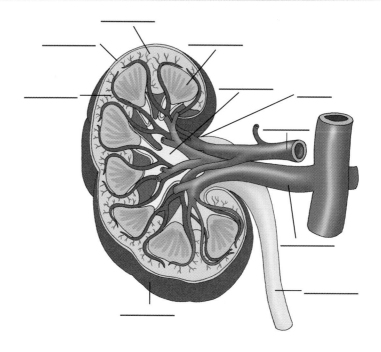

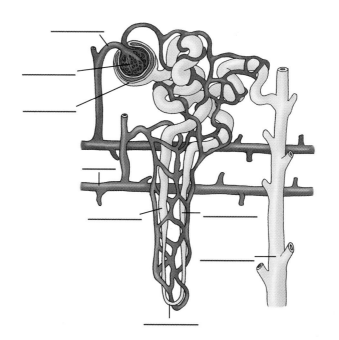

# THE ENDOCRINE SYSTEM 14

Two main communication systems allow the body to identify stimuli and react to internal and external changes. One is the nervous system, which uses electrical impulses and chemicals called neurotransmitters to generate a reaction. The other system is the endocrine system. This system is a collection of ductless glands that secrete chemicals called hormones directly into the bloodstream to control many bodily functions, such as growth, development, protection, and metabolism.

These glands are the pituitary, thyroid, parathyroid, adrenal, pancreas, pineal, thymus, and gonads (see Fig. 14–1). Each gland secretes hormones that control the activities of other systems in the body.

This chapter discusses hormone action and regulation. The structures of the endocrine system and the hormones secreted by each structure are identified.

## Hormones

**Hormones** (to excite) are chemicals secreted by the endocrine glands. The endocrine system produces 30 known hormones. Their purpose is to cause a change in the cells of the body either to produce an action or to slow down or cease an action.

These hormones can be classified into three different types. First are the **steroid hormones**, which are made from cholesterol. Steroid hormones are water-soluble and travel in the bloodstream. These hormones can cross through cell membranes.

The second type of hormone is the **nonsteroid hormones**. These hormones are made of amino acids and also travel in the bloodstream. Nonsteroid hormones are not water-soluble, so they cannot pass through a cell membrane.

The third type of hormone is the **prostaglandins**. They are made of cholesterol and are found within cell membranes.

### Actions of Hormones

Hormones generate changes in a cell or a whole organ. The cell or organ the hormone interacts with is called a target cell or a target organ. Because each hormone type has a different composition, it has a different means of interacting with its target (see Fig. 14–2).

## Key Terms

androgens

corticosteroids

endocrine gland

epinephrine

estrogens

exocrine gland

glucagon

hormones

insulin

negative feedback

nonsteroid hormones

norepinephrine

pituitary gland

prostaglandins

steroid hormones

thyroid hormone

*Flashpoint*

The endocrine system maintains homeostasis in the body by controlling the functions of all other body systems.

*Flashpoint*

The term hormone was first used by the British biochemists Bayliss and Starling in 1904.

**247**

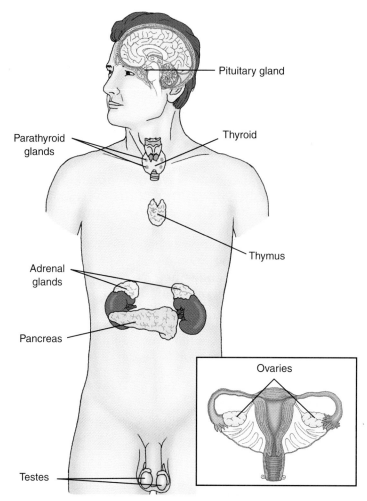

FIGURE 14–1  **Location of endocrine glands.** (From Eagle S. *Medical Terminology in a Flash!* Philadelphia, PA: FA Davis; 2006:198.)

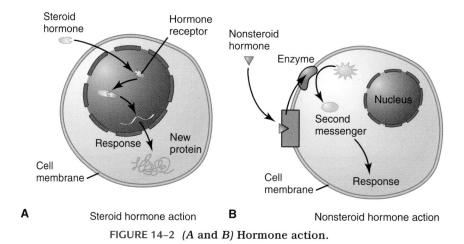

A        Steroid hormone action    B        Nonsteroid hormone action

FIGURE 14–2  *(A and B)* **Hormone action.**

Steroid hormones can move through a cell membrane. When inside the membrane of a target cell, the hormone enters the nucleus of that cell. Here it binds to a receptor for that particular hormone. This binding of the hormone to the receptor activates the cell.

Nonsteroid hormones cannot pass through a cell membrane. These hormones cause a cellular response by binding to receptors on the outside of the cell membrane. When the hormone binds to the receptor, it triggers the response of enzymes within the cell. The enzymes cause the response of the cell. This action is referred to as a second messenger because it is not directly caused by the hormone.

## Regulation of Hormones

Hormones are secreted by the endocrine glands only as they are needed by the target cells or organs. The endocrine glands respond to a change in the body that signals a particular gland to increase or decrease secretion, depending on the need of the target organ. A hormone is secreted only until the signal to which it is responding stops. The hormone level then decreases until it receives a signal to be secreted again.

This action is called **negative feedback**. This means the hormone is secreted only until the action of the hormone resolves the need of the target cell or organ. As the cell or organ changes because of the actions of the hormone, the signal it was sending out decreases so the hormone decreases as well. The gland then waits until it receives the stimulus again to begin secretion. This is why it is a negative effect: The action of the hormone itself causes the stimulus to reverse and decrease its secretion.

If the glucose level in the blood is above normal, a signal is sent to the pancreas to secrete more insulin. As the insulin carries the glucose to the cells, the blood glucose levels decrease. When the glucose level returns to normal, the need for insulin decreases, so the signal for insulin decreases causing the pancreas to secrete less insulin.

## Endocrine Glands

The body contains two types of glands: **exocrine** (secretions without) **glands** that secrete hormones through ducts to the external body, and **endocrine** (secretions within) **glands** that secrete hormones internally directly into the bloodstream. The glands of the endocrine system influence the functioning of every body system and include the pituitary gland, thyroid gland, parathyroid gland, adrenal gland, pancreas, pineal gland, thymus, and gonads.

## Pituitary Gland

The **pituitary gland** hangs by a stalk from the hypothalamus in the interior of the brain. It is called the "master gland" because it regulates the functions of the other glands (see Fig. 14–3). The pituitary gland is composed of two parts: the anterior lobe and posterior lobe. Both lobes are part of hormone secretion, but the posterior lobe is actually a storage area for hormones made by another

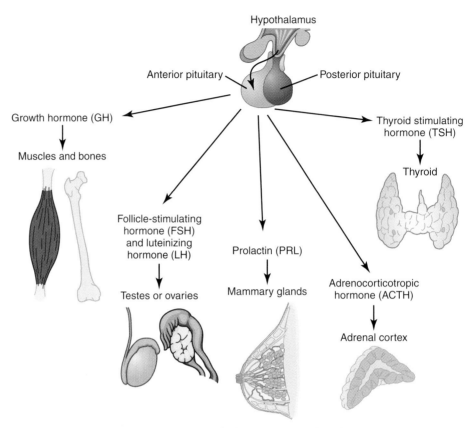

FIGURE 14–3  Hormones of the pituitary gland and their target organs.

structure of the brain called the hypothalamus. Secretions of the anterior lobe control the functions of the other glands: growth hormone, adrenocorticotropic hormone, prolactin, thyroid-stimulating hormone, follicle-stimulating hormone, and luteinizing hormone. The posterior lobe secretes oxytocin and antidiuretic hormone. See Table 14–1 for a description of the pituitary hormones.

- *Growth hormone* (GH) is a metabolic hormone that controls the growth of muscles and bones. It stimulates amino acids to be made into proteins and causes most cells to grow and divide.
- *Adrenocorticotropic hormone* (ACTH) stimulates the cortex of the adrenal gland to make steroid hormones.
- *Prolactin* (PRL) stimulates the mammary glands to produce milk during pregnancy. After delivery, prolactin levels increase and remain high as long as the mother continues to breastfeed. During weaning or if breastfeeding does not occur, prolactin levels decrease, slowing and eventually ceasing milk production.
- *Thyroid-stimulating hormone* (TSH) regulates the growth of the thyroid gland and stimulates secretion of the thyroid hormones.
- *Follicle-stimulating hormone* (FSH) stimulates follicle development for egg maturation in the ovaries of the female and begins sperm development in the testes of the male.
- *Luteinizing hormone* (LH) causes ovulation or release of a mature egg from the ovary of the female and stimulates production of the hormone testosterone by the testes of the male.

**TABLE 14–1**

**HORMONES**

**Hormones of the Pituitary Gland**

| Hormone<br>*Anterior Pituitary* | Function |
| --- | --- |
| Growth hormone (GH) | Affects growth of skeletal muscles and long bones |
| Prolactin (PRL) | Stimulates breast growth and milk production after childbirth |
| Adrenocorticotropic hormone (ACTH) | Regulates functions of the adrenal gland |
| Thyroid-stimulating hormone (TSH) | Regulates functions of the thyroid |
| Follicle-stimulating hormone (FSH) | Specific gonadotropic hormone that stimulates follicle development in the ovaries and sperm production in the testes |
| Luteinizing hormone (LH) | Stimulates ovulation, which causes estrogen and progesterone to be produced in the ovary and testosterone production in the testes |
| *Posterior Pituitary* | |
| Oxytocin | Stimulates uterine contractions during childbirth and milk ejection when breastfeeding |
| Antidiuretic hormone (ADH) | Inhibits urine production preventing water loss or dehydration |

**Hormones of the Thyroid Gland**

| | |
| --- | --- |
| Thyroxine ($T_4$) and triiodothyronine ($T_3$) | Increases metabolism and energy production |
| Calcitonin | Decreases reabsorption of calcium from bones to the blood |

**Hormones of the Parathyroid Gland**

| | |
| --- | --- |
| Parathyroid hormone (PTH) | Increases reabsorption of calcium from bone to the blood<br>Increases absorption of calcium in the small intestine<br>Activates vitamin D |

**Hormones of the Adrenal Glands**
*Adrenal Cortex*

| | |
| --- | --- |
| Aldosterone | Increases reabsorption of $Na^+$ ions by the kidneys back to the blood |
| Cortisol | Increases fat metabolism for energy<br>Blocks effects of histamine |
| Sex hormones | Secretes small amounts of male and female hormones in both genders |
| *Adrenal Medulla* | |
| Norepinephrine | Causes vasoconstriction throughout the body |
| Epinephrine | Increases heart rate, blood pressure, and respiration<br>Slows digestion |

*Continued*

| TABLE 14–1 | |
|---|---|
| **HORMONES—cont'd** | |
| **Hormones of the Pancreas** | |
| Insulin | Increases glucose transport to the cells<br>Increases conversion of excess glucose to glycogen in the liver |
| Glucagon | Increases conversion of glucose to glycogen |
| **Hormones of the Pineal Gland** | |
| Melatonin | Regulates the sleep cycle |
| **Hormones of the Thymus** | |
| Thymosin | Stimulates T-lymphocyte maturation |
| **Hormones of the Gonads** | |
| Estrogens | Stimulates menstrual cycle<br>Responsible for development of secondary female sex characteristics |
| Androgens | Stimulates testes to produce sperm.<br>Responsible for development of secondary male sex characteristics |

Flashpoint

Pituitary tumors, or adenomas, are a common tumor and account for 15% of all brain tumors. Pituitary adenomas can be either hormone producing and interfere with hormone levels or non-hormone producing and cause compression of the pituitary gland or other brain structures.

- *Oxytocin* is released in high amounts during pregnancy. During childbirth, it stimulates uterine contractions and milk release during breastfeeding. Synthetic oxytocin is used to induce labor or quicken labor if contractions slow.
- *Antidiuretic hormone* (ADH) increases or decreases urine production by causing the kidneys to reabsorb more water from the urine to increase blood volume and decrease urine output. ADH can also increase blood pressure by constricting the arterioles. Because of this function, ADH is sometimes called vasopressin.

## Thyroid Gland

The *thyroid gland* is butterfly-shaped and located at the base of the throat (see Figure 14–4). It consists of two lobes joined at the center by tissue. It produces two hormones: thyroid hormone and calcitonin.

The *thyroid hormone* is actually two hormones called *thyroxine* (T$_4$) and *triiodothyronine* (T$_3$). These hormones are metabolic hormones and control the rate at which glucose is used by the body. Both of these hormones need iodine to be produced. Without enough iodine in the diet, the thyroid must work harder to make hormones, so it enlarges. An enlarged thyroid gland is called a *goiter*. Iodine is found naturally in soil, but is lacking in mountainous regions where the soil is poor in nutrients. A child who lacks sufficient iodine or born to a mother who lacked sufficient iodine in her diet has a condition called *cretinism*. This condition causes stunted growth and mental retardation. To prevent goiters and other diseases caused by lack of iodine, salt manufacturers

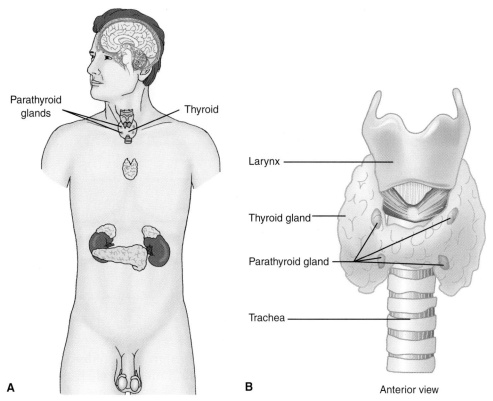

Parathyroid glands

Thyroid

Larynx

Thyroid gland

Parathyroid gland

Trachea

A

B

Anterior view

FIGURE 14–4 *(A and B)* Thyroid and parathyroid glands.

iodize, or added iodine to, salt to ensure sufficient amounts would be ingested by the population.

The thyroid also produces the hormone ***calcitonin***, which causes free-floating calcium in the blood to deposit in the bones. This hormone is antagonistic to a hormone produced by the parathyroid gland.

## Parathyroid Glands

***Parathyroid glands*** are small circular masses about the size of a grain of rice located on the posterior surface of the thyroid gland. Commonly, there are two masses on each lobe, but more have been found on some individuals. These glands secrete ***parathyroid hormone*** (PTH), which performs the opposite function of calcitonin. If blood calcium levels decrease, it stimulates the bones to release calcium into the blood. A low level of blood calcium is called ***hypocalcemia***. PTH causes bone to release calcium by stimulating osteoclasts, or bone breaking cells, to break down the bone matrix. PTH can also stimulate the kidneys to reabsorb more calcium and stimulate the intestines to absorb calcium that has been released by digested food.

## Adrenal Glands

The ***adrenal glands*** are triangular structures that sit atop each kidney (see Fig. 14–5). Hormones are produced by the outer layer of the gland, called the ***adrenal cortex***, and by the inner layer, called the ***adrenal***

Flashpoint

There are several diseases of the parathyroid gland, but parathyroid cancer is very rare. Most physicians have no experience treating it.

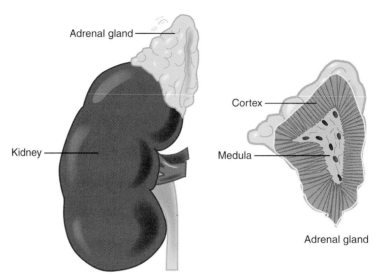

**FIGURE 14–5  Adrenal glands.**

*medulla*. The adrenal cortex makes three different groups of steroid hormones collectively called **corticosteroids**: mineralocorticoids, glucocorticoids, and sex hormones.

- *Mineralocorticoids* regulate the mineral content of the body. One of these hormones is *aldosterone*. It increases the reabsorption of Na$^+$ ions in the kidney so that more Na$^+$ ions return to the blood. This causes more K$^+$ ions to be flushed out with the urine.
- *Glucocorticoids* promote cellular metabolism. *Cortisol* is a glucocorticoid that is also called the "stress hormone" because it is secreted in stressful situations, such as injury, emotional distress, exercise, or hunger. It increases the use of fat as an energy source instead of glucose. This process saves glucose that may be in short supply for the brain so that it can continue functioning efficiently. Another glucocorticoid hormone is *cortisone*. It is also an anti-inflammatory that counters the effects of histamine, which causes swelling of tissue during injury or allergy.
- *Sex hormones* produce, regardless of gender, small amounts of estrogens, which are female sex hormones, and androgens, which are male sex hormones.

The adrenal medulla produces two hormones collectively called *catecholamines*. One is *epinephrine*, also called adrenaline, which speeds up heart rate, increases blood pressure, and increases breathing when the body reacts to stress. This activity increases the movement of oxygen and glucose into the organs, especially the brain, heart, and skeletal muscles. Secretion of epinephrine depends on the sympathetic nervous system. Release of this hormone allows a quick response in a stressful situation, often called the "fight or flight" response.

The other catecholamine is *norepinephrine*, also produced by the neurons as a neurotransmitter. Norepinephrine slows the epinephrine reaction and returns heart rate and blood pressure back to normal. This hormone also maintains the organ functions when the body is at rest.

Flashpoint

The EpiPen contains epinephrine, and it is injected during an allergic reaction to prevent shock.

## Pancreas

The *pancreas* is found in the abdominal cavity behind the lower stomach (see Fig. 14–6). This gland is an exocrine and an endocrine gland. As part of the digestive system, it is an exocrine gland that uses ducts to carry pancreatic juices to the stomach to aid in digestion. As an endocrine gland, it secretes insulin and glucagon into the bloodstream. These hormones are made in an area of the pancreas called the pancreatic islets, also called the islets of Langerhans. *Insulin* is secreted by cells called beta cells (see Box 14–1). This hormone carries

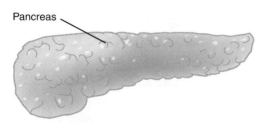

Pancreas

**FIGURE 14–6  Pancreas.**

## Box 14–1 Diabetes

Of all the endocrine system diseases and disorders, one of the most common is diabetes. There are three different forms of diabetes: diabetes mellitus, diabetes insipidus, and gestational diabetes.

Diabetes mellitus comes in two forms: Type 1 and Type 2. Type 1, also called juvenile diabetes or insulin-dependent diabetes, occurs when the pancreas, because of illness, injury, or defect, stops producing the hormone insulin. This hormone is needed to carry glucose from the bloodstream to the cells. If insulin is not produced, blood glucose levels increase, and the patient has increased thirst, weight loss, increased urination, and fatigue. Prolonged elevated glucose levels in the blood can cause mental confusion, unconsciousness, and coma. Treatment for Type 1 diabetes is injection of synthetic insulin several times a day to regulate the blood glucose levels.

Type 2, often called adult-onset diabetes or non–insulin-dependent diabetes, occurs when insulin is being produced by the pancreas, but is not being used correctly by the body. Type 2 diabetes can have a slow onset and is linked to lifestyle. Overweight, a poor diet, and lack of exercise all contribute to Type 2 diabetes. Treatment begins with increased exercise and weight loss. Prescription oral medications can also be taken to reduce blood glucose levels.

Diabetes insipidus causes increased thirst, increased fluid intake, and increased urination. Urine production increases, so urine does not concentrate and it appears pale or colorless. The most common reason for diabetes insipidus is a lack of vasopressin, a hormone produced by the kidney that controls the output of urine. Treatment with synthetic vasopressin relieves symptoms.

Gestational diabetes occurs during pregnancy and is a result of changing hormones and rapid weight gain. The insulin being produced by the mother's pancreas is not made in sufficient amounts to remove the excess glucose from the blood. High blood glucose levels can affect the fetus by causing high birth weight, low blood glucose, and breathing problems. Treatment includes diet restrictions and exercise. If glucose levels cannot be regulated with conservative treatment, insulin injections are prescribed.

glucose to the cells to be used as energy. A higher-than-normal level of blood glucose is *hyperglycemia*. *Glucagon* is released by alpha cells. It is the antagonist to insulin and is produced as a substitute if blood glucose levels become too low. A low blood glucose level is called *hypoglycemia*.

## Pineal Gland

The *pineal gland* is a small cone-shaped gland that hangs from the roof of the interior brain. The full function of the pineal gland is unknown, but it has been found to secrete a hormone called melatonin. *Melatonin* regulates the sleep cycle and causes drowsiness at night when levels increase and wakefulness during the day when levels decline.

## Thymus Gland

The *thymus gland* is located posterior to the sternum. It is the storage area for T lymphocytes, or T cells, and secretes *thymosin*, which causes the T lymphocytes to mature. The thymus gland is large at birth, but shrinks with age as the production of new T lymphocytes decreases.

## Gonads

The *gonads* are the general term for the female and male reproductive organs. In the ovaries, female hormones collectively called **estrogens** are produced. Individually, they are estrogen and progesterone. Both hormones regulate the menstrual cycle. Estrogen also stimulates the development of the female secondary sex characteristics.

The testes produce the male hormones called **androgens**. Testosterone is the most abundant and influential of these hormones. It is responsible for development of the male secondary sex characteristics and stimulates sperm production.

## Hormones Produced by Other Organs

Some other tissues and organs that are not a part of the endocrine system produce hormones. These organs include the kidney, heart, and stomach.

The kidneys secrete *erythropoietin*. This hormone stimulates blood cell production in the bone marrow. *Atrial natriuretic peptide* (ANP) is produced by the heart in response to an increase in blood pressure. ANP stimulates the kidney to release $Na^+$ in the urine and decrease blood pressure. The stomach produces *gastrin*, which stimulates the glands to secrete hydrochloric acid (HCl) for digestion.

Another structure that produces hormones is the placenta. This is a temporary organ that acts as the lifeline between a developing fetus and the mother. When implantation of the embryo occurs in the wall of the uterus, the placenta forms and secretes the hormone *human chorionic gonadotropin* (HCG). This hormone stimulates the corpus luteum of the ovary to continue making progesterone to maintain the uterine lining. After the third month of gestation, the ovary stops hormone production, and the placenta secretes estrogen and progesterone instead. These hormones are needed to maintain the uterine lining and suppress release of another egg.

See Table 14–2 for a summary of pathological disorders of the endocrine system.

## TABLE 14–2
### PATHOLOGY TERMS FOR THE ENDOCRINE SYSTEM

| | |
|---|---|
| Acromegaly | Enlargement of the extremities caused by production of growth hormone in adulthood after full growth has been reached |
| Addison disease | Adrenal glands cease producing sufficient amounts of steroid hormones; symptoms begin gradually and include fatigue, weight loss, and muscle weakness; advanced symptoms include nausea, diarrhea, hypoglycemia, sweating, and hyperpigmentation of the skin and mucous membranes; untreated, the disease can be fatal; treatment includes replacing the hormones the adrenal glands are not producing |
| Cretinism | Mental retardation caused by congenital deficiency of thyroid hormones |
| Diabetes | Disease in which the pancreas does not produce insulin or does not use it correctly, resulting in increased blood glucose levels; there are three forms: Type 1 where insulin is not being produced, Type 2 where insulin is not being used efficiently by the body, and gestational that occurs during pregnancy |
| Gigantism | Excessive height caused by increased amounts of growth hormone during childhood before the growth plates in the bones have closed; most often caused by a tumor on the pituitary gland; also known as giantism |

Pituitary gigantism.

| | |
|---|---|
| Goiter | Enlarged thyroid gland as a result of thyroid insufficiency because of lack of iodine in the diet |
| Graves disease | Autoimmune disease that causes overproduction of thyroid hormones; more common in women older than 20 yr; causes bulging of the eyes (exophthalmos), increased heart rate, and increased metabolism; treatment includes shrinking the thyroid with radioactive iodine or removal of the gland |

*Continued*

**TABLE 14–2**

**PATHOLOGY TERMS FOR THE ENDOCRINE SYSTEM—cont'd**

| Pituitary dwarfism | Decreased height and growth because of insufficiency of growth hormone before the growth plates in the bones have closed |

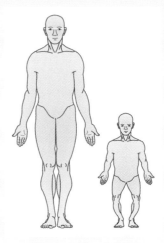

Pituitary dwarfism.

# Practice Exercises

## Multiple Choice

1. Thyroxine and triiodothyronine are hormones excreted by the _____.
   a. thalamus
   b. thymus
   c. thyroid
   d. throat

2. Cortisol is a _____.
   a. mineralocorticoid
   b. sex hormone
   c. glucocorticoid
   d. cortisone

3. The hormone that is an antagonist to insulin is _____.
   a. glucagon
   b. glucose
   c. glycogen
   d. glycerol

4. The hormones produced by the adrenal medulla are the _____.

   a.   catecholamines

   b.   mineralocorticoids

   c.   androgens

   d.   glucocorticoids

5. Human chorionic gonadotropin is secreted by the _____.

   a.   ovary

   b.   uterus

   c.   placenta

   d.   breast

## Fill in the Blank

1. The _____ gland is the storage area for T lymphocytes.

2. The "master gland" is the _____ gland.

3. The chemicals secreted by endocrine glands are called _____.

4. Metabolism is controlled by the _____ gland.

5. Regulation of hormones is done by _____.

6. The _____ is an endocrine and exocrine gland.

7. Melatonin is secreted by the _____ gland.

8. Male hormones are collectively called _____.

9. The pituitary gland is divided into a _____ and _____ lobe.

10. _____ is a neurotransmitter and a hormone.

## Matching

1. _____ Oxytocin

2. _____ Prolactin

3. _____ Thymosin

4. _____ Epinephrine

5. _____ Calcitonin

6. _____ Insulin

7. _____ Norepinephrine

8. _____ Thyroxine

9. _____ Melatonin

10. _____ Estrogen

a. Stimulates maturation of the T lymphocytes

b. Regulates the sleep cycle

c. Carries glucose to the cells

d. Female hormone

e. Stimulates uterine contractions during childbirth

f. Speeds up heart rate and blood pressure

g. Causes calcium to be stored in the bones

h. Stimulates breast development

i. Regulates heart rate when the body is at rest

j. Metabolic hormone

## Short Answer

1. **List the endocrine glands and their location in the body.**

2. **What is the difference between an endocrine gland and an exocrine gland?**

## Labeling

*Fill in the blanks with the appropriate anatomical terms.*

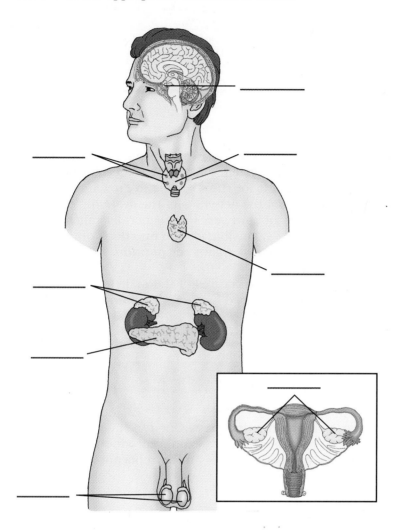

# 15

# THE REPRODUCTIVE SYSTEM

## Key Terms

blastocyst

dilation

embryo

expulsion

fertilization

fetus

gamete

gonad

human chorionic
gonadotropin

meiosis

menarche

menopause

menstrual cycle

mitosis

oogenesis

ovulation

ovum

prepuce

semen

sperm

### Flashpoint

The reproductive system contributes to homeostasis by secreting sex hormones that maintain the male and female body so that they are able to reproduce.

The ability of an organism to create new organisms is known as reproduction. In humans, the reproductive system makes the sex cells that carry genetic information, provides a means for the sex cells to grow and change, and produces hormones that control the activities of the system.

The reproductive organs of both sexes are generally called genitalia. The structures of the genitalia responsible for the functions of the reproductive system are the primary reproductive organs, or **gonads**. The gonads produce sex cells and secrete hormones.

This chapter discusses the structures of the male and female reproductive systems and the sex cells produced by each. Pregnancy and fetal development are also described.

## Types of Reproduction

Two different types of reproduction exist. One type is mitosis, or asexual reproduction. The other type is meiosis, or sexual reproduction. The human body uses both of these to replicate its cells and to replicate itself.

### Mitosis

**Mitosis** is known as asexual reproduction because it is how the cells of the body replicate (see Fig. 15–1).These cells reproduce by dividing themselves into two new cells. Mitosis has several different phases: interphase, prophase, metaphase, anaphase, and telophase. During these different phases, the cell organelles replicate, and the chromosomes in the nucleus become visible and align themselves in the middle of the cell. The chromosome strands split as they pull apart, and the cell separates, taking half of the DNA strand and half of the organelles with it. Eventually, the cell splits creating two identical cells.

Division by mitosis increases cell numbers for growth or repair of a cell and replaces cells that have died. Cells replicate themselves only a limited number of times; the number is different for different cells. At this point, the cell becomes specialized, so it does not need to divide further, such as a nerve cell, or it dies.

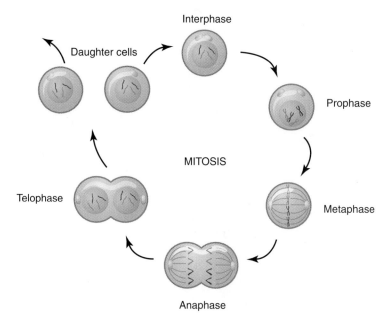

FIGURE 15–1 **Stages of mitosis.**

## Meiosis

**Meiosis** is sexual reproduction, and it is how sex cells or gametes are created (see Fig. 15–2). **Gametes** carry the genetic material that combine with gametes of the opposite gender to create a new organism. In humans, gametes each carry 23 chromosomes—half of the 46 chromosomes in the body. The process of meiosis differs between the male and female, but both reproductive systems produce cells that contain half the genes of the organism.

## Male Reproductive System

Organs of the male reproductive system produce sex cells, transport the cells, and secrete male hormones, collectively called **androgens**, that support the body. The male reproductive system has primary reproductive organs or gonads called testes, which are supported by accessory reproductive organs that include external and internal structures (see Fig. 15–3). Some reproductive structures of the male are also shared with the urinary system.

## External Reproductive System

The external male genitalia are the scrotum, testes, and penis. These structures are involved in making gametes and provide a means for them to be introduced in the female.

Males have two **testes**, which are the gonads, and they create gametes called sperm. **Sperm** contain the genetic material of the male.

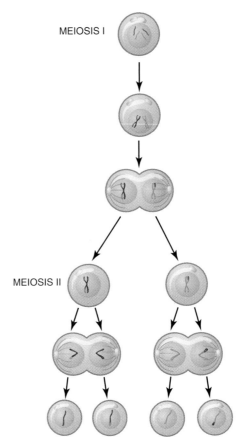

FIGURE 15–2  Stages of meiosis.

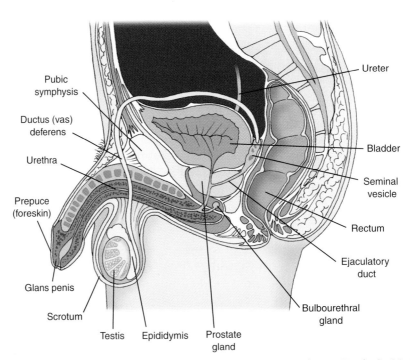

FIGURE 15–3  Internal and external male reproductive system. (From Eagle S. *Medical Terminology in a Flash!* Philadelphia, PA: FA Davis; 2006:171.)

The testes are located in a skin sac called the *scrotum*. Sperm prefer a temperature less than that of the body to mature. The scrotum enables the testes to hang away from the body so that they maintain a cooler temperature. The skin found between the scrotum and anus is the perineum.

Within each testis are tightly coiled ducts called *seminiferous tubules*. The stem cells that develop into immature sperm called spermatids are stored here.

The seminiferous tubules join to the *epididymis*, which is another coiled tubule that sits atop each testis. In the epididymis, the spermatids mature into sperm that are capable of swimming. The epididymis is also a temporary storage area for sperm. If the sperm are expelled or ejaculated, they enter into a duct called the *vas deferens*, or ductus deferens. The vas deferens joins to the epididymis externally, then enters the body to begin the internal structure of the reproductive system.

The *penis* is the organ that allows *semen*, which is the fluid containing sperm, to be introduced into the female reproductive system. The *shaft* of the penis is composed of erectile tissue, which is capable of filling with blood and becoming erect. The head of the penis is the *glans penis* and is covered by the *prepuce*, or foreskin. The *prepuce* attaches just under the glans penis to a ridge of skin called the *corona*. Often the prepuce is removed shortly after birth by a procedure called circumcision. The urethra opens at the tip of the glans penis, and the opening is referred to as the *meatus*.

Flashpoint

If the seminiferous tubules were stretched out, they would be longer than a football field.

## Internal Reproductive System

The internal structures and glands of the male reproductive system provide a means for sperm to be expelled from the body, and the glands provide nutrients and protection for the sperm. These structures are the vas deferens, urethra, seminal vesicles, prostate gland, and bulbourethral gland.

The vas deferens from each testis enters into the inguinal region of the pelvis and loops over the urinary bladder. The two ducts join here and become the urethra, which extends through the penis.

The *urethra* is the tube through which semen and urine leave the body, although both never pass at the same time. When ejaculation occurs and semen enters the urethra, the internal sphincter of the urinary bladder constricts so urine cannot leave the bladder and semen cannot enter.

In addition to sperm, semen comprises fluids that are received from three different glands located along the vas deferens. First are the *seminal vesicles* located at the base of the bladder where the vas deferens join to form the urethra. The seminal vesicles produce most of the fluid volume of semen. This fluid is a thick, yellowish secretion that contains sugar, vitamin C, prostaglandins, and other nutrients that activate and energize the sperm. The urethra begins as it enters through the second gland called the prostate gland.

The *prostate gland*, which encircles the urethra, is located just below the bladder and is about the size of a walnut. It secretes a milky fluid that further activates the sperm.

The third gland is the *bulbourethral gland*, which sits just below the prostate gland and attaches to the urethra by a duct. This gland secretes thick, clear mucus that drains into the urethra before semen is released. The mucus coats the urethra protecting the sperm from the acidic residue of urine and acts as a lubricant during sexual intercourse.

Flashpoint

Prostate cancer affects one in six men in the United States and occurs most commonly in men older than age 75.

increased height, increased body hair, and deepening of the voice. Men produce testosterone and sperm for the remainder of their lives, although the levels of both decrease with age.

# Female Reproductive System

The organs of the female reproductive system produce sex cells, transport those cells, secrete female hormones collectively called *estrogens*, and support and maintain a growing fetus. The primary sex organs, or gonads, of the female reproductive system are the ovaries, and they are supported by external and internal accessory structures. In contrast to the male, the gonads of the female are located within the pelvic cavity.

## External Genitalia

The external reproductive structures of the female are collectively called the *vulva* (see Fig. 15–7). The vulva consists of the mons pubis, labia majora, labia minora, and clitoris. These organs are not involved in gamete production or fetal development, but provide a means for a fetus to be expelled from the body, provide protection, and provide sexual stimulation.

The **mons pubis** (pubic mound) is a fleshy mound of adipose located just above the genitalia that protects the pubic bone. Continuous with the flesh of the mons pubis are large outer folds of skin called the *labia majora* (large lips). The mons pubis and labia majora are covered in pubic hair. Within the labia majora are smaller folds of skin called the *labia minora* (small lips). Between the labia minora is the *clitoris*, which is a small button-shaped piece of tissue that is equivalent to the glans penis. This structure is not directly related to reproduction, but gives pleasurable sensations during sexual intercourse. Below the clitoris is the urethral opening, and inferior to this is the vaginal opening. The vaginal opening is partially covered by a membrane called the *hymen*. This membrane is torn away by such things as trauma, use of tampons, or sexual intercourse. The *perineum* is the skin between the vagina and the anus.

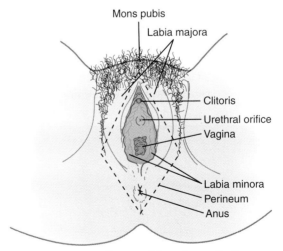

FIGURE 15–7 **External female genitalia.**

## Internal Genitalia

The internal female reproductive structures are involved in production of the gametes and provide an environment that supports the growth of a fetus. These structures include the vagina, cervix, uterus, fallopian tubes, and ovaries.

The internal structures start with the *vagina* (see Fig. 15–8). The vagina is a muscular tube 3 to 6 inches in length that lies between the bladder and the rectum. It is the receiving passage for the penis during intercourse and is the passageway for the delivery of an infant and for the flow of menstrual blood to leave the body.

Above the vagina is a small, funnel-shaped muscle called the *cervix* that connects the vagina to the uterus. The cervix is covered with mucus that slows the rate sperm enter the uterus except during the time that an egg is available for fertilization. This mucus also protects a fetus from microorganisms that may cause an infection.

The *uterus* is a pear-shaped hollow organ whose purpose is to receive a fertilized egg and retain and grow the developing fetus. The uterus is made of three layers of tissue: the *endometrium* (within the uterus), which lines the inside; the *myometrium* (muscle of the uterus), which is the thick muscle of the organ itself; and the *perimetrium* (around the uterus), which is the thin layer of muscle on the exterior.

Attached to either side of the uterus is a thin tube called the *fallopian tube*. Also called the uterine tube or oviduct, this tube acts as a passageway for an egg to reach the uterus and acts as the site for fertilization of an egg.

The egg is received from one of the two *ovaries* that are the primary female reproductive organs. The eggs carry the genetic material of the female. Ovaries are round structures located outside the fallopian tubes. The tubes are not attached to the ovaries, but have finger-like projections called *fimbriae* that create a current that carries the released egg into the tube.

*Flashpoint*

The fallopian tubes are named after Gabriele Fallopio, who was a 16th century anatomist that described the tubes and the other reproductive organs of both sexes.

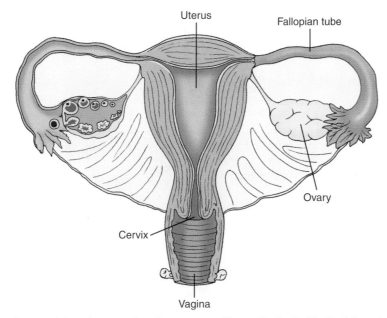

**FIGURE 15–8  Internal female reproductive system.** (From Eagle S. *Medical Terminology in a Flash!* Philadelphia, PA: FA Davis; 2006:172.)

## Egg Production

The process of creating egg cells is called oogenesis (see Fig. 15–9). In contrast to the male, this process starts in the womb when the ovaries are being formed. Within the ovaries are stem cells called ***oogonia***. These cells go through mitosis and form immature eggs cells called primary ***oocytes***. All primary oocytes are formed at about 20 weeks of gestation, and the ovaries contain approximately 7 million oocytes at birth. These oocytes remain dormant until puberty, but they decline in number as the female ages. After puberty, less than 800 of these oocytes mature over the course of a reproductive lifetime.

Similar to sperm, the gametes carry 23 of the 46 original chromosomes. In contrast to the gametes of the male, which have either an X or a Y chromosome, all eggs carry only an X chromosome.

Within the ovaries are follicles called ***graafian follicles*** that house the individual oocytes. At puberty, luteinizing hormone and follicle-stimulating hormone stimulate the ovaries, which trigger the graafian follicles to mature. Within the follicle, the primary oocyte divides several times until it becomes a secondary oocyte. Several follicles begin to mature simultaneously, although usually only one egg or ***ovum*** is released. After release of the egg, the empty follicle is now a ***corpus luteum*** (hollow body). This structure produces the female hormones estrogen and progesterone. These hormones change in levels throughout a 28-day cycle, and they influence the ovary and the uterus simultaneously (see Table 15–2).

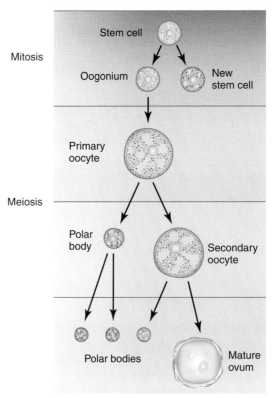

FIGURE 15–9  **Oogenesis.**

**TABLE 15–2**

**FEMALE REPRODUCTIVE HORMONES**

| Hormone | Function | Secreted by |
| --- | --- | --- |
| Follicle-stimulating hormone (FSH) | Stimulates ovaries to develop egg follicles; stimulates follicles to produce estrogen | Anterior pituitary |
| Luteinizing hormone (LH) | Causes ovulation; stimulates corpus luteum to secrete progesterone | Anterior pituitary |
| Estrogen | Causes maturation of egg follicles; promotes growth of uterine lining; responsible for female secondary sex characteristics | Ovary (follicle) |
| Progesterone | Causes increase in uterine lining | Ovary (corpus luteum) |
| Prolactin | Stimulates milk production in the breasts | Anterior pituitary |
| Oxytocin | Causes uterine contractions; stimulates release of milk by the breasts | Posterior pituitary |

# Menstrual Cycle

The **menstrual cycle** refers to the effect of the female hormones progesterone and estrogen on the reproductive system over a recurring 28-day cycle (see Fig. 15–10). The menstrual cycle is divided into four phases: menstruation, proliferative, ovulation, and secretory.

The first menstruation is called **menarche** and is a sign of the onset of puberty. Puberty begins in girls around age 12 to 15 years, although it may start in girls age 10 depending on weight, nutrition, level of body fat, and genetics. The female hormones are also responsible for the other effects of puberty, such as breast growth, widening of the hips, and the formation of fat deposits on the hips, buttocks, and thighs.

The menstrual cycle stimulates maturation and release of an egg. The first phase is the menstrual phase, and lasts for the first 4 or 5 days. At this time, the uterine lining is shed because no egg was implanted.

The second phase of the menstrual cycle is the proliferative, or follicular, phase and covers days 5 to 13 of the cycle. At this time, the ovary is producing estrogen at increasing levels, and progesterone is maintained at an even level. **Estrogen** stimulates the maturation of the graafian follicle.

Estrogen levels peak around day 14, and the egg erupts from the follicle to create the phase called **ovulation**. When the egg is released, there is an abrupt decline in the level of estrogen, which remains at a low level through the rest of the cycle.

The fourth phase is the secretory, or luteal, phase, which covers the rest of the cycle from day 15 to 28. During this phase, the empty graafian follicle becomes a structure called the corpus luteum (hollow body). For the next 14 days, the corpus luteum produces **progesterone**, which increases the thickness of the uterine lining in anticipation of implantation of a fertilized egg. If implantation does not occur, the corpus luteum heals and leaves scar tissue. This abrupt decrease in progesterone causes the uterine lining to be shed, which once again begins the menstrual phase (days 1 to 4). This cycle repeats itself throughout the reproductive years. **Menopause** occurs when a woman reaches an age at

Flashpoint
A normal menstrual flow produces about 2 to 3 oz of blood.

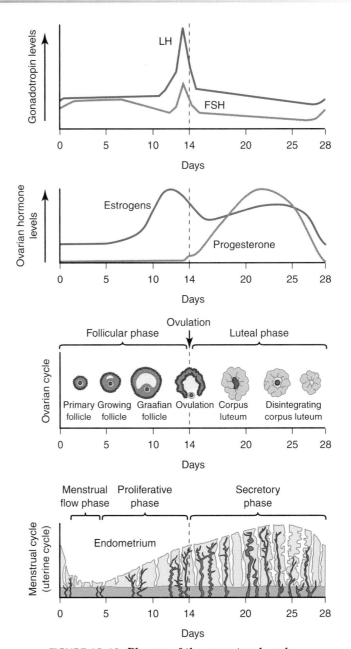

FIGURE 15–10  **Phases of the menstrual cycle.**

which the ovaries produce less hormone, and the menstrual cycle eventually stops altogether. Average age for menopause is between 45 and 55 years.

## Pregnancy

When a single sperm penetrates an egg, it is now fertilized. Fertilization, often called conception, most often occurs in the fallopian tube. Conception results in *pregnancy*, which is the state of a woman carrying a developing fetus within her body until its delivery. Human pregnancy lasts 40 weeks, or 9 calendar months. This time is also known as gestation, and the time is divided into trimesters, which are three phases of 3 months each. Each of these trimesters marks a different developmental stage of the fetus.

## Fetal Development

When fertilization occurs, the chromosomes from the sperm and egg combine to create a cell called a ***zygote***. The zygote begins cellular mitosis. After about 3 days of division, the zygote forms into a ***blastocyst***, which contains cells that separate to form two different structures—the placenta and the fetus. The blastocyst is responsible for implantation by sticking onto and then burrowing into the uterine lining. This occurs 5 to 7 days after conception. After implantation, the blastocyst is now an ***embryo*** and remains so until the eighth week of pregnancy. After the eighth week, the embryo is called a ***fetus*** (see Fig. 15–11).

The growth of the fetus is rapid, developing from one cell to an organism in 40 weeks (see Fig. 15–12). Growth in the first trimester or first 14 weeks is the most rapid. After implantation, the neural tube, which becomes the brain and spinal cord, and the heart develop. The heart beats at about week 5. By week 7, the fetus has arm and leg buds and developing internal organs. Next, cartilage starts to develop in the limbs, and the fetus can move by week 9. By the end of

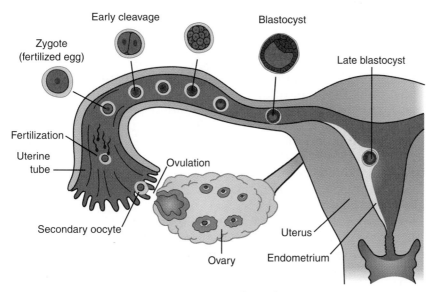

FIGURE 15–11  **Implantation.**

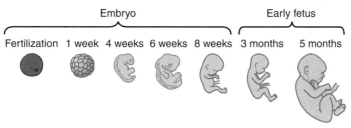

FIGURE 15–12  **Fetal development.**

the first trimester, all organs are present, and some are functional. The hands and feet are also fully developed.

The second trimester comprises weeks 15 to 28. At week 18, the vocal cords are functional, and the fetus can cry. Hair appears on the head at about week 20, and the sex organs are visible. In the later weeks of the second trimester, the lungs begin to develop. By the end of week 28, the fetus can recognize voices. The fetus now weighs about 2.2 lb, and muscle mass is increasing.

In the third trimester, weeks 29 to 40, the mass of the fetus increases quickly. Fat is deposited under the skin, and muscle becomes denser. Bone is quickly replacing the cartilage. By week 30, red blood cells are produced in the bone marrow. The rate of development slows in week 31. During week 33, the neurons grow rapidly forming the nervous system. At week 34, the fetus can blink and closes the eyes to sleep and opens them when awake. The fetus now looks like a newborn, and it can survive outside the uterus if necessary. A fetus is considered term at 37 weeks, but uses the last few weeks to gain weight and develop the lungs further. The fetus now weighs about 6 lb and gains a few more pounds by week 40.

## Placenta

After implantation, the blastocyst also forms a structure called a *placenta*, or umbilical cord, which is the lifeline between the fetus and the mother. Here the fetus exchanges oxygen, nutrients, antibodies, and wastes with the maternal blood that flows into and out of the placenta. A sac called the *amnion* forms around the embryo, and it floats in a protective fluid called *amniotic fluid*.

The placenta secretes a hormone called **human chorionic gonadotropin** (HCG), which inhibits the pituitary gland from secreting follicle-stimulating hormone and luteinizing hormone. This inhibition occurs so that the ovaries do not produce another egg. HCG stimulates the corpus luteum so that progesterone is still produced to maintain the uterine lining and prevent it from being expelled. HCG is the "pregnancy hormone" and is detectable in the urine and blood about 2 weeks after implantation. The levels increase for about 2 months after conception, then recede for the next 4 months and disappear altogether before birth.

## Birth

When a fetus has reached full development, hormone levels within the woman change and cause physical adjustments in her body. These changes allow the fetus to be born. *Birth*, or delivery, is initiated by the secretion of the hormone oxytocin, which stimulates uterine contractions and causes thinning and widening of the cervix. This stage is known as **dilation**. When the cervix dilates to 10 cm, the fetus can move into the birth canal or vagina. The abdominal muscles contract and push the fetus out. This is the stage of **expulsion**. After the fetus is delivered, the placenta pulls away from the uterus and is expelled as tissue called *afterbirth*.

*Flashpoint*

The word twin comes from the German word twine, which means "two together."

*Flashpoint*

Amniocentesis is a procedure in which a needle is inserted into the amnion, and a small amount of amniotic fluid is withdrawn. This fluid contains fetal cells that can be examined for genetic abnormalities.

# Breasts

In females, the **breasts** or mammary glands are an accessory organ of the female reproductive system and serve as a means of nourishing a newborn (see Fig. 15–13). Breasts are located above the pectoralis major muscles and start at about the third rib and extend to about the sixth rib; they extend laterally from the sternum to the axillae. On the tip of each breast is a nipple surrounded by an area of pigmented skin called an **areola**. Breasts comprise lobes that contain glands and ducts. Milk-producing ducts within the lobes connect to the nipple. The lobes are separated by dense connective tissue and adipose that support the breasts and attach them to the pectoral muscles. Estrogen causes enlargement of breast tissue during puberty. During pregnancy, the hormone **prolactin** causes milk to be secreted in the ducts. Male mammary glands are similar to mammary glands of the female, but do not develop during puberty.

For a summary of diseases and disorders of the reproductive system, see Table 15–3 and Box 15-1..

*Flashpoint*

Male breast cancer is a rare condition, accounting for only 1% of breast cancers. Most cases of male breast cancer occur in men 60 to 70 years old.

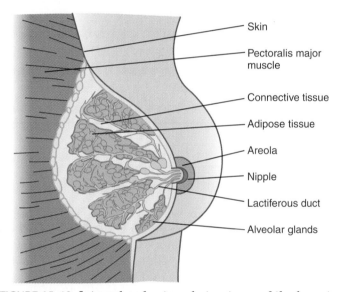

- Skin
- Pectoralis major muscle
- Connective tissue
- Adipose tissue
- Areola
- Nipple
- Lactiferous duct
- Alveolar glands

**FIGURE 15–13  Internal and external structures of the breast.**

## TABLE 15–3

### PATHOLOGY TERMS FOR THE REPRODUCTIVE SYSTEM

| | |
|---|---|
| Amenorrhea | Absence of menstruation; may be due to endocrine disorders, low body weight, excessive exercise, or medications |
| Anorchidism | Failure of one or both testes to develop |
| Benign prostatic hypertrophy | Enlargement of prostate gland; commonly occurs in men >60 years old |
| Breast cancer | Malignant neoplasm of the breast; found most often in milk ducts or lobules that produce milk; risk increases with age for all women, and there is a genetic link that increases risk in some women |

*Continued*

**TABLE 15-3**

**PATHOLOGY TERMS FOR THE REPRODUCTIVE SYSTEM—cont'd**

| | |
|---|---|
| Abruptio placentae | Result of placenta pulling away from uterine wall leaving the fetus without a supply of oxygen or nutrients and causing severe bleeding in the mother |
| Breech birth | Delivery of the fetus in a position other than head first |
| Cervical cancer | Malignant neoplasm of the cervix; most often caused by some strains of human papillomavirus (HPV) |
| Cryptorchidism | Failure of the testes to descend into the scrotum |
| Eclampsia | Seizures during pregnancy usually caused by preeclampsia |
| Ectopic pregnancy | Implantation of a fertilized egg in a place other than the uterus, most commonly in the fallopian tube; symptoms include stabbing pain in the abdomen, dizziness, and unusual vaginal discharge; if caught early, a dose of methotrexate allows the body to absorb the embryo; in later stages, laparoscopic surgery is needed to remove embryo; untreated, fallopian tube ruptures causing hemorrhage and possibly death |
| Endometriosis | Growth of uterine tissue outside the uterus; most common symptom is pelvic pain during menstruation; laparoscopic surgery is done to remove excess tissue; hysterectomy may be done in severe cases |
| Ovarian cyst | Fluid-filled sacs on ovary that may cause pain, abnormal bleeding, and cramping; most cysts heal without treatment |
| Preeclampsia | Hypertension, vision changes, and headaches during pregnancy; may progress to eclampsia |
| Testicular cancer | Malignant neoplasm of the testis; occurs most commonly in men 20-34 years old |

## Box 15-1 Sexually Transmitted Diseases

Sexually transmitted diseases (STDs), or venereal diseases, are also called sexually transmitted infections (STIs), to reflect the potential for someone to be infected and spread the infection, but not show symptoms of the disease. STDs are caused by bacteria, viruses, and other microorganisms. It is estimated that 19 million people are infected with STDs each year, and 50% are 15 to 24 years old.

Gonorrhea is caused the bacterium *Neisseria gonorrhoeae,* which grows in the mucous membranes, in the genital area, and inside the uterus. There are 700,000 new cases each year in the United States. Gonorrhea is spread through contact with an infected penis, anus, vagina, or mouth. Pregnant women can pass it to the fetus. This infection is most active in teenagers. Women may have no symptoms. If symptoms appear, they include painful or burning urination, increased vaginal discharge, and bleeding between periods. Men also may not show symptoms, but if present they include burning during urination, green discharge, and swollen testicles. For men and women, anal gonorrhea causes itching, soreness, bleeding, or painful bowel movements. In the throat, it causes a sore, burning throat. If untreated in women, gonorrhea can lead to pelvic inflammatory disease, which damages the fallopian tubes and increases the chance of ectopic pregnancy. In men, it can cause epididymitis, which can lead to infertility. In a fetus, it can cause eye infections that may cause blindness. Gonorrhea is treated with antibiotics.

## Box 15–1 Sexually Transmitted Diseases—cont'd

Syphilis is caused by the bacterium *Treponema pallidum*. There are about 36,000 new cases per year in the United States, and it tends to occur in people 20 to 39 years old. There are three phases of the infection. The first phase is the appearance of chancres or open sores on the mouth and genitals. They heal in 1 to 5 weeks. If the person has not been diagnosed with syphilis, the infection goes to the second phase, which can start several months after the first phase. This phase causes a round, copper-colored rash on the feet and lower legs called "copper penny rash," patchy hair loss, and development of hard white warts on the genital area. The third phase of syphilis can develop months or years after infection. In this stage, the bacteria have spread to the nervous system and heart. The bacteria cause dementia, blindness, and heart damage, and can cause large ulcers on the face that destroy the nose and lips. Syphilis spreads through contact with the sores and fluids from those sores. In the first stage, syphilis can be cured with an injection of penicillin. Later stages can be cured with several doses of penicillin, but the damage to the nervous system and heart cannot be undone.

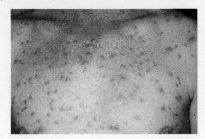

Copper penny rash from syphilis. (From *Taber's Cyclopedic Medical Dictionary Edition*. 21st ed. Philadelphia, PA: FA Davis; 2009:2264.)

Chlamydia is caused by the bacterium *Chlamydia trachomatis*. It is the most common STD in the United States with more 2 million individuals 14 to 39 years old infected each year. The numbers are so high because about 75% of infected women and 50% of infected men do not show symptoms, so they do not know they are infected. Symptoms in women are abnormal vaginal discharge, painful urination, bleeding between periods, lower back pain, and pain during intercourse. The bacteria spread to the fallopian tubes, causing scarring and infertility. Men may have a discharge and painful urination. Some may experience burning or itching around the opening of the urethra. In the rectum of men and women, chlamydia can cause pain, discharge, and bleeding. Bacteria in the throat cause soreness. A pregnant woman can pass the infection to a fetus resulting in eye and respiratory infections and premature birth. Treatment is a single dose of antibiotic. Reinfection with chlamydia is more common than with other STDs.

Herpes simplex virus (HSV) affects approximately 67 million people, or one out of four individuals, in the United States. There are two types of virus: HSV-1 infects the mouth, and HSV-2 infects the genitals. About 500,000 new cases of both types are reported every year. HSV causes sores or ulcers on the skin. On the mouth, these ulcers are referred to as "cold sores"; they take 2 to 21 days to heal. Genital herpes may appear asymptomatic, meaning no ulcers may appear after infection. When the first infection occurs, the virus moves to the sensory nerves in the area and remains dormant or resting. Stress, other infections, diet, and other irritations to the sensory nerves trigger another cycle of ulcers, and this continues for the life of the infected person. Herpes of the mouth is not considered an STD, but both types are spread by skin-to-skin contact and contact with the open sores or infected body fluids.

*Continued*

## Box 15–1 Sexually Transmitted Diseases—cont'd

Genital herpes can be spread when no sores are present. There is no cure for the virus, but medication such as valacyclovir can lessen the time of an outbreak and increase the time between outbreaks. Patients taking the medication are still contagious and capable of spreading the disease to his or her partner.

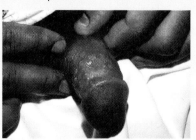

Genital herpes. (From *Taber's Cyclopedic Medical Dictionary Edition.* 21st ed. Philadelphia, PA: FA Davis; 2009:1069.)

Human papillomavirus (HPV) affects the skin and mucous membranes. About 20 million people are infected, and 6 million become newly infected each year. There are more than 40 different strains of HPV that can cause infections of the genitals of men and women. HPV causes genital warts, although 90% of infected individuals do not have the warts. If warts appear, they are usually in groups, and they can be flat or raised or resemble cauliflower. The warts can appear on the thighs, vagina, cervix, penis, scrotum, and anus of the infected person. This virus is spread through skin contact with an infected individual. Some types of HPV that infect the cervix can cause cervical cancer. Others increase the chances of penile cancer. There is no cure for HPV. A vaccine has become available to prevent some strains that cause cervical cancer. It has been approved for use in girls and women 11 to 26 years old.

About 1 million people are infected with human immunodeficiency virus (HIV) in the United States. It is spread through contact with body fluids, such as semen, blood, and vaginal secretions. It can enter the body through unprotected sex or a needle stick, and at one time it was transmitted through blood transfusions. Donated blood is now screened for HIV and is considered safe. There are three stages of HIV infection. The first stage begins with flu-like symptoms that appear 10 to 14 days after infection with the virus. These symptoms are fever, swollen glands, and fatigue. These symptoms last 1 week to 1 month. The second stage of infection is when the virus continues to spread throughout the cells of the body. HIV targets and destroys T lymphocytes, so it decreases the body's ability to protect itself. As the immune system is destroyed, infected individuals begin to have symptoms of weight loss, fatigue, persistent yeast infections or urinary tract infections, skin rashes, and short-term memory loss. This phase can take years to progress. When all the T lymphocytes are destroyed, the infected person has progressed to acquired immunodeficiency syndrome (AIDS). Patients do not die of AIDS; they die of opportunistic infections that would not harm people with normal immune systems. Symptoms of AIDS are pneumonia, tumors, mental confusion and dementia, vision loss, skin sores and ulcers, lack of coordination, and seizures. HIV can be passed to a fetus from an infected mother. HIV infection in children progresses the same as in adults, but children may not become infected with the same opportunistic infections. Children tend to have recurrent childhood illnesses, such as ear infections, conjunctivitis, and tonsillitis.

# Practice Exercises

## Multiple Choice

1. An embryo becomes a _____ after 8 weeks of gestation.
   a. zygote
   b. fetus
   c. neonate
   d. blastocyst

2. Milk production is stimulated by the hormone _____.
   a. estrogen
   b. progesterone
   c. prolactin
   d. oxytocin

3. The _____ connects the embryo to the uterus.
   a. placenta
   b. blastocyst
   c. fetal cord
   d. fallopian tube

4. The stage of _____ is when the uterus contracts and the cervix opens.
   a. ovulation
   b. dilation
   c. expulsion
   d. contraction

5. The _____ gland produces fluid that activates the sperm.
   a. prostate gland
   b. seminal
   c. bulbourethral
   d. pituitary

6. Afterbirth is the name of the _____ when it is expelled after delivery.
   a. fetus
   b. placenta
   c. amniotic fluid
   d. uterine lining

7. An empty egg follicle is called a _____.

   a. corpus luteum

   b. graafian follicle

   c. ovary

   d. oocyte

8. The coiled tubule that sits on top of each testis is the _____.

   a. urethra

   b. epididymis

   c. seminal tubule

   d. vas deferens

9. Male hormones are collectively called _____.

   a. androgens

   b. testosterones

   c. estrogens

   d. progesterones

10. Another term for sex cells is _____.

   a. spermatids

   b. oocytes

   c. gametes

   d. gonads

## True or False

1. True   False   A blastocyst becomes a fetus after 2 weeks.

2. True   False   HCG is an indicator of pregnancy.

3. True   False   Immature egg cells are called oocytes.

4. True   False   The cervix connects the uterus to the vagina.

5. True   False   A fertilized egg implants in the fallopian tube.

6. True   False   The medical term for foreskin is prepuce.

7. True   False   A human pregnancy lasts for 42 weeks.

8. True   False   Fimbriae are finger-like projections at the end of the vas deferens.

9.  True    False    The fetus floats in amniotic fluid.

10. True    False    Ovulation is the release of an ovum from the ovary.

## Fill in the Blank

1.  The production of sperm is _____.

2.  The hormones _____ and _____ control the menstrual cycle.

3.  The _____ follicles of the ovaries hold an oocyte.

4.  Sperm mature in a coiled tubule on the testis called the _____.

5.  The production of eggs is _____.

6.  _____ is the first menstrual cycle.

7.  Testes make the hormone _____.

8.  Sexual reproduction is also called _____.

9.  A general term for the female genitalia is _____.

10. _____ is the stoppage of the menstrual cycle because of decrease in hormones.

## Short Answer

1.  **List the steps of spermatogenesis.**

2.  **List the steps of oogenesis.**

## Labeling

*Fill in the blanks with the appropriate anatomical terms.*

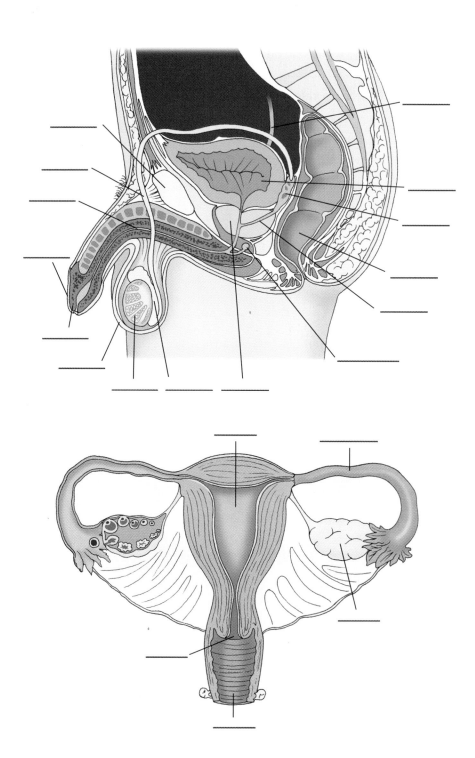

# A

**abdominal cavity:** Space located below the diaphragm and under the abdominal muscles that contains the internal organs.

**absorption:** Action of nutrients entering into the tissues of the small intestine by finger-like structures called microvilli.

**accommodation:** Changes that occur in the eye when light entering the eye from a close object causes the light to scatter so that the lens must shorten and bulge slightly to get the light into a tighter form to correct the image.

**action potential:** Change in a cell from a state of rest to that of activity and back to rest.

**active immunity:** Type of immunity in which the body must find and recognize a foreign antigen and create an antibody against it.

**active transport:** Form of cell transport that needs to use energy to move substances in and out of a cell.

**adipose:** Connective tissue found in the subcutaneous layer of the skin; composed of adipocytes and collagen, and connects the skin to the muscle beneath.

**aerobic respiration:** Process of breaking down glucose into energy by the use of oxygen.

**agglutination:** Immune response that causes the clumping of blood cells secondary to mixing incompatible blood types.

**alimentary canal:** Continuous tube from the mouth to the anus; also called the gastrointestinal tract.

**allergy:** Overreaction of the immune system to a substance that is perceived as a threat but actually is harmless. The body produces IgE and eosinophils, which stimulate the release of histamine. The histamine causes vessels to become leaky, resulting in a runny nose, watery eyes, and itching, reddened skin.

**amphiarthroses:** Slightly movable joints.

**anabolism:** Process of metabolism that forms or binds together smaller molecules to make larger ones.

**anaerobic respiration:** Process of breaking down glucose into energy without the presence of oxygen.

**anaphylaxis:** Condition that results when an allergen enters the bloodstream and causes a rapid immune response, which includes constriction of the airway, dilation of the blood vessels resulting in rapid collapse of circulation, and a sudden decrease in blood pressure. Death can occur quickly, often within minutes.

**anatomical position:** The body when standing erect with the face front and arms at the sides and palms facing forward.

**anatomy:** Study of the structure of the body.

**androgens:** Collective name for the male hormones produced by the testes.

**antagonist:** Muscles that have an opposite function.

**antibody:** Made by B cells in response to foreign antigens in the body. They attach to and destroy the foreign antigens; also called immunoglobulins.

**antigen:** Identifying marker on the surface of a cell.

**aorta:** Largest artery of the body, which is attached to the heart at the left ventricle; responsible for taking oxygenated blood to the body.

**aortic semilunar valve:** Structure between the left ventricle and the aorta that acts as a doorway to keep blood in the aorta.

**appendicular skeleton:** The bones of the appendages or limbs.

**artery:** Vessels that carry oxygenated blood. They pulse in time with the heartbeat to push blood into smaller vessels.

**articulated:** The act of the bones of the skeleton being in their proper location and joined together at the joints.

**ATP (adenosine triphosphate):** The energy created by the mitochondria of the cell.

**atria:** Two upper chambers of the heart.

**atrioventricular (AV) node:** Second node in the intrinsic conduction system located at the entrance to the right ventricle.

**autograft:** Transplant that involves moving tissue from one area to another in the same person.

**autoimmune disease:** Occurs when cells or tissues of the body come under attack by T cells because they are mistakenly identified as foreign.

**autonomic nervous system:** Part of the peripheral nervous system that controls involuntary bodily functions.

**axial skeleton:** Bones that make up the axis of the body or the main point from which the limbs are joined.

## B

**basal cell carcinoma:** Form of skin cancer that results in the cells of the basal layer being unable to keratinize and rising to the surface of the skin to form shiny nodules; most often found on the face and ears. Survival rate is 99%.

**bicuspid valve:** Structure found between the left atrium and left ventricle of the heart that acts as a doorway to prevent blood from flowing backward.

**bile:** Substance made by the liver and stored in the gallbladder; responsible for emulsification of fat.

**blastocyst:** Stage of fetal development after the zygote stage where the rapidly dividing cell forms a mass that implants in the uterine lining and will become the embryo and placenta.

**bolus:** Mass of chewed food and saliva formed in the oral cavity.

**brain:** Organ found within the skull that acts as control center of the body; part of the central nervous system.

**bulk transport:** Form of active transport that causes a change in the cell membrane to move a substance in and out. Endocytosis and exocytosis are forms of bulk transport.

**bundle of His:** Conductive tissue located in the septum of the heart.

## C

**callus:** Raised area that forms around the break in a bone as a result of osteoblasts creating cartilage to repair the break.

**carbohydrate:** Nutrient that is the preferred source of fuel for cells to make ATP. Carbohydrates are digested into their simplest form, which is glucose.

**cartilage:** Fibrous tissue found between bones; acts as a cushion to prevent bone grinding against bone.

**catabolism:** Process of metabolism that breaks down substances into smaller ones

**cell:** First functional level for living things.

**cell-mediated immunity:** Immunity created by the T lymphocytes that is responsible for recognizing the body's own antigens as being different from foreign antigens.

**cell membrane:** Skinlike outer covering of the cell. It is semipermeable, allowing some substances in while keeping others out.

**cellular respiration:** Process of cells creating energy to power the muscles.

**cellular transport:** General term for moving substances back and forth between the cell and the environment.

**central nervous system (CNS):** Comprises the brain and spinal cord, and oversees the entire nervous system.

**cerebrospinal fluid:** Protective fluid found in the ventricles of the brain and surrounding the spinal cord.

**cerebrum:** Largest section of the brain. It is separated into two hemispheres and controls all learned information, logic, speech, and interpretation of stimuli.

**chemical level:** First structural level. This level is composed of atoms that form molecules.

**chemoreceptors:** Receptors that respond to chemical changes in the body.

**cholesterol:** Lipid made by the liver and ingested through diet. It is used in transportation and is a component of cell membranes.

**chromosome:** Genetic material that carries the codes that make up an organism.

**chyme:** Semiliquid that forms when the bolus is broken down by enzymes and acids in the stomach.

**cilia:** Long hairlike projections on the surface of some cells that move substances across the surface of the cell.

**codon:** Three base pairs on a strand of DNA that form an amino acid during protein synthesis.

**colony-stimulating factor:** Substance that stimulates the bone marrow to produce white blood cells.

**compact bone:** Bone that has a dense and heavy structure; found in the bones that need strength to hold the body upright.

**concentration gradient:** Range of a concentration from lowest to highest.

**conduction:** Process of sound traveling through the structures of the outer, middle, and inner ear.

**cones:** Color receptors found in the retina of the eye.

**contraction:** Shortening of a muscle, which is the basis for body movement.

**corticosteroids:** Collective name of the three different groups of steroid hormones produced by the adrenal cortex—mineralocorticoids, glucocorticoids, and sex hormones.

**cranial cavity:** Cavity that contains the brain and is part of the dorsal cavity.

**cranial nerves:** Twelve pairs of nerves attached to the brain that control movement and stimuli of the head, neck, and abdomen.

**cytoplasm:** Collectively, fluid and organelles inside of the cell membrane.

**cytosol:** Semifluid substance in which cell organelles are suspended.

## D

**defecation:** Act of removing solid waste from the body.

**depolarization:** Part of the action potential when a cell is stimulated and capable of producing an action.

**dermis:** Second layer of the skin, which consists of blood vessels, nerves, hair follicles, and glands.

**diaphysis:** Shaft of a long bone.

**diarthroses:** Freely movable joint.

**diastole:** Relaxation phase of the heart created by the release of the Purkinje fibers on the ventricles.

**diffusion:** Movement of molecules from a higher concentration to a lower concentration across a concentration gradient.

**digestion:** Act of breaking down food into nutrients that can be used by the body.

**DNA (deoxyribonucleic acid):** Genetic material found in the nucleus of a cell; carries all information needed to make a new organism.

**dorsal cavity:** Cavity that contains the cranial cavity and spinal cavity.

## E

**embryo:** Stage of fetal development after implantation until the eighth week of gestation.

**emulsification:** Act of bile breaking down fat contained in the chyme.

**endocardium:** Smooth epithelial tissue lining the inside of the heart.

**endocrine gland:** Duct-less glands that secrete hormones directly into the bloodstream.

**endoplasmic reticulum:** Cell organelle that provides a transportation system to take proteins from the ribosomes to the Golgi bodies.

**epicardium:** Outer layer of the heart.

**epidermis:** Outer layer of the skin made of epithelial tissue; contains no blood vessels or glands.

**epigastric region:** Abdominal region directly above the umbilicus.

**epinephrine:** Catecholamine produced by the parasympathetic nervous system that speeds up heart rate, dilates pupils, and increases respiration in response to stress; also called adrenaline.

**epiphysis:** End of a long bone; the site of bone growth.

**equilibrium:** State of balance. In a concentration gradient, it is when there is no longer a more or less concentrated area.

**erythrocytes:** Red blood cells (RBCs) that carry oxygen.

**erythropoietin:** Hormone that stimulates the bone marrow to produce red blood cells.

**estrogens:** Collective name for the female sex hormones produced by the ovaries. Individually, estrogen stimulates the development of secondary female sex characteristics, controls the start of menstruation, and maintains the menstrual cycle.

**excretion:** Elimination of substances.

**exocrine gland:** Glands that secrete hormones through ducts to the external body.

**expiration:** Exhalation, or the releasing of breath.

**expiratory reserve volume:** Amount of air that is expired with one maximum breath. This is a breath that forces air out of the lungs longer than a normal expiration. On average, 1200 mL of air can be forced out of the lungs.

**external respiration:** Action that occurs only in the lungs when an expiration releases the carbon dioxide from the body and an inspiration brings oxygen in. Air is brought in from the external environment and returned to the external environment.

**extracellular fluid:** Fluid found outside the cells.

**facilitated diffusion:** Use of enzymes to carry molecules from a higher concentration to a lower concentration across a cell membrane.

## F

**fat:** Nutrient used for energy production; is a component of cell membranes and is stored for insulation and cushioning. Fat stores can also be used in place of glucose if none is available. Fats are a type of lipid and are broken down into triglycerides.

**fertilization:** Act of a sperm penetrating an egg and beginning the division of the cells to create an embryo; also called conception.

**fetus:** Stage of fetal development; an embryo becomes a fetus after 8 days of gestation. This is the time of organ development and growth.

**filtration:** Process of bringing blood into the glomerulus of the nephron for separating soluble wastes.

**fixator:** Muscle that holds one bone in place while a more distal bone moves.

**flagellum:** Single projection on some cells that moves the cell by propelling it forward.

**fontanel:** Cartilage found between the skull bones in newborns.

**frequency:** Number of vibrations in a sound wave; measured in Hertz (Hz).

**frontal plane:** Plane that separates the body into a ventral and dorsal section.

**full-thickness burn:** Burn where skin appears blackened and charred, and damage can go to the muscle and bone; also called third-degree burn.

## G

**gamete:** General term for the male and female sex cells, called an ovum in females and sperm in males.

**gene:** Section of DNA that codes for a single protein.

**gland:** Cells or organs that secrete a substance that has some effect on another cell or organ.

**Golgi body:** Organelles that wrap proteins in membranes and send them to wherever they are needed inside or outside the cell.

**gonads:** General term for the primary sex organs, called the ovary in females and the testis in males.

**granulocytes:** Leukocytes that have granules in the cytoplasm.

**growth hormone (GH):** Metabolic hormone secreted by the anterior pituitary that controls the growth of muscles and bones; also stimulates amino acids to be made into proteins and causes most cells to grow and divide.

**gyri:** Folds of the cerebrum.

## H

**hematopoiesis:** Production of blood cells in the red bone marrow.

**hemolytic disease of the newborn:** Destruction of fetal red blood cells that occurs when an Rh⁻ mother is pregnant with an Rh⁺ fetus, and maternal Rh antibodies attack the fetal cells.

**hemostasis:** Blood stoppage because of a clot formed by platelets and fibrinogen.

**homeostasis:** When the body maintains a stable state in response to changes in the internal and external environment.

**hormones:** Chemicals secreted by the exocrine glands that create a change in the body.

**human chorionic gonadotropin (HCG):** Hormone released by an embryo and then by the placenta. It causes the corpus luteum to continue to produce progesterone to maintain the uterine lining. It is detectable in urine and blood about 2 weeks after conception.

**humoral immunity:** Immunity created by B cells that circulate in the blood searching for and destroying foreign antigens, such as bacteria and mold.

**hypochondriac region:** Region of the abdomen found on the left and right sides just under the ribs.

**hypogastric region:** Region of the abdomen located under the umbilicus.

## I

**iliac region:** Region of the abdomen found on the right and left sides of the pelvic area.

**immunity:** Protection of the body by the lymphatic system by creation of either a nonspecific or a specific defensive response to foreign substances.

**immunoglobulin:** Made by B lymphocytes in response to foreign antigens in the body. They attach to and destroy foreign antigens; also called antibodies.

**inflammatory response:** Pain, redness, heat, and swelling that occur when the skin has been broken. This response prevents foreign substances from entering.

**ingestion:** Act of taking food into the mouth.

**insertion:** Site where a muscle attaches to a moving bone.

**inspiration:** Act of inhalation or breathing in.

**inspiratory reserve volume:** Amount of air breathed into the lungs past the normal inspired volume; range 2000 to 3200 mL.

**insulin:** Hormone secreted by the pancreas that binds to glucose in the blood and transports it to the cells.

**internal respiration:** Action that occurs within the cells of the body when oxygen and carbon dioxide are exchanged within the capillaries.

**intracellular fluid:** Fluid found within the cells.

**isograft:** Transplant graft performed between identical twins. Tissue types are the same in identical twins, so antigens on the tissues are identical.

**isometric contraction:** Causes tension on the muscle, but does not produce movement.

**isotonic contraction:** Causes shortening of the muscle to produce movement.

# J

**joint:** Place where two bones come together.

# K

**keratinize:** Hardening or thickening of cells by the protein keratin.

# L

**left atrium:** Chamber of the heart that receives oxygenated blood from the lungs.

**left ventricle:** Chamber of the heart that contracts to push oxygenated blood into the aorta.

**leukocytes:** White blood cells (WBCs) that protect the body and fight infection.

**ligament:** Connective tissue that joins bone to bone at a joint.

**lobe:** Area of the brain named for the cranial bone under which it is located.

**lumbar region:** Lateral to the umbilical region.

**lymphocytes:** Agranulocytic leukocytes that increase in response to foreign substances and provide immunity; also called B and T cells.

**lysosomes:** Organelles that collect and digest any debris in the cell.

# M

**malignant melanoma:** Form of skin cancer that results from damage to the melanocytes. It appears as a brown splotch on the skin and can spread quickly to the lymph nodes and other areas of the body. Survival rate is 50%.

**mastication:** Act of breaking down or chewing of food.

**matrix:** Substance composed of nonliving materials in which the cells that form the different types of connective tissue are suspended.

**mechanoreceptors:** Receptors that detect changes in movement or pressure.

**median plane:** Sagittal plane that divides the body into equal right and left parts; also called the mid-sagittal plane.

**meiosis:** Sexual reproduction; through a series of divisions, stem cells become immature gametes that carry half the chromosomes of the organism.

**melanin:** Black, brown, green, or yellow pigment that gives color to skin, hair, and the iris of the eye.

**melanocytes:** Cells that produce black, brown, yellow, or green pigment. These cells give color to the skin, hair, and iris of the eyes.

**membrane:** Thin layers of tissue that cover structures and line cavities.

**menarche:** First menstrual cycle.

**meninges:** Tissues that cover the brain and spinal cord.

**menopause:** Age at which the ovaries cease producing hormones, and the menstrual cycle stops.

**menstrual cycle:** Recurring 28-day cycle in women in which the effects of estrogen and progesterone on the ovaries and uterus cause an egg to mature and be released and the uterine lining to thicken and be expelled if implantation does not occur.

**metabolism:** General term for all the chemical reactions that occur in the body.

**microvilli:** Finger-like projections lining the small intestine that increase the surface area and aid in the absorption of nutrients.

**micturition:** Process of urination.

**mineral:** Inorganic substances needed in small or trace amounts by the body.

**mitochondria:** Organelles that are called the "powerhouse" of the cell because they take nutrients and turn them into an energy source called ATP.

**mitosis:** Asexual reproduction; the process of cells splitting into two new cells identical to the original.

**muscle fibers:** Found in skeletal and smooth muscle and have an elongated, cylindrical shape; also called muscle cells.

**muscle tone:** Slight state of contraction a muscle always maintains.

**myocardium:** Thick middle layer of the heart muscle.

# N

**nares:** Another term for nostrils.

**natural flora:** Bacteria that live normally in and on the body.

**negative feedback:** An action that regulates hormone levels. Hormones are secreted by the endocrine glands only as they are needed by the target cells or organs. The endocrine glands respond to a change in the body that signals a particular gland to increase or decrease secretion depending on the need of the target organ. Secretion of a hormone occurs until the signal to which it is responding stops. The hormone level then decreases until the hormone receives a signal to be secreted again.

**nephron:** Structures inside the kidney that filter waste and produce urine.

**neuroglia:** Collective name for the cells that aid the nervous system.

**neuron:** Nerve cell.

**neurotransmitters:** Chemicals produced by the axon terminals that pass a stimulus across the synapse to the next neuron. Different chemicals control specific bodily functions or responses.

**nitrogenous wastes:** Soluble wastes found in urine that are the by-products of the breakdown of nitrogen; include urea and uric acid

**nonspecific immunity:** Type of immunity that comprises the defenses with which we are born; also called natural or innate immunity.

**nonsteroid hormones:** Hormones that are not water soluble and need to bind to receptors on the cell membrane to cause a response in the cell.

**norepinephrine:** Catecholamine produced by the sympathetic nervous system that aids epinephrine by increasing heart rate and releasing glucose stores to be used for energy to fuel the skeletal muscles.

**nucleus:** Organelle that holds the DNA or the genetic material of the cell.

**nutrients:** Essential substances the body needs to grow, repair, and sustain life functions.

# O

**olfactory receptors:** Sensory receptors in the nose that detect odors.

**oogenesis:** Creation of egg cells or ova in the primary sex organs of the female by meiosis.

**organ:** Structural level formed by two or more different tissues that perform the same function.

**organelle:** Structures within a cell that perform the processes that keep a cell alive.

**organism:** The highest structural level formed by different systems working together.

**origin:** Site where a muscle attaches to a stationary bone.

**osmosis:** Form of diffusion that moves water from a place of high concentration to a lower concentration.

**osseous tissue:** Type of connective tissue that forms the skeleton; also called bone tissue.

**ossification:** Process of cartilage turning to bone.

**osteoblasts:** Cells that create bone.

**osteocytes:** Individual bone cells.

**ovulation:** Act of a mature egg being released by the graafian follicle in the ovary owing to changes in levels of progesterone and estrogen; usually occurs at day 14 of the menstrual cycle.

**ovum:** Egg cell.

# P

**pain receptors:** Sensory receptors in the skin that detect tissue damage.

**parasympathetic nervous system:** Part of the autonomic nervous system responsible for controlling internal functions when the body is at rest.

**partial-thickness burn:** Burn that is painful, blisters, and involves the dermis; also called a second-degree burn.

**passive immunity:** Type of immunity in which the body does not have to detect a foreign antigen and make an antibody before immunity can occur, such as a fetus receiving immunoglobulins across the placenta and through breast milk.

**pelvic cavity:** Part of the ventral cavity located within the pelvic bones.

**pericardium:** Membrane that surrounds the heart.

**periosteum:** Protective tissue that surrounds a long bone.

**peripheral nervous system (PNS):** The nerves surrounding the brain and spinal cord, or central nervous system.

**peristalsis:** Wavelike movement that moves a bolus through the esophagus.

**peroxisomes:** Organelles that contain enzymes that break down fatty acids, break down amino acids, and detoxify alcohol.

**photoreceptors:** Receptors that respond to changes in light.

**physiology:** Study of how the body functions.

**pitch:** Sensation of sound entering the ear; related to frequency in that the higher the frequency, the higher the pitch, and the lower the frequency, the lower the pitch.

**pituitary gland:** Gland located in the hypothalamus of the brain. It is the master gland that controls the function of the other endocrine glands.

**planes:** Imaginary flat surfaces that pass through an object. The human body has three planes.

**plasma:** Fluid portion of whole blood.

**polarization:** Part of the action potential when a cell is at rest.

**primary response:** Response of the immune system when the body first comes in contact with a foreign antigen. B lymphocytes recognize that the antigen is foreign and change to plasma cells, which make antibodies. IgM is the first antibody to be made, but it lasts only a few days. IgG is made several days after IgM, and it continues to fight the foreign antigen after IgM cells die. IgG lasts several weeks to several months after the initial contact. Memory B lymphocytes are made after the initial response, and they remain in the bloodstream to recognize the foreign antigen if it returns.

**prime mover:** Muscle that plays more of a role in movement in a group of synergistic muscles.

**process:** Outcropping of bone that provides a place for muscle or ligament attachment.

**prostaglandins:** Type of hormone made of cholesterol and found within cell membranes.

**protein:** Nutrient found throughout the body. The simplest form of a protein is an amino acid.

**protein synthesis:** Protein manufacture in the ribosomes done by changing the genetic code in each sequence of DNA into individual proteins.

**pulmonary artery:** Structure that carries deoxygenated blood from the right ventricle to the lungs.

**pulmonary semilunar valve:** Structure that acts as a doorway between the right ventricle and pulmonary artery to keep blood in the artery.

**pulmonary veins:** Vessels that bring oxygenated blood back from the lungs to the left atrium.

**pulmonary ventilation:** Process of air moving into and out of the lungs so that the alveoli are constantly exposed to air for gas exchange to occur; also called breathing.

**Purkinje fibers:** Last structures of the intrinsic conduction system that surround the heart ventricles like a net. When an impulse reaches them, they pull upward causing a strong contraction in the ventricles.

## Q

**quadrant:** One of the four sections of the abdominal cavity created by a transverse and sagittal plane that cross at the umbilicus. This term is used to provide a general location of internal organs.

## R

**reabsorption:** Process of the proximal convoluted tubule that allows some substances to return to the body and keeps the waste.

**red marrow:** Found in spongy bone; the site for blood cell production.

**reflex:** Rapid, involuntary, and predictable responses of the nervous system. There are two types of reflexes: somatic reflexes, which control body responses, and autonomic reflexes, which control involuntary responses. Reflexes can use neurons in the brain and spine or just spinal neurons for an even faster response.

**refraction:** Bending of light as it enters the lens of the eye.

**region:** One of nine sections that divide the abdominal cavity. This term is used to provide a more specific location of the internal organs.

**renal filtrate:** Fluid filtered from the blood found in the proximal convoluted tubule.

**repolarization:** Part of the action potential where a cell changes from an active state back to resting.

**residual volume:** Amount of air always present in the lungs regardless of how much air is expelled, about 1200 mL.

**respiratory cycle:** Cycle of one inspiration and one expiration; also equal to one breath.

**ribosomes:** Organelles that produce proteins.

**right atrium:** Upper chamber of the heart that receives deoxygenated blood from the body.

**right ventricle:** Lower heart chamber that contracts to push blood into the pulmonary artery.

**RNA (ribonucleic acid):** Single strand of nucleotides that is responsible for protein synthesis.

**rods:** Structures found in the retina that aid in distinguishing shadows.

**rule of nines:** Determination of how much of the body surface is burned based on different body parts being equal to 9%.

## S

**sagittal plane:** Vertical plane that divides the body into ventral and dorsal sections.

**sebaceous gland:** Type of gland found in the dermis of the skin that produces oil.

**sebum:** Oil produced by sebaceous glands.

**secondary response:** Response of the immune system when a foreign antigen returns. Memory B lymphocytes recognize it and organize a faster response because antibodies have already been made for this antigen. IgM reacts within 1 or 2 days and remains active for up to a few weeks. IgG also reacts faster and is ready within 3 or 4 days.

**secretion:** Process of ions leaving the distal convoluted tubule to maintain blood pH and water added or released to the fluid that is now urine.

**selectively permeable:** Ability of the cell membrane to allow some substances to flow through the membrane while keeping other substances out.

**sensation:** Stimuli that different receptors transmit to the brain for interpretation.

**sensorineural:** Type of hearing begins in the hair cells located inside the cochlea. These cells take the stimulus of the sound wave and convert it to an electrical impulse, and the impulse travels via the vestibulocochlear nerve to the brain.

**septum:** Thick wall of tissue between the right and left half of the heart.

**sinoatrial (SA) node:** First conductor of electrical impulses in the intrinsic conduction system; also called the pacemaker of the heart or the sinus node.

**skeletal muscle:** Consciously controlled muscle attached to bones that move by shortening or contraction of the muscle; also called voluntary muscle.

**smooth muscle:** Muscle found in the organs that is not consciously controlled; also called involuntary.

**somatic nervous system:** Part of the peripheral nervous system that maintains voluntary functions.

**somatosensory receptors:** Sensory receptors in the skin that detect pain, heat, cold, pressure, and vibration.

**specific immunity:** Type of immunity that is not inborn, so the body must first come in contact with a foreign substance before defenses can be made against it; also called acquired immunity.

**sperm:** Male gametes produced by the testes.

**spermatogenesis:** Creation of sperm by the testes, which are the primary sex organs of males.

**spinal cavity:** Cavity that contains the spinal cord and is part of the dorsal cavity.

**spinal cord:** Conductive tissue protected by the vertebral column that takes impulses to and from the brain; part of the central nervous system.

**spinal nerves:** Thirty-one pairs of nerves attached to the spinal cord that make up the peripheral nervous system.

**spongy bone:** Bone that is lighter and more porous than compact bone. It is found in bones that do not need to be as heavy, such as the skull and ribs.

**squamous cell carcinoma:** Second most common form of skin cancer; affects the middle layer of the epidermis and forms scaly patches that ulcerate and scab over.

**steroid hormones:** Water-soluble hormones that can pass through the cell membrane to create a response within the cell.

**stratum basale:** Innermost layer of epithelium closest to the dermis where new epithelial cells are made.

**stratum corneum:** Outermost layer of epithelium made of keratinized epithelial cells.

**subcutaneous:** Third layer of skin composed of adipose tissue that acts as insulation and protection.

**sudoriferous gland:** Type of gland found in the dermis of the skin that produces sweat.

**sulci:** Grooves formed by the gyri in the cerebrum.

**superficial-thickness burn:** Type of burn that is red, sore, and hot. Only the epidermis is damaged; also called a first-degree burn.

**surfactant:** Substance that surrounds the alveoli of the lungs and stops them from sticking together after exhalation.

**sutures:** Structures in the skull where the fibrous cartilage that separated the skull bones fused after ossification.

**sympathetic nervous system:** Part of the peripheral nervous system that speeds up heart rate, increases blood pressure, and slows digestion in a "fight or flight" response.

**synarthroses:** Immovable joints.

**synergist:** Groups of muscles that work together.

**system:** Group of organs that perform a common function.

**systole:** Strong contraction created by Purkinje fibers pulling up on the ventricles of the heart.

## T

**tendon:** Connective tissue that joins muscle to bone. This connection creates movement.

**thermoreceptors:** Receptors that detect changes in temperature.

**thoracic cavity:** Part of the ventral cavity located under the rib cage and above the diaphragm; also called the chest cavity.

**thrombocyte:** Clotting cells that aid in stopping blood flow secondary to tissue trauma; also called platelets.

**thrombopoietin:** Hormone that stimulates production of megakaryocytes in the bone marrow.

**thyroid hormones:** Two hormones secreted by the thyroid gland. They are called thyroxine ($T_4$) and triiodothyronine ($T_3$).These hormones are metabolic hormones and control the rate at which glucose is used by the body.

**tidal volume:** Normal amount of air that goes into and out of the lungs with one breath.

**tissue:** Formed by similar cells working together.

**total capacity:** Measurement of all air present in the lungs.

**transcription:** Process of changing DNA into a code that RNA can deliver to the ribosomes during protein synthesis.

**translation:** Process of changing the nucleic acids of DNA into amino acids so that the strand can be copied during protein synthesis.

**transverse plane:** Plane that cuts the body into horizontal sections; also called a cross section.

**tricuspid valve:** Structure located between the right atrium and right ventricle of the heart that acts as a doorway to prevent backflow of blood.

## U

**umbilical region:** Middle section of the abdomen that surrounds the umbilicus.

**urine:** Liquid waste that comprises water and nitrogenous wastes, which is formed and excreted by the kidneys.

**urochrome:** Pigment from the breakdown of red blood cells that gives urine its color.

## V

**vein:** Vessels that carry deoxygenated blood. Blood in the veins is full of the waste product carbon dioxide.

**vena cava:** Largest veins in the body that attach to the heart at the right atrium.

**ventral cavity:** Space found in the front of the body; divided into three cavities-thoracic cavity, abdominal cavity, and pelvic cavity.

**ventricles:** Lower chambers of the heart that contract to cause systole.

**vision:** Means of interpreting light waves and changing them into images the brain can recognize.

**vital capacity:** Normal amount or volume of air within the lungs, which equals about 4000 to 6000 mL.

**vitamin:** Organic molecules needed only in small amounts by the body.

## X

**xenograft:** Transplant grafts where the donated tissue comes from a different animal species.

## Y

**yellow marrow:** Substance found in the shafts of long bones; made of adipose tissue or fat.

## Z

**zygote:** Cell in fetal development that is formed by the combination of the male and female chromosomes during fertilization.

# PATHOLOGY TERMS

## A

**abruptio placentae:** Result of the placenta pulling away from the uterine wall leaving the fetus without a supply of oxygen or nutrients and causing severe bleeding in the mother.

**abscess:** Localized collection of pus; occurs when bacteria have entered the skin through a wound causing infection.

**achondroplasia:** Genetic disease of the connective tissue that results in a normal-sized torso but shortened limbs.

**acne:** Inflammation of the skin resulting in pustular eruptions; caused by overproduction of sebaceous glands in the skin; more common in adolescents.

**acquired immunodeficiency syndrome (AIDS):** Destruction of the cell-mediated immune system by HIV. Patients die of opportunistic infections.

**acromegaly:** Enlargement of the extremities caused by production of growth hormone in adulthood after full growth has been reached.

**Addison's disease:** Adrenal glands cease producing sufficient amounts of steroid hormones. Symptoms begin gradually and include fatigue, weight loss, and muscle weakness. Advanced symptoms include nausea, diarrhea, hypoglycemia, sweating, and hyperpigmentation of the skin and mucous membranes. Untreated, the disease can be fatal. Treatment includes replacing the hormones the adrenal glands are not producing.

**ageusia:** Loss of sense of taste.

**agnosia:** Loss of ability to recognize objects, shapes, sounds, persons, or smells; usually due to brain trauma.

**allergy:** Over-response of the immune system to antigens that would be harmless to the body. Common reaction is sneezing, watery eyes, itching skin, or hives.

**alopecia:** Partial or complete absence of hair; baldness. It can be hereditary, due to a skin condition, or a side effect of a drug.

**amaurosis:** Blindness usually occurring from a lesion in the optic nerve, brain, or spinal cord.

**amenorrhea:** Absence of menstruation; may be due to endocrine disorders, low body weight, excessive exercise, or medications.

**amyotrophic lateral sclerosis (ALS):** Progressive weakness and wasting of the muscles caused by degeneration of the motor neurons. Eventually the muscles become paralyzed; usually begins as weakness in the muscles of the arms and muscles involved in swallowing and speech; also called Lou Gehrig disease.

**anacusis:** Total deafness.

**anemia:** General name for several different conditions; can be a result of decrease in number of red blood cells, deficiency in hemoglobin, or lack of iron in the diet.

**angina pectoris:** Chest pain and discomfort that occurs when the heart is not receiving enough blood, usually caused by arteriosclerosis or atherosclerosis.

**anorchidism:** Failure of one or both testes to develop.

**anosmia:** Loss of sense of smell.

**anuria:** Lack of urine production or inability to void urine.

**aphasia:** Defective or absent language functions resulting from disease or injury of Broca area in the frontal lobe of the brain.

**arrhythmia:** Abnormal or irregular heartbeat.

**arteriosclerosis:** Thickening of the arteries that slows blood flow.

**ascites:** Accumulation of serous fluid in the peritoneal cavity; most often due to liver disease or trauma.

**asthma:** Chronic attacks of dyspnea caused by spasms of the bronchi; usually starts in childhood, but can begin at any age. Symptoms include wheezing, tightness of the chest, and shortness of breath. The exact cause is unknown, although it has been linked to genetics, respiratory infections, and airborne irritants such as dust and cigarette smoke.

**ataxia:** Motor dysfunction secondary to disease or injury to the brain causing loss of coordination and unsteady gait.

**atherosclerosis:** Plaque called atheroma builds up in the arteries and slows blood flow.

**atrophy:** Deterioration of muscle because of disease, injury, or disuse.

## B

**benign prostatic hypertrophy:** Enlargement of the prostate gland; commonly occurs in men older than 60.

**bradycardia:** Slow heartbeat (<60 bpm).

**breast cancer:** Malignant neoplasm of the breast; found most often in the milk ducts or the lobules that produce milk. Risk increases with age for all women, and for some women there is a genetic link that increases risk.

**breech birth:** Delivery of the fetus in a position other than head first.

**bronchitis:** Inflammation of the bronchi; can be caused by bacterial or viral infection. Chronic bronchitis is due to inhaled irritants, such as cigarette smoke.

## C

**cervical cancer:** Malignant neoplasm of the cervix; most often caused by some strains of human papillomavirus (HPV).

**chronic obstructive pulmonary disease (COPD):** General term for obstruction of the lung tissue resulting in loss of air flow.

**color blindness:** Inability to perceive some or all colors; most often due to a genetic defect of the X chromosome, so boys are more likely to be affected.

**contracture:** Decrease in mobility of connective tissue because of fibrosis or thickening of the tissue.

**coronary artery disease:** Generalized term for decreased blood supply to the heart caused by either arteriosclerosis or atherosclerosis.

**cretinism:** Mental retardation resulting from congenital deficiency of the thyroid hormones.

**cryptorchidism:** Failure of the testes to descend into the scrotum.

**cyanosis:** Blueness of the skin usually caused by lack of oxygen.

**cystic fibrosis:** Genetic disorder inherited from both parents; causes an overproduction of mucus that clogs the lungs and digestive system. Death occurs from infection or respiratory failure. Life expectancy was previously early childhood, but with antibiotics and other treatments individuals with cystic fibrosis can live well into adulthood.

## D

**dementia:** Progressive loss of cognitive and intellectual function of the brain. Causes include brain injury and depression.

**dermatitis:** General term for inflammation of the skin caused by an irritant, such as soap, perfume, fabric, detergent, sunlight, or medications.

**diabetes:** Disease in which the pancreas does not produce insulin or does not use it correctly resulting in increased blood glucose levels. There are three forms: Type 1, where insulin is not being produced; Type 2, where insulin is not being used efficiently by the body; and gestational, which occurs during pregnancy.

**dislocation:** Displacement of a bone from the joint.

## E

**ecchymosis:** Black and blue mark on the skin caused by blood vessel injury; also called a bruise.

**eclampsia:** Seizures during pregnancy usually secondary to preeclampsia.

**ectopic pregnancy:** Implantation of the fertilized egg in a place other than the uterus, most commonly in the fallopian tube. Symptoms include stabbing pain in the abdomen, dizziness, and unusual vaginal discharge. If caught early, a dose of methotrexate allows the body to absorb the embryo. In later stages, laparoscopic surgery is needed to remove the embryo. Untreated, the fallopian tube ruptures, causing hemorrhage and possible death.

**emphysema:** Irreversible expansion of the alveoli most often secondary to cigarette smoke. Oxygen and carbon dioxide cannot be exchanged because of limited exhalation. Symptoms include COPD, chronic cough, fatigue, and shortness of breath.

**endometriosis:** Growth of the uterine tissue outside the uterus. The most common symptom is pelvic pain during menstruation. Laparoscopic surgery is done to remove the excess tissue. Hysterectomy may be done in severe cases.

**epilepsy:** Group of disorders characterized by recurrent seizures.

**erythema:** Redness of the skin usually resulting from injury or inflammation.

**exophthalmos:** Bulging of the eyes; can result from trauma or from a disease process such as Graves' disease.

## F

**fibrillation:** Type of arrhythmia where the heart is in spasm so it is unable to pump blood.

**flutter:** Lesser form of fibrillation.

## G

**gigantism:** Excessive height caused by increased amounts of growth hormone during childhood before the growth plates in the bones have closed; most often due to a tumor on the pituitary gland; also known as giantism.

**goiter:** Enlarged thyroid gland as a result of thyroid insufficiency because of lack of iodine in the diet.

**Graves disease:** Autoimmune disease that causes overproduction of thyroid hormones; more common in women older than 20; causes bulging of the eyes (exophthalmos), increased heart rate, and increased metabolism. Treatment includes shrinking the thyroid with radioactive iodine or removal of the gland.

## H

**hematoma:** Collection of blood under the skin; also called a bruise.

**hematuria:** Blood in the urine.

**hemophilia:** Inherited disorder. The defect is found on the X chromosome, so it is more common in males. Patients are missing certain clotting proteins, so the blood does not clot.

**hemothorax:** Collection of blood in the pleural cavity that prevents the lungs from expanding during inhalation; most often due to trauma.

**Hodgkin disease:** Tumor of the lymph nodes, spleen, or bone marrow; occurs more often in individuals 15 to 35 years old. With treatment, there is a 90% survival rate.

**hordoleum:** Infection of the sebaceous glands of the eyelid. A yellowish, painful bump develops at the site; also called a stye.

**human immunodeficiency virus (HIV):** Virus that targets and destroys T lymphocytes causing AIDS. It is found in semen, blood, vaginal secretions, and breast milk. The virus is spread through contact with contaminated body fluids that have entered the body through a needle stick, broken skin, or sexual intercourse.

**Huntington chorea:** Inherited disease that causes speech disturbances, muscle tics, and degeneration of the cerebral cortex. Effects start between ages 30 and 50.

**hypertension:** Elevated blood pressure (>140/90 mm Hg).

**hypertrophy:** Abnormal increase in growth of a muscle, organ, or body part.

**hypotrophy:** Abnormal decrease in growth of a muscle, organ, or body part.

## I

**impetigo:** Inflammatory skin disease that results in pustules that crust over and rupture; highly contagious and occurs most often in children.

**ischemia:** Loss of blood supply to a localized area of tissue; associated with coronary artery disease.

## J

**jaundice:** Yellow color of the skin usually a result of liver malfunction.

## K

**kyphosis:** Exaggerated thoracic curve; also called hunchback.

## L

**leukemia:** Cancer of the white blood cells; caused by abnormality in the myeloid cells so that WBCs cannot function normally. Treatment includes chemotherapy, radiation, and bone marrow transplant.

**leukotrichia:** Loss of pigmentation to the hair, or whitening of the hair; most often due to age.

**lordosis:** Exaggerated lumbar curve; also called swayback.

**lymphedema:** Accumulation of lymph fluid in the tissues where the lymph nodes have been surgically removed.

## M

**maple syrup urine disease:** Inherited disorder in which the body is unable to process certain proteins resulting in maple syrup–smelling urine. If untreated, children have seizures, slow growth, and mental delays.

**meningitis:** Inflammation of the covering of the brain and spinal cord because of virus or bacteria.

**motion sickness:** Nausea or dizziness that occurs when the sense of movement and the sense of sight are not in agreement.

**multiple sclerosis:** Autoimmune disease that targets the myelin sheath surrounding motor neurons. This slow degeneration causes various symptoms such as loss of balance and coordination, muscle weakness and pain, visual problems, and speech impairment.

**muscular dystrophy:** General term for many inherited disorders in which the muscle fibers degenerate resulting in muscle weakness.

**myalgia:** Muscle pain.

**myocardial infarction:** Death of the heart muscle because of loss of blood flow; also called heart attack.

**myoclonia:** Irregular muscle twitching resulting from a nervous system disorder.

**myotonia:** General term for muscle spasm or temporary rigidity of a muscle.

## N

**nocturia:** Frequent urination at night.

**nocturnal enuresis:** Involuntary urination while sleeping; usually occurs in children younger than 6 who have not learned to control urination voluntarily; also called bedwetting.

**non-Hodgkin lymphoma:** General name for more than 30 types of lymphoma that are a malignancy of the B or T lymphocytes that have spread to the body tissues; occurs more often in adults 40 to 70 years old. Depending on the type, there is a 70% survival rate after the first year of diagnosis.

## O

**oliguria:** Decreased amount of urine production; decrease in voiding urine. Causes include dehydration, kidney damage, or a blockage.

**osteoarthritis:** Progressive wearing away of the joints because of age or injury. Symptoms include pain and stiffness, which increase during cold, damp weather.

**osteoporosis:** Loss of bone density caused by decreased mineral retention in the bones secondary to a lack of estrogen so that the bones weaken and break easily; commonly affects postmenopausal women.

**ovarian cyst:** Fluid-filled sacs on the ovary that may cause pain, abnormal bleeding, and cramping. Most cysts heal without treatment.

## P

**Paget disease:** Abnormal bone destruction and repair, which creates bone irregularities and deformities; affects middle-aged and elderly adults.

**pallor:** Paleness of the skin.

**Parkinson disease:** Progressive degeneration of the neurons of the brain that causes tremors, stiff joints, and unblinking eyes; usually occurs in adults older than 60.

**pediculosis:** Lice infestation.

**phlebitis:** Inflammation of the veins.

**pituitary dwarfism:** Decreased height and growth because of insufficiency of growth hormone before the growth plates in the bones have closed.

**pleural effusion:** Collection of fluid in the pleural cavity that prevents the lungs from expanding during inhalation; most often due to heart failure or kidney failure.

**pneumonia:** Alveoli become filled with fluid secondary to infection; can be caused by bacteria, viruses, trauma, or mold. Symptoms include fever, chills, productive cough, chest pain when coughing, and shortness of breath.

**pneumothorax:** Collection of air in the pleural cavity that prevents the lungs from expanding during inhalation; most often caused by smoking, lung disease, or trauma; also called collapsed lung.

**polycystic kidney disease:** Genetic disorder in which numerous cysts form in the kidneys resulting in enlarged kidneys and reduction of renal function.

**polyuria:** Increase in urine production; increase in urination. Causes include increased fluid intake, diabetes, or diuretic drugs.

**preeclampsia:** Hypertension, vision changes, and headaches during pregnancy; may progress to eclampsia.

**pruritus:** Itching.

**pyuria:** Pus in the urine; a sign of inflammation in the urinary tract.

## R

**renal calculi:** Hardened mineral deposits that form in the kidneys; also called kidney stones.

**renal failure:** Loss of ability of the kidneys to function; can be due to trauma or a disease process; may be acute or chronic.

**rheumatoid arthritis:** Autoimmune disease in which the immune system attacks the joints mostly of the hands and feet causing deformities of the joints; occurs more often in woman 40 to 60 years old.

## S

**scoliosis:** Lateral curvature of the spine; occurs more often during adolescence.

**severe combined immunodeficiency virus (SCID):** Deficiency of the cell-mediated and humoral immunities. Death occurs within the first few months of life because of infection.

**sickle cell anemia:** Disorder inherited from both parents; more common in people of African ancestry. Red blood cells are sickle-shaped or C-shaped and cannot deliver oxygen efficiently.

**spina bifida:** Congenital malformation in which the spine fails to close. It can range from the occult form, where the spine appears closed from the outside, to the most severe form, where the spinal cord within the meninges is outside the body.

**sprain:** Twisting or tearing of a ligament.

**strabismus:** Inability of the eyes to align so that one or both eyes turn in, out, up, or down; commonly called "cross-eyes."

**strain:** Overuse or overextension of a muscle.

**systemic lupus erythematosus:** Autoimmune disease in which the immune system attacks the connective tissue, usually affecting women of childbearing age.

## T

**tachycardia:** Rapid heartbeat (>100 bpm).

**talipes:** Congenital deformity of the foot where the foot is in a fixed twisted position; also called clubfoot.

**testicular cancer:** Malignant neoplasm of the testis; occurs most commonly in men 20 to 34 years old.

**tetanus:** Bacterial infection that causes the muscles to contract until they spasm resulting in paralysis. The jaw is the first to be affected, sometimes called lockjaw; also a general term for paralysis of a muscle resulting from overcontraction.

**thalassemia:** Inherited disorder from both parents; type of anemia where RBCs are smaller than normal and have reduced amount of hemoglobin; more common in people of Mediterranean ancestry.

**thrombocytopenia:** Decrease in the number of platelets. Reasons for this condition can be a virus, trauma, blood transfusion, medications, or unknown cause.

**tinea pedis:** Fungal infection of the feet; also called athlete's foot.

**tinnitus:** Ringing in the ears secondary to damage to the hair receptors in the inner ear; may be temporary or permanent.

**Tourette syndrome:** Neurological disorder characterized by spasms, tics, uncontrolled vocal sounds, and inappropriate verbal responses.

## U

**uremia:** Urine in the blood caused by urine backing up into the bloodstream because it is unable to leave the body through the urethra.

**urticaria:** Allergic skin reaction that causes itchy, red, elevated patches; also called hives.

## V

**varicose veins:** Swollen and twisted veins most often formed in the legs because of defective valves in the veins; occurs often in elderly adults.

**vertigo:** Sensation of moving or spinning usually a result of disturbance in the inner ear causing a loss of balance.

**vitiligo:** Localized loss of skin pigmentation resulting in white patches.

# ANSWERS TO CHAPTER EXERCISES

## CHAPTER 1

### Multiple Choice

1. C. Trendelenburg
2. a. tissue
3. b. back
4. c. skin
5. d. proximal

### True or False

1. False
2. False
3. True
4. False
5. False
6. False
7. False
8. True
9. True
10. False

### Fill in the Blank

1. mid-sagittal
2. prone
3. superficial
4. superior
5. deep
6. physiology
7. system
8. transverse
9. umbilical
10. anatomy

### Short Answer

1. Lithotomy and dorsal recumbent.
2. Dorsal: Brain and spinal.

Ventral: Thoracic and abdominopelvic.

3. A group of systems working together.
4. Imaginary flat surfaces that pass through the body.
5. When the patient is standing erect with the face forward and arms at the sides with palms facing forward.

### Labeling

See Figure 1–1 Structural levels.

See Figure 1–4 The body planes.

See Figure 1–5 The dorsal and ventral cavities.

See Figure 1–6 (A) The quadrants of the abdominal cavity. (B) The regions of the abdominal cavity.

## CHAPTER 2

### Multiple Choice

1. b. tRNA
2. c. mucous
3. d. reticular
4. c. metaphase
5. a. matrix
6. c. synthesis
7. c. smooth
8. d. cytosol
9. d. gland
10. a. meiosis

### Fill in the Blank

1. mitochondria
2. protein
3. Golgi bodies
4. voluntary
5. epithelial
6. collagen
7. squamous
8. translation
9. stratified
10. nucleus

### Matching

1. d
2. i
3. m
4. n
5. c
6. k
7. l
8. h
9. b
10. a
11. e
12. g
13. j
14. f
15. o

### Short Answer

1. Epithelial tissue: Simple squamous, simple cuboidal, simple columnar, stratified squamous, transitional, ciliated. Connective tissue: Cartilage, bone, blood, adipose, dense connective, reticular, areolar. Muscle tissue: Skeletal, smooth, cardiac. Nervous tissue: Neurons.

2. Mucous membranes line body cavities that open to the outside, and serous membranes line organs and cavities with no outside opening.

3. Bulk transport is a type of active transport used when a substance is too large to pass through the cell membrane. Endocytosis is when the cell membrane envelops the material and brings it into the cell. The two types of endocytosis are phagocytosis, which captures and digests cell debris, and pinocytosis, which envelops fluid droplets.
Exocytosis is when a packaged substance pushes out of the cell forming a bud that breaks, releasing the substance; the hole is filled by the remaining protein packaging.

## CHAPTER 3

### Multiple Choice
1. b. basal cell carcinoma
2. c. third degree
3. a. endocrine
4. c. cortex
5. b. vitamin D

### True or False
1. True
2. False
3. False
4. False
5. False
6. True
7. True
8. True
9. False
10. False

### Fill in the Blank
1. keratinized
2. rule of nines
3. medulla
4. arrector pili
5. matrix
6. epithelial
7. oil
8. lunula
9. eccrine and apocrine
10. superficial

### Short Answer
1. Epidermis: Outer layer made of epithelial tissue; has no veins or glands.
Dermis: Second layer; has hair follicles, sudoriferous and sebaceous glands, and veins.
Subcutaneous: Made of adipose tissue; connects skin to muscle.
2. A—Asymmetry: The two sides of the spot or mole are not the same.
B—Border irregularity: The edges of the spot or mole are not smooth.
C—Color: The spot contains areas of different colors.
D—Diameter: The spot is larger than 6 mm in diameter (size of a pencil eraser).
E—Evolving or extending: The spot has changed or grown quickly.
3. Determination of how much body surface is burned by assigning different body parts 9% of the body surface.

### Labeling
See Figure 3–1 Cross section of the layers of the skin.
See Figure 3–2 Cross section of hair strand.
See Figure 3–3 Cross section of nail structure.

## CHAPTER 4

### Multiple Choice
1. b. masseter
2. c. deltoid
3. a. gluteus maximus
4. c. quadriceps
5. b. brachioradialis
6. c. aerobic
7. a. orbicularis oris
8. b. pectoralis major
9. d. lactic acid
10. a. biceps brachii

### Fill in the Blank
1. origin
2. hypertrophy
3. hamstrings
4. flexion
5. tendon
6. skeletal
7. isotonic
8. synergists
9. abduction
10. achilles

### Matching
1. c
2. g
3. h
4. i
5. a
6. b
7. e
8. f
9. j
10. d

### Short Answer
1. Skeletal: Voluntary, attached to bones, is striated.
Smooth: Involuntary, lines the organs, is spindle-shaped.
Cardiac: Found in the heart, is striated but involuntary.

2. Biceps and triceps and quadriceps and hamstrings.

3. A muscle fiber is surrounded by an endomysium, a fascicle is a bundle of muscle fibers surrounded by a perimysium, and several fascicles make a muscle covered by perimysium.

## Labeling

See Figure 4–2 General structure of skeletal muscle.

See Figure 4–4 Types of muscle movement.

## CHAPTER 5

### Multiple Choice

1. b. epiphysis
2. c. suture
3. c. tibia
4. b. thoracic
5. c. hyoid
6. b. ischium
7. b. ligament
8. d. axial
9. c. vertebral
10. c. heel

### True or False

1. True
2. False
3. True
4. False
5. True

### Fill in the Blank

1. red
2. periosteum
3. fontanel
4. radius; ulna
5. femur
6. epiphyseal plate
7. 12
8. sternum

9. ossification
10. ilium
11. coccyx
12. diaphysis
13. upper
14. diarthrosis
15. patella
16. greenstick
17. amphiarthrosis
18. metacarpals
19. osteocytes
20. shoulder

### Short Answer

1. Synarthroses—immovable; amphiarthroses—slightly movable; diarthroses—freely movable.

2. A comminuted fracture occurs when two or more intersecting breaks meet each other and fragment; an impacted fracture occurs when two bones are forced together and fragment.

3. Ball-and-socket—hip; condyloid—fingers; hinge—elbow; pivot—atlas and axis; plane—wrist; saddle—thumb.

### Labeling

See Figure 5–2 Parts of a long bone.

See Figure 5–14 Types of fractures: simple, compound, greenstick, comminuted, impacted, incomplete.

See Figure 5–15 Types of diarthroses. *(A)* Ball-and-socket. *(B)* Hinge. *(C)* Condyloid. *(D)* Plane. *(E)* Pivot. *(F)* Saddle.

## CHAPTER 6

### Multiple Choice

1. a. cells
2. c. red blood cells

3. d. platelets
4. c. agglutination
5. c. lymphocyte

### True or False

1. True
2. True
3. True
4. False
5. True

### Fill in the Blank

1. recipient
2. water
3. biconcave; discs
4. HDN
5. hematopoiesis; hemopoiesis
6. granulocytes; agranulocytes
7. hemocytoblasts
8. donor
9. antigen
10. bone

### Short Answer

1. Plasma: Water, proteins, glucose.
   Formed elements: Erythrocytes, leukocytes, thrombocytes.

2. Neutrophils: Most numerous, phagocytes.
   Eosinophils: Increase in response to allergies or parasites.
   Basophils: Secrete heparin.
   Monocytes: Largest, phagocytes.
   Lymphocytes: Smallest, provide immunity.

3. An Rh⁻ mother has an Rh⁺ child. Antibodies are made against Rh, so the next Rh⁺ child would have its red blood cells destroyed by the antibodies.

## Labeling

See Figure 6–1 Blood components.

See Figure 6–7 Hematopoiesis.

## CHAPTER 7

### Multiple Choice

1. b. humoral
2. d. IgD
3. c. plasma cell
4. a. IgA
5. c. small intestine

### True or False

1. False
2. False
3. True
4. False
5. True
6. False
7. False
8. False
9. False
10. True

### Fill in the Blank

1. IgM
2. T
3. skin
4. tonsils
5. inflammatory
6. humoral
7. plasma
8. blood
9. lymph
10. secondary

### Short Answer

1. IgG: Second responder to foreign antigens and can cross the placenta to give immunity to the fetus
   IgM: First responder to foreign antigens.

IgD: Found in small amounts. Role is unknown.
IgE: Responsible for allergic reactions and increases in response to parasitic infections.
IgA: Found in body secretions such as breast milk and saliva.

2. Helper T: Interact with B lymphocytes to bring them to a captured antigen.
   Cytotoxic T: Find and destroy cancer cells and foreign tissue.
   Suppressor T: Stop the immune response.
   Memory T: Remember the antigen.

### Labeling

See Figure 7–2 Lymphoid tissues and organs.

See Figure 7–5 Structures of the immunoglobulins.

## CHAPTER 8

### Multiple Choice

1. b. vagus
2. c. fetal
3. d. automaticity
4. a. cardiac
5. b. veins

### True or False

1. True
2. True
3. False
4. False
5. True

### Fill in the Blank

1. septum
2. tricuspid
3. diastole
4. pulse
5. carbon dioxide

6. mediastinum
7. endocardium
8. foramen ovale
9. superior; inferior vena cava
10. SA node

### Short answer

1. If starting at the superior and inferior vena cavae to the right atrium through the tricuspid valve to the right ventricle through the pulmonary semilunar valve to the pulmonary artery to the lungs, back from the lungs, blood goes through the pulmonary veins to the left atrium through the bicuspid valve to the left ventricle through the aortic semilunar valve to the aorta, then to the arterioles, then the capillaries back to the venules, then the veins returning to the superior and inferior vena cavae.

2. Pericardium: Membrane that surrounds the heart.
   Myocardium: The heart muscle.
   Endocardium: Smooth epithelial tissue lining the heart.

### Labeling

See Figure 8–2 (A) Exterior view of the heart. (B) Interior view of the heart.

See Figure 8–7 Intrinsic conduction system of the heart.

## CHAPTER 9

### Multiple Choice

1. b. vital capacity
2. c. uvula
3. a. larynx
4. b. external
5. b. parietal

## Fill in the Blank

1. oxygen; carbon dioxide
2. eupnea
3. respiratory cycle
4. vocal cords
5. mouth; pharynx
6. alveoli
7. ATP
8. carbon dioxide
9. residual volume
10. 3; 2

## Matching

1. h
2. b
3. e
4. a
5. d
6. c
7. g
8. j
9. i
10. f

## Short Answer

1. Tidal volume: Amount of air taken in a normal single breath.
   Expiratory reserve volume: Amount of air expelled in one maximum breath past normal exhalation.
   Residual volume: Amount of air left in the lungs after maximum expiration.
   Total capacity: Total amount of the residual volume and vital capacity.
   Vital capacity: Amount of air exchanged during normal breathing.
   Inspiratory reserve volume: Amount of air taken in past the normal inhalation.

## Labeling

See Figure 9–1 Respiratory system.

See Figure 9–2 Oral cavity, pharynx, and larynx.

# CHAPTER 10

## Multiple Choice

1. c. ingestion
2. a. glucose
3. a. liver
4. b. rugae
5. c. deciduous
6. a. microvilli
7. b. vitamins
8. a. uvula
9. c. liver
10. d. proteins

## True or False

1. True
2. True
3. False
4. True
5. True
6. True
7. False
8. True
9. False
10. True

## Fill in the Blank

1. rugae
2. nutrients
3. bolus
4. emulsification
5. appendix
6. liver; gallbladder
7. peristalsis
8. chyme
9. pyloric
10. ingestion

## Matching

1. g
2. a
3. f
4. j
5. b
6. i
7. e
8. c
9. d
10. h

## Short Answer

1. Pancreas, liver, appendix, gallbladder
2. Ingestion, digestion, absorption, excretion

## Labeling

See Figure 10–1 Structures and organs of the alimentary canal.

See Figure 10–2 *(A)* Adult teeth. *(B)* Deciduous teeth.

# CHAPTER 11

## Multiple Choice

1. b. microglia
2. c. synapse
3. d. dura mater
4. a. occipital
5. b. hypothalamus
6. b. pons
7. a. astrocytes
8. b. reflexes
9. c. neurotransmitters
10. a. cerebellum

## True or False

1. False
2. True
3. False
4. False
5. False

6. False
7. True
8. True
9. True
10. False

## Fill in the Blank

1. sensory; motor
2. synapse
3. cell body
4. gyri; sulci
5. sympathetic; parasympathetic
6. dendrites
7. ependymal cells
8. cerebrospinal fluid
9. sensory
10. myelin

## Short Answer

1. The sympathetic nervous system controls "fight or flight" response—increases heart rate, respiration, and blood pressure; uses epinephrine. The parasympathetic nervous system slows sympathetic response and controls body when at rest; uses acetylcholine.

2. The autonomic nervous system controls involuntary responses.
The somatic nervous system controls voluntary responses.

## Labeling

See Figure 11–1 Structure of a neuron. *(A)* Sensory neuron. *(B)* Motor neuron.

See Figure 11–5 Divisions of the nervous system.

## CHAPTER 12

### Multiple Choice

1. b. iris
2. c. chemoreceptor
3. a. cochlea

4. c. static
5. d. lens

### True or False

1. False
2. True
3. False
4. True
5. False
6. True
7. False
8. True
9. False
10. False

### Fill in the Blank

1. cones; rods
2. lens
3. taste buds
4. sensory
5. pinna; auricle
6. umami
7. cochlea
8. lacrimal
9. sclera
10. somatosensory

### Short Answer

1. Sweet taste buds are found on the tip of the tongue. Sour taste buds are found on the sides of the tongue. Taste buds for bitter are found on the back of the tongue. Salt taste buds are scattered over the tongue. Umami taste buds are scattered over the tongue.

2. Pain receptors, chemoreceptors, thermoreceptors, photoreceptors, mechanoreceptors.

### Labeling

See Figure 12–2 Internal structures of the eye.

See Figure 12–6 Structures of the ear

## CHAPTER 13

### Multiple Choice

1. a. renal capsule
2. a. ureter
3. c. trigone
4. b. renin
5. c. urochrome
6. c. proximal convoluted tubule
7. a. distilled water
8. a. urethra
9. b. renal cortex
10. b. distal convoluted tubule

### True or False

1. True
2. True
3. True
4. True
5. False

### Fill in the Blank

1. ADH
2. micturition
3. glomerulus
4. trigone
5. filtration
6. ureter
7. renal medulla
8. reabsorption
9. hilus
10. nitrogenous wastes

### Short Answer

1. Glomerulus: Filters blood.
Glomerular capsule: Holds the glomerulus.
Proximal convoluted tubule: Reabsorption of substances the body needs.
Loop of Henle: Bend of the tubule.
Distal convoluted tubule: Secretion, makes urine.
Collecting ducts: Carries urine to ureters.

## Labeling

See Figure 13–1 Organs of the urinary system.

See Figure 13–2 Sagittal view of the kidney.

See Figure 13–3 Structures of the nephron.

## CHAPTER 14

### Multiple Choice

1. c. thyroid
2. c. glucocorticoid
3. a. glucagon
4. a. catecholamines
5. c. placenta

### Fill in the Blank

1. thymus
2. pituitary
3. hormones
4. thyroid
5. negative feedback
6. pancreas
7. pineal
8. androgens
9. anterior; posterior
10. norepinephrine

### Matching

1. e
2. h
3. a
4. f
5. g
6. c
7. i
8. j
9. b
10. d

### Short Answer

1. Pituitary and pineal—brain; thyroid—throat; thymus—chest; pancreas—abdomen; tonsils-throat; Peyer patches—small intestine.
2. Endocrine: Ductless glands secrete chemicals into the bloodstream.
   Exocrine: Have ducts to take secretions to outside the body.

### Labeling

See Figure 14–1 Location of endocrine glands.

## CHAPTER 15

### Multiple Choice

1. b. fetus
2. c. prolactin
3. a. placenta
4. b. dilation
5. a. prostate gland
6. b. placenta
7. a. corpus luteum
8. b. epididymis
9. a. androgens
10. c. gametes

### True or False

1. False
2. True
3. True
4. True
5. False
6. True
7. False
8. False
9. True
10. True

### Fill in the Blank

1. Spermatogenesis
2. estrogen; progesterone
3. graafian
4. epididymis
5. oogenesis
6. menarche
7. testosterone
8. meiosis
9. vulva
10. menopause

### Short Answer

1. Spermatogonia, spermatocyte, spermatid, sperm.
2. Oogonia, oocyte, ovum.

### Labeling

See Figure 15–3 Internal and external male reproductive system.

See Figure 15–8 Internal female reproductive system.

Sickle cell anemia, 110t
Sight, 208–217
  blindness, childhood causes of, 221
  process of vision, 211, 212f, 213
  reflexes of the eye, 215, 216f, 216t, 217
  structures of the eye, 208–211, 209f–210f
Sigmoid colon, 174, 174f
Simple (closed) fractures, 91f, 91t
Simple columnar epithelial tissue, 31, 31t
Simple cuboidal epithelial tissue, 31, 31t
Simple epithelial tissue, 30f, 31
Simple squamous epithelial tissue, 31, 31t
Sims position, 9f
Sinoatrial (SA) node, 142f, 143
Sinuses, 84
Skeletal muscle, 34, 34f, 58–59
Skeletal system, 3f, 77–94
  bone repair, 89–91, 90f–91f, 91t
  bones, 77–79, 78f
    classification, 78–79
    structure of long bones, 79, 79f
    types, 77–78
  diseases and disorders, 94t
    childhood, 82
  overview, 6, 77
  skeleton, 80–89
    divisions, 80–81, 82f–83f, 84–85, 85f–90f, 87–89
    fetal skeleton, 80, 81f
    overview, 80
  types of joints, 92–93, 92f–93f, 93t
Skin cancer, 50–52, 51f–52f, 52t
Skin lesions, 51f, 52t
Skull, 80, 83f
  fetal, 81f
SLE (systemic lupus erythematosus), 125
Small intestine, 171, 172f
Smell, 222–223, 222f
  structure of the nose, 222–223
Smooth muscle, 34f, 34–35, 59
Sneezing, 161
Snellen chart, 213–214
Sodium-potassium pump, 23f, 24
Soleus, 69, 71f, 71t
Somatic nervous system, 200
Somatic reflexes, 202
Sound, 218
Specific immunity, 119–121, 120f, 121t, 122f, 123
Sperm, 263, 267f
Spermatids, 266f, 266–267
Spermatocytes, 266, 266f
Spermatogenesis, 266, 266f
Spermatogonia, 266, 266f
Spermatozoa, 266f
Sperm production, 266–268, 266f, 266t
Sphenoid bone, 83f
Spina bifida, 203t

Spinal cavity, 10
Spinal column, 84
Spinal cord, 200
  ascending tract, 200
  descending tract, 200
  spinal nerves, 200, 201f
Spinal nerves, 200, 201f
Spindle fibers, 28–29
Spleen, 116f, 117
Spongy bone, 78
Sprain, 72t
Squamous cell carcinoma, 50, 53t
Squamous epithelial tissue, 30, 30f
Stapes, 217f, 218
Static equilibrium, 221
STDs (sexually transmitted diseases), 276–278
Stem cells, 105, 105f, 266, 270
Sternocleidomastoid, 66f–67f, 67, 68t
Sternum, 84, 86f
Steroid hormones, 247, 248f
STIs (sexually transmitted infections), 276
Stomach, 168–170, 169f–170f
Strabismus, 226t
Strain, 61, 72t
Stratified epithelial tissue, 30f, 31
Stratified squamous epithelial tissue, 31, 31t
Stratum basale, 42
Stratum corneum, 42
Stratum granulosum, 42
Stratum lucidum, 42
Stratum spinosum, 42
Styloid process, 83f
Subcutaneous layer of skin, 45
Sudoriferous glands, 45
Sulci, 195f, 197
Superficial-thickness burn, 48, 49f
Supination, 63f, 64, 64t
Supine position, 9f
Surfactant, 155
Sutures, 81
Sympathetic nervous system, 200
Synapse, 190, 190f
Synarthroses, 92
Synergistic muscles, 63
Syphilis, 277
System, 2–2f
Systemic circulation, 140, 141f
Systemic lupus erythematosus (SLE), 125, 127t
Systole, 143

**T**

Tachycardia, 148t
Talipes, 82, 94t
Tarsals, 89, 90f
Taste, 223–224, 223f
  structure of the tongue, 223–224
Taste buds, 223, 223f, 224t
Teeth, 167, 168f

Temporal bone, 81f, 83f
Temporalis, 67, 67f, 68t
Temporal lobes, 197f, 198
Tendons, 62
Testes, 263, 264f
Testicular cancer, 276t
Testosterone, 266, 267t, 267–268
Tetanus, 72t
Thalamus, 195f, 196–197
Thalassemia, 110t
Thermoreceptors, 225, 225f
Thoracic cavity, 10, 12f
Thoracic vertebrae, 84, 85f
Thrombocytes, 103
Thrombocytopenia, 106, 110t
Thrombocytosis, 106
Thrombopoietin, 106
Thymosin, 252t, 256
Thymus, 116f, 117, 252t, 256
Thyroid gland, 251t, 252–253, 253f
Thyroid hormone, 252
Thyroid-stimulating hormone, 250, 250f, 251t
Thyroxine, 251t, 252
Tibia, 89, 89f
Tidal volume, 159, 159f, 160t
Tinea alba, 69
Tinnitus, 226t
Tissues, 1–2f, 30–36
  connective tissue, 32–34, 33t
  diseases and disorders, 36t
  epithelial tissue, 30–32
    classification, 30–32, 30f, 31t
    glands, 32
  membranes, 35
  muscle tissue, 34–35, 34f
  nervous tissue, 35–35f
  overview, 30
T lymphocytes, 121, 122f, 123
Tongue, 166, 167f, 223–224
Tonsils, 116f, 117, 154, 154f
Torso and back, muscles of, 68–69, 70f, 70t
Total lung capacity, 159, 159f, 160t
Touch, 224–225, 224t–225t
Trachea, 153f–155f, 155
Transcription, 26
Transitional epithelium, 31t, 31–32
Translation, 26–27
Transport, cellular, 21–25, 23f, 25f
Transverse colon, 174, 174f
Transverse plane, 10, 11f
Trapezius, 69, 70f, 70t
Trendelenburg position, 10f
Triceps brachii, 66f, 67, 68f
Tricuspid valve, 133, 134f
Trigone, 234
Triiodothyronine, 251t, 252
Tuberculosis, 160
Tussis, 161
Tympanic membrane, 217f, 218
Tympanometry, 220